hairdressing

with barbering

hairdressing

with barbering

Gilly **Ford**
Helen **Stewart**

www.heinemann.co.uk
✓ Free online support
✓ Useful weblinks
✓ 24 hour online ordering

01865 888058

Heinemann
Inspiring generations

Heinemann Educational Publishers
Halley Court, Jordan Hill, Oxford OX2 8EJ
Part of Harcourt Education

Heinemann is the registered trademark of
Harcourt Education Limited

© Helen Stewart and Gilly Ford, 2003

First published 2003

08 07 06 05 04 03
10 9 8 7 6 5 4 3 2 1

British Library Cataloguing in Publication Data is available
from the British Library on request.

ISBN 0 435 45647 4

Designed, typeset and illustrated by Hardlines, Charlbury, Oxon
Original illustrations © Heinemann Educational Publishers,
2003

Printed in Spain by Edelvives.

Cover photo: © Getty

Acknowledgements
Every effort has been made to contact copyright holders
of material reproduced in this book. Any omissions will
be rectified in subsequent printings if notice is given to
the publishers.

Tel: 01865 888058   www.heinemann.co.uk

Contents

Acknowledgements

To Ade, Paul and Michael for their love and support.

The authors and publishers would like to thank the following individuals and organisations for their invaluable input into the production of this book:

Judith Hughes, our African Caribbean expert, without whose help these units wouldn't have been possible.

Dr. Ali.N Syed, master chemist and president of Avlon Inc. – for his help and advice with the African Caribbean units.

Yvonne Davies – for her advice on African Caribbean styling.

Dave Parr – for providing advice on Health and Safety issues.

Sterling Hairdressing and Beauty Equipment Supplies – for the supply of materials used during the photoshoot.

Clynol/Schwarzkopf – for providing artwork used within the book.

Harry Callaghan, MIT – for providing specific information relating to hair and skin diseases and disorders; and always being able to answer our questions.

John Mason, MIT – for answering some of those quirky questions only a trichologist can answer.

Rebecca May, Lesley Faulkner and Katie Woodman – for reading through copious amounts of text and giving us constructive assistance and inspiration.

Sue Cressy who thought we may enjoy the challenge of writing a book and has offered us the benefit of her wisdom as an established author.

Michael John Training, Manchester – for allowing us to use their premises for the photo shoot, which ran over on most days!

Sophie Drake Thomas and Richard and Byron Calame of R&B Cuts, 289 Chester Road, Manchester.

Thanks also to the following people for giving up their valuable time to offer a wealth of superb hairdressing skills, all of which have contributed to the visual content of the book:

Gemma Abdullah, Sophie Brown, Lesley Faulkner, Judith Hughes, Donnette Julien, Keisha Mason, Natalie Mitchell and Katie Woodman.

A big thank-you must go to all the photo shoot models and make-up artists for their time and patience:

Nita Blackwell, Rachael Brady, Janine Brown, Salome Brown, Sue Cressy, Waheed Chowan, Emma Fairfield, Ammarron Fredrick, Louise Fogg, Rachel Gear, Samantha Higgins, Amanda James, Meleika Lawrence, Emma Leary, Rebecca Leary, Kathy McQuade, Louisa Morgan, Ashley Morris, Lynsey O'Callaghan, Adeela Rathore and Jenny Sealy.

Thanks to L'Oreal, The John Carne Hairdressing Group, Babylis UK Ltd, Goldwell and Black Like Me for kindly providing photographs used in the book, as well as Wella UK and Wesley Ricketts from Avlon for providing photographs used within the book and products used during the photoshoot.

We would also like to thank the following for their input into various units:

Harry Cabello (Trichologist), Jackie Gordon (African Caribbean), Ian Littlewood (Marketing) and Joanna Okpoti (African Caribbean).

The following organisations generously provided important information and realia used in the book:

Clynol, Whal UK, G.E. Betterton & Co. Ltd., The Commission for Racial Equality (CRA), The Equal Opportunities Commission (EOC) and The Disability Rights Commission (DRC).

Use of HABIA unit titles and element headings by kind permission of HABIA:

Fraser House
Nether Hall Road
Doncaster
South Yorkshire DN1 2PH
Tel: 01302 380000
Fax: 01302 380028
Email: enquiries@habia.org.uk
Website: www.habia.org.uk

We would also like to acknowledge all the people who have helped us in some way that we may have unwittingly forgotten.

Photo acknowledgements

The authors and publishers would like to thank the following individuals and organisations for permission to reproduce photographs:

American Crew: page 324.

Anita Cox: page 118.

Avlon: pages 335, 349, 356, 358 & 359.

Mayk Azzato: page 127 (left).

Babyliss: page 278 (rows 1, 3 & 7).

Paul Baker: page 126.

Bella Hair: page 279.

Black Like Me: pages 347 & 363.

Gareth Boden: pages 8, 18, 32, 36, 46, 47, 70, 75, 85, 86, 127 (left), 153 (left & middle), 157, 159, 160–5, 168, 176 (left & middle), 179, 181 (row 1 & 3), 183 (top), 187-8, 189, 191, 196, 207 (rows 2 & 4), 209 (rows 1, 2 & 4–6), 210–13, 218, 221, 224, 232–3, 234, 235, 248, 250, 261, 262, 271, 289, 290, 291 (top row), 296, 303, 306, 311, 317, 318–9, 322–3, 328, 330, 331 (sectioning clips), 340–1, 346, 357, 360–1, 365, 374, 376–7 & 378–9.

Camera Press: pages 373, 375 & 380.

Clarins: page 308.

Corbis: page 173.

Croydon College: pages 255, 265, & 286.

Goldwell: pages 1 (middle & right), 5 (left), 73, 98, 122 (left), 150, 194, 206, 207 (row 3), 217, 228, 229 (top), 239 & 257.

Keith Hall: pages 61, 253 & 268.

Chris Honeywell: pages 1 (left), 6, 30, 34, 71, 117 (right), 153 (right), 156, 171, 180, 183 (bottom), 184 (bottom), 197, 207 (rows 1 & 5), 209 (row 3), 270, 278 (rows 2 & 4–6), 281, 293, 302 (right), 314, 331 & 332.

The John Carne Hairdressing Group: pages 5 (middle), 84, 117 (left), 122 (right), 127 (top), 132, 176, 226 & 283.

Lakmé: pages 21, 242 & 263.

Mediscan: pages 55 (row 2) & 53 (row 2).

Derek Murray: page 135.

Photodisc: page 188 (bottom).

Science Photo Library: pages 48, 51, 52, 53 (rows 1 & 5), 54 (rows 2 , 3, 5 & 6), 55 (rows 1 & 4) & 23.

Scissors: page 74.

Trip: pages 125 (bottom) & 291 (bottom).

WAHL: pages 155, 181 (row 2 & 4), 184 (top) & 302 (left).

Wella: pages 5 (left), 102, 107, 110 (top), 117 (middle), 216, 229 (bottom) & 281 (top & bottom).

Wellcome Trust: pages 53 (rows 3 & 4), 54 (row 1) & 55 (row 3).

INTRODUCTION

Introduction

This book has been written to help you achieve your S/NVQ Level 3 qualification in Hairdressing and Barbering. It has been designed to provide you with all the information you need in an accessible format including all the necessary technical guidance with illustrations to support the text.

Throughout the book, reference is made to maintaining, improving and personalizing your professional skills, as this is an essential part of your vocation. Each technical unit is supported by step-by-step photographs, to help you both understand the content and give you ideas to help develop your current skills.

Key features

In the salon – includes case studies based on real-life events that you may face in the salon. They are designed to allow you to consider how you would respond in situations that may actually arise. Questions are provided to enable you to explore the key issues and decide on your own course of action.

Keys to good practice – tips and suggestions for promoting good practice in the salon and in your working methods.

Check it out – provides activities to help you to apply theory to practical situations. These can also be used to provide evidence for your portfolio, key skills or customer service.

Remember – highlights specific areas that you need to pay particular attention to and to remind you of the important legal and professional issues within the hairdressing business.

Knowledge check – a set of questions to check your knowledge at the end of each unit.

Hairdressing is an ever-changing industry that requires creativity, confidence and inspirational ideas. The Level 3 standards reflect that current direction; nothing short of perfection is good enough and this should be reflected in your passion to be the best! We wish you every success in achieving your S/NVQ Level 3 in Hairdressing and Barbering.

About the NVQ

What is an NVQ?

NVQ stands for **National Vocational Qualification**. This means that it is a nationally recognised qualification in a vocational area. The NVQ Level 3 in Hairdressing is written jointly by representatives from industry, trainers and teaching staff, HABIA and several awarding bodies. It is approved by the Qualifications and Curriculum Authority.

How to gain an NVQ

In order to gain an NVQ, you will need to collect the evidence required for each unit. Many forms of evidence are acceptable including observed work, oral questions, witness statements and assignments.

To achieve a Level 3 NVQ in Hairdressing, candidates must be able to:

- show competence in a broad range of hairdressing skills and activities e.g. cutting and restyling, and be able to perform in a wide variety of contexts, including non-routine tasks;
- demonstrate considerable responsibility for their work and the ability to work independently;
- guide and train others, as is required of the job.

Who is the qualification for?

This qualification is designed for hairdressers who work independently in the salon and support others in their role. You may have already achieved NVQ Levels 1 and 2 in Hairdressing. However, if you have sufficient practical experience working as a hairdresser but have not yet achieved a formal qualification, you may also be at the right stage to study at Level 3.

How the qualification is structured

To complete the full award you must achieve a total of nine units. These nine units are made up of four mandatory units and five optional units, chosen from the two option groups. The path you wish to follow in your hairdressing work will determine which optional units you choose.

A **unit** is the term given to each separate area of competence, whether that is a technical or non-technical area, e.g. cutting, thermal styling, consultation, or health and safety.

Each unit is broken down into **outcomes**, which describe in further detail the skills and knowledge required to prove competence.

Each outcome has a set of **performance criteria** that set out what should be performed in order to demonstrate competence. **Range** statements set out the various circumstances under which the performance criteria must be achieved.

Essential knowledge and understanding requirements are fulfilled by various methods e.g. assignments, oral questions and test papers. This is the knowledge that you must acquire to demonstrate your understanding of the various hairdressing skills and tasks you will undertake as part of your job.

Assessment of the qualification

You may provide a range of sources of evidence to prove competence as listed below; however, most of your evidence will be derived from direct observation of your work by your assessor/s. All of the evidence must be recorded in your candidate logbook and a portfolio of evidence should be built over time to prove your competence.

Types of evidence

Observation: Direct observations by your assessor watching you produce the work.

Witness testimony: A detailed record of the work you have produced which must be signed by both yourself and a witness.

Oral questions: Questions asked directly by your assessor to check your understanding.

Written questions: Questions that you must answer to in order to check your understanding of the subject area.

Assignments: A piece of written work that must be produced to assess your knowledge of the subject area.

Mandatory written test paper: A written test that must be taken under controlled conditions.

Product evidence: Any evidence that is a product of the assessment, for example, a consultation sheet or record card.

Simulation: Simulation of an activity may be used only under specific circumstances and for particular units.

Accreditation of prior learning: This enables you to claim knowledge and skills you have already acquired from previous work or study. Evidence must be produced to prove your competence and knowledge in a particular area. This could be statements from employers and clients, or photos of work you have completed.

Assessment and quality

While you are working towards your NVQ Level 3 Hairdressing, you may be assessed by all or just a few of the above methods. Your assessor/s will judge your competence against the standards as written and you have a right to appeal against any assessment decision made. The quality of assessment is controlled by measures which are set in order to standardise assessment decisions, and these are regularly checked and monitored by internal verifiers and external verifiers employed by the awarding body.

the workplace
ENVIRONMENT

Ensure your own actions reduce the risks to health and safety

Unit G1

Introduction

Health and safety is an essential aspect of any workplace environment and especially so within the hairdressing salon. Without a thorough understanding of the importance of health and safety in your work and working practices, you could become a danger to yourself and those around you. This unit covers the health and safety legislation that relates to salon owners and their employees, and looks at ways to ensure your own safety in the salon as well as the safety of others.

Health and safety should be a key factor when preparing for a service

What you will learn
• Health and safety legislation
• Identify the hazards and evaluate and reduce the risks to health and safety in your workplace

You the stylist

As a stylist, you should have a good awareness of health and safety to ensure that your working practices are sound and comply with current legislation. To do this you need to be aware of the everyday hazards that are present in your place of work and also the ones that may occur more infrequently. However, being aware of such hazards is not enough; you must be able to decide how much of a threat they pose and act accordingly, e.g. whether you should deal with the hazard yourself, delegate the task to another member of staff, or report it to the person in your salon who is responsible for health and safety.

Health and safety legislation

Before you begin to address issues such as hazards and risks, it is helpful to first define a few key terms. This will help you to clarify how they relate to your salon environment.

Hazard – a hazard is anything that has the potential to cause harm, for example, a hairdryer flex, water on the floor, or a heavy box that needs moving.

Risk – a risk is the chance, either high or low, that the harm caused by the hazard will occur.

Control measure – something that reduces and/or controls the risks to health and safety.

Workplace – the workplace refers to all areas of the business premises including the staff rooms, toilets, and so on. This means every area of the salon and not just the part where hairdressing is carried out.

It is vital that you are aware of current health and safety legislation and how it relates to you and your responsibilities within the salon. Your working life is controlled by

Check it out
Have a look around your workplace and see if you can identify any hazards. If you can, what are the potential risks to health and safety?

two sets of external laws known as acts and regulations. An **act** is laid down by Parliament and, after going through the parliamentary process, becomes law. It usually contains general objectives that employers, employees and others must achieve. A **regulation** is a statutory instrument – in other words, a detailed means of meeting the general objectives of an act.

The Health and Safety at Work Act 1974

Most health and safety law is derived from the Health and Safety at Work Act 1974. This Act requires employers to:

- provide and maintain a safe working environment
- provide adequate welfare facilities
- provide safe systems of work
- provide information, training and supervision
- ensure the safe handling, storage and transportation of goods and materials
- provide and maintain safe equipment.

These requirements are also included in other regulations, some of which will be discussed later in this unit.

The enforcement of health and safety regulations is carried out by inspectors who are employed by the Health and Safety Executive (HSE), a government appointed body. Inspectors may enter and inspect a workplace at any reasonable time, following an accident or complaint, and can do so without forewarning. For example, they may:

- offer informal advice
- offer informal advice supported by a formal letter
- issue an improvement notice
- issue a prohibition notice
- recommend prosecution.

An improvement notice will recommend actions to be completed by the employer within a certain period of time, whereas a prohibition notice will require immediate action and may well involve the removal of a process or item of equipment until these actions have been completed. Failure to comply with either of these notices will result in a criminal prosecution in either a Magistrates or Crown Court, depending on the gravity of the offence. Courts have the power to fine or even imprison for such offences.

As an employee, you also have duties under this Act. You must:

- not endanger yourself or others by your acts or omissions
- co-operate with your employer in order for their duties to be fulfilled
- not misuse anything provided in the interests of health and safety
- report all accidents, incidents and unsafe conditions or practices.

As you progress through this unit, you will see that many of your workplace activities relate to this Act.

Electricity at Work Regulations 1989

These regulations are concerned with ensuring safety when using electrical equipment. Your employer must ensure:

- all electrical equipment is properly maintained and in good working order
- regular tests are made by a qualified electrician on each piece of equipment, as appropriate

Check it out

What welfare facilities are provided in your salon?

- records are kept regarding the testing of all electrical equipment and may be provided for inspection purposes if required.

As an employee, it is your responsibility to co-operate with your employer to comply with these regulations.

Personal Protective Equipment at Work Regulations 1992

These regulations require an employer to provide their employees with protective equipment if they may be exposed to any risk to health or injury during their working hours. The risks will have been assessed during the risk assessment your employer has to carry out under related regulations.

It is your employer's responsibility to:

- assess the need for the use of personal protective equipment
- supply protective clothing or equipment free of charge
- train staff in the use of personal protective equipment
- ensure the equipment is properly maintained
- ensure it is fit for purpose.

Wearing PPE ensures that both you and your client are protected

Personal protective equipment for you may include gloves, an apron and a facemask for asthmatics when mixing powder bleach, but not of the 'dust free' variety. Personal protective equipment for your clients includes a gown, towels and plastic capes. These should be used to ensure the client's skin and clothes are protected.

Check it out

Look at the statements that outline your responsibilities within the Electricity at Work Regulations. What should you be doing to fulfill your obligations relating to this piece of legislation?

Keys to good practice

- It is your responsibility to look after personal protective equipment and report its loss or demise to your employer so it can be replaced.
- It should be noted, however, that personal protective equipment is considered to be a last resort when implementing measures designed to reduce or control an identified risk. It is essential that other control measures be used before, or in addition to, the provision of such items.

Check it out

What are your responsibilities within the Personal Protective Equipment at Work Regulations?

Control of Substances Hazardous to Health Regulations (COSHH) 2003

In the salon you will use many substances that may put your health at risk. The COSHH regulations require your employer to assess the health risks that arise from the use of hazardous substances within your workplace and to provide the controls that will be most effective in protecting you and members of the public. The regulations apply to substances that have been classified as corrosive, explosive, harmful, highly flammable, irritant, oxidising or toxic. The COSHH classification symbols are shown opposite.

Your employer is required to:

- assess the risk to your health from the use of hazardous substances at work and what precautions are needed
- design and introduce appropriate measures to prevent or control your exposure to hazardous substances
- ensure that you follow the control measures and safety procedures, and use your protective equipment when appropriate
- monitor your exposure to hazardous substances and carry out appropriate forms of surveillance to ensure you maintain good health
- inform and instruct you about the risks and precautions you need to take and train you to work in a safe way when dealing with hazardous chemicals.

Storage of hazardous chemicals

Products that are identified as hazardous must be stored in a cool dark place, with good ventilation and away from direct sunlight. Always read the manufacturer's instructions with regard to storing hazardous substances.

Handling and using hazardous substances

When using hazardous products, for example, colour, perm lotion, neutraliser or relaxing products, disposable gloves and an apron (personal protective equipment) must be worn. Some cleaning materials are classed as hazardous products and therefore gloves and an apron may be necessary. Look out for the COSHH classification symbols on the bottle or packaging and always read the labels to ensure your own safety.

Aerosols should be used away from any source of heat, especially from a lit cigarette or naked flame. Many styling and finishing products are classed as flammable substances and should not be used near any heat source.

 (a) Corrosive

 (b) Explosive

 (c) Harmful

 (d) Highly flammable

 (e) Irritant

 (f) Oxidizing

 (g) Toxic

COSHH classification symbols

Disposal of hazardous substances

Hazardous substances may cause harm to our environment and other people if they are not disposed of in the correct way. Always read the manufacturer's instructions regarding the safe disposal of these substances. If you have any doubts, you can telephone the manufacturer and they will advise you on safe methods of disposal. Your salon may have its own policy for disposing of salon waste – ask the designated person within your salon.

Cosmetic Products (Safety) Regulations 1996

These regulations are specifically concerned with the ingredients contained within hairdressing preparations and their safe usage. The regulations state that hair products supplied to the salon must comply with the UK Cosmetic Products (Safety) Regulations. Under the Health and Safety at Work Act 1974, product manufacturers are required by law to supply health and safety information on any products used in a hairdressing salon that contain potentially hazardous substances. They must also provide information on the precautions to be taken to reduce any risks. This information can be found in the booklet *A Guide to Health and Safety in the Salon*.

10A Hair Colorant – Semi-Permanent (Non-Aerosol)

Composition
Solutions of direct dyestuffs in a shampoo base which may be liquid, cream or gel.

Ingredients

Dyestuffs	up to 10%
Solvents (e.g. glycols or glycol ethers)	up to 10%
Ethanol	up to 50%

Hazards Identification
Refer to manufacturer's pack for list of declarable dyestuffs which, if present, may require a sensitivity test before use. May be flammable.

First Aid measures
Eyes: Rinse eyes immediately with plenty of water. If irritation persists seek medical advice.
Skin: Wash skin immediately (mainly to avoid staining).
Ingestion: Drink 2–3 glasses of water or milk. Seek medical advice immediately.

Accidental Release Measures
Use plenty of water to dilute and mop up spillages.

Fire-fighting Measures
Use carbon-dioxide or dry powder extinguisher.

Handling & Storage
Avoid contact with eyes and face. Do not use on abraded or sensitive skin. Store in a cool place away from direct sunlight and other sources of heat. Use away from sources of ignition.
Liquid products may contain alcohol which makes the product flammable; keep small quantities in the salon for immediate use only.

Exposure Controls/Personal Protection
Apply in a well-ventilated area. Always wear suitable protective gloves.

Disposal
Do not incinerate. Wash down the drain with plenty of water.

Check it out

Why is it important to read and follow the manufacturer's instructions when storing, using or disposing of hazardous substances?

Check it out

Do you have a copy of the booklet, *A Guide to Health and Safety in the Salon*? If not, you can order a copy from The Hairdressing and Beauty Suppliers Association, tel. 020 7836 4008, www.hbsa.uk.com

Check it out

Look at a selection of hair care products in your salon. Are there any COSHH classification symbols on the packaging? If so, what do they mean?

COSHH Requirements
With regard to the Wella Product Range
As at 1st July 2002

The following information should be read in conjunction with the booklet "A Guide to Health & Safety in the Salon" (Sixth Edition). If you do not already have a copy of this booklet, contact our Customer Service Department on 01256 320202. For further details regarding our products, contact our Technical Advisory Helpline on 0345 045775. Alternatively email us on hair@wella.co.uk.

Product		Page No.	Section No.	Reference Section
Accord	Coloured Styling Mousse	19	10B	Hair Colourant – Semi-Permanent (Aerosol)
	Styling Lotion/Coloured Setting Lotion	22	12	Setting Lotion – Inc Coloured Setting & Blow Dry Lotion
Back to Basics	All Shampoos	7	–	Unlikely Hazards
	All Conditioners and conditioning balm	7	–	Unlikely Hazards
	Texturising Lotion	7	–	Unlikely Hazards
	Thickening Serum	25	14	Hair Styling gel
	Smoothing Elixir	7	–	Unlikely Hazards
	Volume Spray	21	11B	Hairspray inc Treatment Sprays (Aerosol)
	Firm Hold Gel	25	14	Hair Styling Gel
	Finishing Hairspray	21	11B	Hairspray inc Treatment Sprays (Aerosol)
	Leave in Conditioning and Detangling Spray	20	11A	Hairspray inc Treatment Sprays (Non-Aerosol)
	Crème Mousse	24	13B	Styling Mousse/Foam – Inc Setting/Cond. Mousse (Aerosol)
	Firm Hold Hairspray	21	11B	Hairspray inc Treatment Sprays (Aerosol)
Blondor	Special Cream	8	1	Bleach Powder and Emulsion
	Coco	8	1	Bleach Powder and Emulsion
	Creative Colors	18	10A	Hair Colourant – Semi-Permanent (Non-Aerosol)
	Special Dust Free Powder	8	1	Bleach Powder and Emulsion
Color Fresh		18	10A	Hair Colourant – Semi-Permanent (Non-Aerosol)
Color Touch	Color Touch	15	8A	Hair Colourant – Permanent, Oxidation type (Non-Aerosol)
	4% Crème Lotion (Intensive)	9	2	Hydrogen Peroxide Solution
	1.9% Crème Lotion (Original)	9	2	Hydrogen Peroxide Solution
	Sunlights	15	8A	Hair Colourant – Permanent, Oxidation type (Non-Aerosol)
Cuticin		22	12	Setting Lotion – Inc Colour Setting & Blow Dry Lotion
EOS		18	10A	Hair Colourant – Semi Permanent (Non-Aerosol)
Fashion Fix		9	2	Hydrogen Peroxide Solution
Fashion Form		10	3	Perm – Alkaline Type
Headlines	Fixing Lotion/Crème Fixative	9	2	Hydrogen Peroxide Solution
	Forming Lotion/Creme	10	3	Perm – Alkaline
Herbal Antioxy		7	–	Unlikely Hazards

Beautiful hair needs an expert.

Ordering – www.welladirect.co.uk
Website – www.wella.co.uk (user name; salon: password; wella)

Example of a COSHH data sheet

In addition to the booklet, your product manufacturer should also supply your salon with a list of their products that specifies which section of the booklet is relevant to each individual product.

These regulations ensure that products sold in the UK are safe when used correctly. The products covered include:

- hair tints and bleaches
- products for waving, straightening and fixing
- setting products
- cleansing products (shampoos, powders, lotions)
- conditioning products (lotions, creams and oils)

- hairdressing preparations (lotions, lacquers and brilliantines)
- shaving products (creams, foams and lotions).

These regulations have a direct link with COSHH legislation and should be used by your employer when carrying out a COSHH risk assessment.

Manual Handling Operations Regulations 1992

These regulations are concerned with the manual handling of loads, for example, equipment or stock. This includes the way we lift things and move them from place to place. Your employer has specific duties under these regulations which involve assessing the risks when manually handling loads. To do this, the employer must look at:

- the task to be undertaken
- the capabilities and limitations of the staff (e.g. pregnant women or staff who have recently returned to work after an illness may not be back to full strength)
- the type of load to be handled
- the working environment (if the atmosphere is damp, your hands may be wet and the load may slip).

Once your employer has assessed the risks, it is necessary to put systems in place to control the likelihood of them occurring. Training and information should be provided to all staff that are involved in manual handling activities.

You also have responsibilities as follows:

- To take reasonable care for your own and others' health and safety who may be affected by your actions.
- To co-operate with your employer so that they can carry out their health and safety duties.
- To use any equipment provided by your employer to enable you to move or handle loads – this could include a sturdy stepladder for placing stock on a high shelf or a trolley device for moving heavy boxes.
- To follow the safe systems of work that your employer has laid down.

> **Check it out**
>
> What are the potential risks of carrying a heavy box with smaller boxes balanced on the top? Practise good manual handling techniques in the salon.

Fire Precautions Act 1971

The Fire Precautions Act 1971 is concerned with fire prevention and the provision of escape routes in the event of an evacuation. The employer is responsible for fire safety in the workplace and ensuring the workplace complies with the fire regulations. Your employer should have a fire certificate if:

- there will be more than twenty people working on the premises at any one time
- there are more than ten people working anywhere other than the ground floor.

Fire Precautions (Workplace) Regulations (Amendment) 1999

Your employer is responsible for undertaking an assessment of the fire risks on the premises, to produce an emergency plan, and to inform, instruct and train you about the fire precautions in your workplace. Your employer should also nominate a designated person to help them.

You also have responsibilities to ensure your own health and safety and that of your colleagues and others who may be affected by your actions.

- You should co-operate with your employer to enable them to be able to carry out their statutory duties.
- You must inform your employer/health and safety representative of any situation within the workplace that you feel may constitute a risk to health and safety.
- You must use all equipment correctly, following the training and instruction guidance you have received.

Health and Safety (First Aid) Regulations 1981

These regulations require your employer to provide adequate and appropriate equipment, facilities and personnel to enable first aid to be given to you if you are injured or become ill at work. The minimum first aid provision within a hairdressing salon is a suitably stocked first aid box and an appointed person to take charge of first aid arrangements.

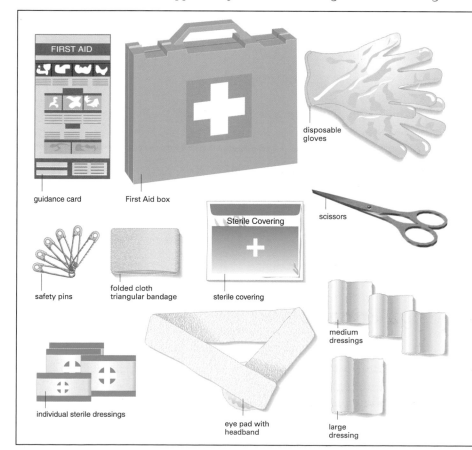

guidance card

First Aid box

disposable gloves

safety pins

folded cloth triangular bandage

sterile covering

scissors

individual sterile dressings

eye pad with headband

medium dressings

large dressing

The first aid box at work should, as a minimum, contain:

- a first aid guidance card
- twenty individually wrapped adhesive sterile dressings
- two sterile eye patches
- four individually wrapped triangular bandages
- six safety pins
- six medium sized (approximately 12cm × 12cm) sterile individually wrapped unmedicated wound dressings
- two large (approximately 18cm × 18cm) sterile individually wrapped unmedicated wound dressings
- one pair of disposable gloves.

Tablets or medicine should not be kept in the first aid box.

Your employer should have chosen an appointed person within the salon to take charge when someone is injured or becomes ill at work (this includes calling an ambulance if necessary). The appointed person should look after the first aid equipment and ensure the first aid box is restocked at regular intervals. He or she should not give first aid unless they have been trained and hold a current first aid at work certificate. As there should be an appointed person in the workplace at all times, your employer may have chosen two people to carry out this role to ensure there is always one appointed person in the salon.

Check it out

If you want to obtain a First Aid qualification, do you know where you could find an appropriate course?

Reporting of Injuries, Diseases and Dangerous Occurrences Regulations (RIDDOR) 1995

These regulations are the responsibility of your employer, but also include self-employed people. Your employer, or self-employed person, must report:

- a death or major injury
- an over-three day injury
- a dangerous occurrence
- a work-related illness, which may include dermatitis, skin cancer and occupational asthma.

All workplace accidents or incidents, however trivial they may seem at the time, should be reported to your employer. In addition, under the RIDDOR regulations, employers have a legal duty to report any workplace accidents, diseases or dangerous occurrences to the Health and Safety Executive (HSE). This information enables the HSE and local authorities to identify where and how risks arise, and investigate any serious accidents.

Environmental Protection Act 1990

This Act is relevant to hairdressers, as you have to dispose of waste products, including chemicals. The part of this Act that affects you is concerned with your duty of care when disposing of waste. All salon waste should be disposed of in a manner that will not pollute the environment or cause harm to others.

Your employer's responsibilities within this Act are to:

- dispose of all waste in a safe manner
- provide training for all employees in the safe disposal of waste
- contact product manufacturers for information regarding the safe disposal of products, including out-of-date stock.

Your employer should have a commercial waste contract, which should include sharps.

Check it out

What is the correct procedure for disposing of sharps?

Local Government (Miscellaneous Provisions) Act 1982

The Local Government (Miscellaneous Provisions) Act 1982 has its own set of by-laws relating to hairdressers and barbers. These may also be referred to as 'local by-laws' and are specific to the area where the business is situated. Both you and your employer have responsibilities under this Act.

The Act is primarily concerned with cleanliness and hygiene. It covers the salon, tools and equipment, and people working there. If you do not comply with these regulations, you could be liable to a fine.

The Management of Health and Safety at Work Regulations 1999

These regulations are considered to be the most important legislation relating to health and safety since the Health and Safety at Work Act 1974. This is because they legally require all employers to effectively manage the health and safety within their business.

Your employer is obliged to:

- carry out risk assessments to determine what health and safety measures are needed to protect you, the employee, and others who may enter the business premises
- plan, implement, and control whatever measures are deemed necessary
- review these measures on a regular basis
- provide health and safety training to all employees.

The Provision and Use of Work Equipment Regulations 1998

Under these regulations your employer is required to prevent or control the risks to your health and safety from any equipment you use at work. This applies to both new and second-hand equipment. The regulations state that equipment used at work must be:

- suitable for use and used for the purpose for which it is intended
- maintained in a safe condition for use
- inspected on a regular basis, by a competent person, and records kept
- used only by people who have been trained and instructed in its correct usage.

Written instructions must be provided if and when necessary.

Workplace (Health, Safety and Welfare) Regulations 1992

Your employer should ensure your workplace complies with the requirements of these regulations by:

- maintaining the workplace and all equipment and systems used there
- ensuring adequate ventilation
- keeping the workplace at a reasonable temperature (minimum 16°C)
- making sure you have sufficient light to work comfortably
- keeping your workplace clean and tidy
- ensuring you have enough room to work comfortably
- keeping floor and 'traffic routes' in a reasonable condition (no holes, slopes or uneven surfaces)
- ensuring the workstations and seating are suitable
- providing you with suitable washing and toilet facilities (with soap and a means of drying your hands)
- making sure you have accommodation for clothing (worn at work) and changing facilities

Check it out

Contact your local authority to get a copy of the Local Government (Miscellaneous Provisions) Act 1982, relating to hairdressers and barbers, if your salon does not already have one.

Check it out

How often does your salon give health and safety training?

- providing you with facilities for resting and eating (if meals are to be eaten on the premises)
- providing you with clean drinking water and cups
- removing waste materials on a regular basis
- keeping you safe from falling objects
- making sure all doors and gates are suitably constructed and fitted with any necessary safety devices
- making sure windows are protected against breakage and incorporate signs (or similar) where there is a danger of someone walking into them
- making sure escalators and moving walkways have safety devices fitted so they can be stopped in an emergency.

Identify the hazards and evaluate and reduce the risks to health and safety in your workplace

In this section, we will identify the hazards in your workplace, evaluate the risks and look at ways to reduce them.

A hazard is something that can cause harm. You must remain alert to the presence of hazards in the workplace to help prevent accidents or damage to property. Under the Health and Safety at Work Act 1974, you have a duty of care not to intentionally harm yourself, your colleagues, or other people by your acts or omissions. You must be vigilant at all times and act accordingly when you identify a hazard.

Hazards occur in all areas of everyday life, from crossing the street to boiling the kettle. All you need to do is look around the workplace and see how many things have the potential to harm you or other people around you. Stairs or steps in the salon could be deemed a hazard, but what is the likelihood of anyone actually falling? If the stairs are well maintained and have a handrail, the likelihood of an accident is reduced. However, if the stairs are wet after mopping or the handrail becomes loose, the risk would be much higher.

The backwash area may also be classed as a hazardous area, as there is the possibility of spillages, which would leave the floor wet and slippery. However, if immediate action is taken, the risk will be reduced.

Check it out

Look at the table below. How could you prevent the hazards from becoming risks?

Identify the hazard	What is the risk?	What should I do?
Water on the floor	Slipping	Inform everyone in the salon. Cone off the area and wipe up the spillage. Do not remove the cones until the floor is dry.
Perm lotion on the floor	Slipping	As above, but the spillage must be diluted first and PPE worn.
Shampoo on the floor	Slipping	Inform everyone in the salon. Cone off the area and wipe up the spillage. Mop the floor using a detergent to remove any slippery residue. Do not remove cones until the floor is dry.
Mirror smashed on floor	Cuts from broken glass	Carefully pick up the glass and either: **1** Wrap in several layers of newspaper and place into a cardboard box. Seal the box and label it with 'broken glass'; or **2** Place the glass into the sharps box. On completion, sweep the floor to make sure there are no shards of glass left on the floor

Hazards in the workplace

'Staff only' areas in the workplace are often forgotten when it comes to health and safety as the clients do not see this part of the business premises.

Some of the substances used in the salon are hazardous, especially those used for chemical treatments, for example, colours, bleach or relaxers. These products are potentially very dangerous. However, if used with protective equipment, good training and following the manufacturer's instructions, they should not pose a threat. Used in untrained hands, the outcome could be very different – the client could suffer chemical burns to the scalp or skin.

As part of your job role you will be carrying out numerous activities, including chemical work, styling hair (using electrical equipment, sharps and styling/finishing products) and stock control. Within each of these areas there is an element of risk. However, if policies and control measures are followed, it should greatly reduce the risks involved.

Your employer will have various procedures and policies in place, all of which are there to protect you, your colleagues, and others who enter your place of work. The policies should cover:

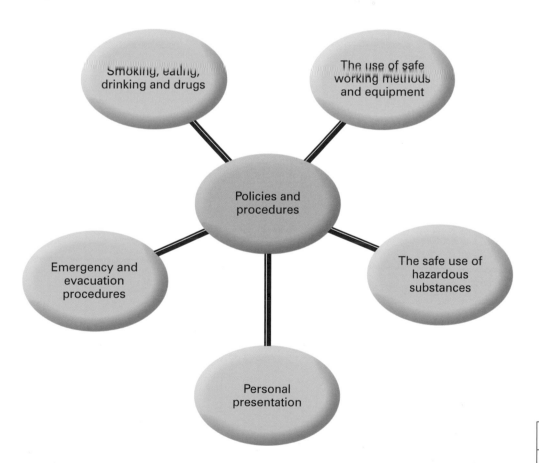

Firstly, you need to establish who is responsible for health and safety in your salon, as certain hazards will need to be reported to this person. If you do not know who to report to, how can these problems be rectified? Secondly, you will need to find out who is the appointed person for first aid and who acts as designated person in the event of an evacuation. This is usually the owner, but it could be the salon manager, the senior stylist, or even you!

Check it out

Look around your staff room. Using the same format as in the table opposite:

1   Identify any additional hazards.
2   State the risk involved.
3   What should you do about it?
4   How could you prevent the hazard from becoming a risk?

Check it out

Within your salon, identify who is responsible for the following:

*   health and safety
*   first aid
*   evacuating the premises in the event of an emergency.

The use of safe working methods and equipment

Sterilisation

It is vital that you look after your equipment by keeping it clean and well maintained. One way of doing this is to ensure that equipment is sterilised. Sterilisation is the complete destruction of living organisms to prevent cross-infection. All tools should be cleaned before sterilising to remove traces of hair, dirt and dust. Brushes, combs and rollers should be cleaned with hot soapy water. Scissors and razors should be wiped with alcohol or spirit.

A chemical jar

Chemical sterilisers

Many salons sterilise tools in a chemical jar. The chemicals must be prepared according to the manufacturer's instructions, using PPE if stated. Tools must be completely immersed in the chemical for the specified length of time for sterilisation to take place. Check with the manufacturer that fluid is suitable for metal tools, otherwise they may rust. Remember that the fluid will need to be changed periodically to ensure it is of the correct strength.

Ultra-violet radiation cabinet

This is used in many salons as a means of sterilisation. The ultra-violet light rays come from the top of the cabinet and will sterilise the surfaces that they hit. You must remember to turn the tools over to ensure all surfaces are sterilised. Each side of your tools should be sterilised for at least twenty minutes.

A U.V. cabinet

Moist heat sterilisation

Towels and gowns should be washed on a hot wash cycle. The temperature of the water should reach 95°C.

Autoclave

The autoclave is the most effective method of sterilisation. The principle is the same as a pressure cooker. Sterilisation takes place as the water inside the autoclave is heated to 121°C (due to a build up of pressure).

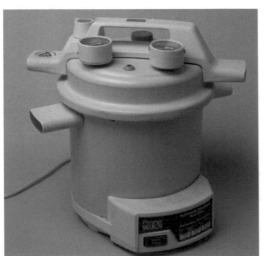

An autoclave

Check it out

Why should all tools be clean and sterilised before use? What kind of infection could be carried on unsterilised tools?

Risk of infection

As part of your duty of care towards your clients, you must be aware of the risk of infection when using sharps. Think about the implications of accidentally cutting your client with dirty scissors. What if your client has the HIV virus or hepatitis B or C, which is passed through body fluids such as blood? Can you afford to take the risk?

Identify the hazard	What is the risk?	What should I do?	
Use of sharps	• Cutting the client • Cross-infection	• Check cutting tools prior to use and only use cutting tools you have been trained to use.	• Use extreme care • Dispose of sharps in the 'sharps bin'. • Ensure all tools are sterile before use.

To evaluate the risks, think of the worst thing that could possibly happen. This will help you to decide whether the hazard presents a high, medium or low risk. Once you have established this, you need to decide how to reduce the risk, remove it completely, or report it to the designated person for them to take action.

Safe working methods

You need to look at all aspects of your job role and decide whether your working methods are safe or a liability. For example, you may be responsible for ordering and receiving stock. The stock may arrive in a large heavy box, which you then need to move to the stockroom. This could prove to be hazardous; if you try to lift the box, you may drop it on your foot, causing bruising or possibly broken bones. It may cause disc or ligament injuries, which would necessitate you taking time off work. The situation may be avoided by using a mechanical device, for example, a trolley, to move the box. If you do not have access to such a device, then unpack the box and move the stock in workable loads. This may take longer, but the risk of injury should lessen considerably. You could ask a colleague for help and between you it may be possible to move the box.

Remember

If moving objects manually, remember to bend your knees, keep your back straight and stand up using the muscles in your legs, rather than those in your back.

1 Think about the lift. Where is the load to be placed? Do you need help? Are handling aids available?

2 Get ready to lift. Stand with your feet apart.

3 Bend the knees. Keep the back straight. Tuck in your chin. Lean slightly forward over the load to get a good grip.

4 Get a good grip on the load and lift smoothly.

Identify the hazard	What is the risk?	What should I do to prevent the hazard from becoming a risk?
Moving heavy or awkwardly shaped boxes of stock	• Overstretching muscles, possibly straining back, shoulders and arms. Disc or ligament injuries. • Dropping the box onto feet or toes.	• Unpack box until you are able to lift it comfortably and then lift using your leg muscles, keeping your back straight. • Ask for help from a colleague. • Use a trolley or other mechanical device.
Storing/reaching stock on a high shelf	• Overstretching muscles, possibly straining back, shoulders and arms. • Dropping stock, causing breakages and/or spillages.	• Use a sturdy stepladder. • Store frequently used stock at eye level or below.

When undertaking any task within the salon, your posture is important. Many hairdressers suffer with back problems due to incorrect posture, stooping or leaning over the client. This is most common in taller people and can be avoided by using hydraulic chairs, which can be adjusted in height to accommodate the stylist. As your work requires you to stand for long periods of time, you need to ensure you are standing correctly with your weight evenly distributed. This will prevent unnecessary stress and strain on your body and should help to prevent fatigue.

Using electrical equipment

You will use a number of electrical appliances in the salon. Electricity can kill so do not take unnecessary risks. Using electrical equipment for its intended purpose should minimise the risk of damage. Before using any piece of electrical equipment you should have received training or instruction on its usage. If you know how to use the equipment safely, the risk of accidents is reduced. Check that an appropriate person has tested the equipment so you know it is safe to use.

Visually check each piece of equipment prior to use. You should check the plugs and sockets are not cracked or broken. You could be electrocuted if you touch something live. Ensure the flex is not worn or that bare wires are showing. This will prevent electrocution.

> ### Keys to good practice
> - Do not use too many electrical appliances from one socket; this could lead to overloading and possibly fire.
> - Check the air filter on hand dryers to ensure they are free from dust and debris, as they could overheat.
> - Ensure straightening irons or tongs are cool before storing. The heat from the irons or tongs may wear the flex, leaving the bare wires on show.
> - Electrical appliances should be switched off and unplugged after use.
> - If your salon policies differ in any way to those of the manufacturer, you must report it to your employer or designated person immediately, as there could be significant risks attached.

Any risk that you consider to be high risk should be reported to the designated person for health and safety in your salon.

Electrical equipment, such as a hairdryer, roller ball or kettle, can present risks if they are not well maintained and checked regularly. For example, a hairdryer used near water or with wet hands has the potential to cause harm. However, if it is used properly, away from the water and with dry hands, the risk will be considerably less. A hairdryer with trailing wires is also a hazard, as people may trip and hurt themselves, or the plug may become loosened in the socket, which could leave the pins exposed.

> ### In the salon
>
> Lisa was new to the salon. Her client was having bleached highlights using the cap. She applied the bleach and went to get the climazone, but another stylist was already using it, so she decided to use the old steamer in the back room. She had never used a steamer before, but she sort of knew how to use it as she had seen one being used a few years ago when she was training. She filled the glass bottle to the brim, put it into the steamer and switched it on. It took a little while to heat up, but she was busy with her next client so she was not too worried. The client under the steamer let out a cry and when Lisa turned around the steamer was 'spitting' boiling water onto her client. The client suffered scalding to her neck and has decided to sue the salon for negligence.
>
> - What went wrong?
> - How could this situation have been avoided?

The table below identifies a few hazards associated with using electrical appliances.

Identify the hazard	What is the risk?	What should I do to prevent the hazard from becoming a risk?
Cracked plugs/frayed flexes	Electric shock/electrocution	• DO NOT USE. • Report to designated person.
Trailing flexes	Trip hazard and possibility of electrocution	• Use another socket to avoid trailing the flex. • Take the flex around the outside of the room, thus removing the hazard.
Curling tongs left on worktop and switched on after use	• May burn someone • May be knocked off the worktop and broken	• Isolate the power after use and unplug the appliance. • Allow to cool and then store safely where applicable.
Heated electrical styling tools	Burning the client	• Keep the heated styling tool away from client's face and protect skin/scalp by placing comb underneath (where possible), thus keeping the heat source away from the skin. • Use extreme care.

Use of materials and hazardous substances

In the salon you will use numerous substances that are considered to be hazardous to health. When using chemical substances, ensure you read and follow any instructions the manufacturer gives. If your salon policies differ in any way from the manufacturer's instructions, you must inform your employer or designated person immediately, as there could be significant risks involved.

When dealing with chemicals it is essential that you use the personal protective equipment that has been supplied to you by your employer. This is to prevent marking your clothes and, more importantly, to protect your hands. If your hands become irritated and sore, this will affect your ability to work. Dermatitis is a common complaint amongst hairdressers and in some cases may end a promising career. It is suggested that some colouring products may be carcinogenic (cancer causing) and prolonged use of such chemical products without the appropriate protection may have very serious consequences.

Chemical products should not be used on skin with cuts or abrasions, or be allowed to come into contact with the eyes or face. As some of these products are caustic, for example, relaxers used on African-Caribbean hair, they may burn the eyes, which may lead to scarring of the delicate tissue in the eye, causing temporary or permanent blindness. In addition, relaxers, if used incorrectly without due care or without sufficient training, can cause skin/scalp burns and hair loss.

Make sure you follow the manufacturer's instructions when using chemical products

Keys to good practice

- A skin test is required when using quasi and permanent colouring products. This is to safeguard your client from the possibility of an allergic reaction and should be carried out 24–48 hours prior to the colour application. Other pre-service tests should be carried out where applicable to ensure the safety of your client.
- Store chemicals in a cool, dry place away from direct sunlight or heat source.
- When applying P.W. lotion, do not flood the scalp as this may cause chemical burns. The excess will drip onto the floor and may cause someone to slip.
- Do not mix chemicals together unless stated by the manufacturer. They may give off heat or dangerous fumes.
- Look out for the COSHH symbols on items such as hairspray or even the disinfectant you use to clean the toilet. If the product is stored, handled, used and disposed of correctly, the risk of accident or injury is significantly reduced.

Identify the hazard	What is the risk?	What should I do to prevent the hazard from becoming a risk?
Storing H_2O_2 in a lemonade bottle	Someone may drink it	• Never use food or drink containers to store chemicals. • If transferring chemicals to another bottle, ensure it is properly labelled.
Storing H_2O_2 near aerosols	In the event of a fire, the oxygen from the H_2O_2 will feed the fire and the aerosols may explode	Move the stock to ensure the H_2O_2 is not stored near the aerosols. If this is not within the scope of your job role, report it to the designated person.
Use of styling and finishing products	• Product in client's eyes • Fire, if used near naked flame	• Use extreme care. • Use a face shield if possible when using finishing sprays. • Do not use near naked flame or lit cigarette.

Smoking, eating, drinking and drugs

Smoking

When you are working in the salon it is important that your behaviour does not pose a risk to anyone. Smoking in the salon, apart from being unprofessional and unpleasant for others, has health and safety implications. The biggest problem associated with smoking in the workplace is the effect of passive smoking, that is, inhaling smoke from other people's cigarettes. There has been a considerable amount of research into passive smoking and the effect that is has on non-smokers. In the short term the effects may be:

- eye irritation
- headache
- cough
- sore throat
- nausea
- a decline in lung function in people with asthma.

Your employer has a duty under the Health and Safety at Work Act 1974 to protect non-smoking employees from the hazards of tobacco smoke. Their duty of care also extends to clients and other people who enter the salon.

Eating

Eating in the salon is unprofessional and gives a poor impression to clients. The lingering smell of food can be off-putting for clients, especially food that has a strong smell. Food that is dropped on the floor makes the floor slippery and therefore the hazard becomes a risk. The risk becomes greater if you have, for example, a client with impaired sight; the client may not see what is visible to others and slip.

Drinking

Providing drinks in the salon carries its own set of risks. A hot drink may be accidentally spilled onto a client causing scalding or it may be spilled onto the floor, making it slippery and creating a hazard. The effects of alcoholic drinks on the body make them unacceptable within the working environment. Even in low doses, alcohol will:

- aid relaxation
- reduce tension
- lower inhibitions
- impair concentration
- slow reflexes
- reduce co-ordination.

Even drinking alcohol in small quantities can reduce your effectiveness at work. A few drinks will lower your inhibitions, leaving you open to mistakes. A hangover will also affect your ability to work effectively.

Drugs

Using drugs whilst working in the salon is not recommended. The taking of drugs, depending on the type of drug, may have an effect on your ability to work safely. If you are taking prescribed drugs, it is important that you read the warning information specific to the medication. For example, tranquilisers may leave you slightly drowsy the following day and impair your ability to concentrate. Prescribed or non-prescribed medication for conditions such as hay fever may also affect your ability to work. You should inform your employer of any potential side effects from the medication you are taking and, if necessary, they may adjust your workload accordingly.

The side effects from the use of such drugs are varied and include:

- extreme over-activity (hyperactivity)
- fatigue (resulting from an inability to sleep)
- unexpected changes in mood or behaviour
- a deterioration in performance at work.

It is important to remember that taking recreational drugs is illegal in the U.K. and, if you have taken recreational drugs the night before, they may still be affecting your actions for up to 48 hours. This has obvious implications for the salon. Firstly, there is the likelihood of an accident or incident occurring due to one of the above contributory factors. Secondly, there is the impact on the business resulting from poor performance and increased absence.

Check it out

If you are a smoker, how much time have you needed to take off work due to smoking-related illnesses, chest infections etc.?

In the salon

The junior stylist comes to work with a slightly glazed look and smiling much more than usual. She is usually quite morose and sullen. You notice an unusual 'sweet' smell on her breath and clothing. The salon owner asks her to carry out a trim on an elderly client with long hair, a task she is more than capable of carrying out. When you look round, the client's hair is three centimetres long at the back. The junior stylist does not seem concerned in any way and is ready to start on the top.

- What do you think may have happened?

There are other practices in the salon that may be classed as unsafe. The table below identifies a few hazards associated with unsafe practices.

Identify the hazard	What is the risk?	What should I do?
Running in the salon	Slip, trip or fall	Don't run!
Water spray fights	Water on the floor, someone may slip	• Mop up the water immediately and allow the floor to dry. • Remember your duty of care.

Risks from environmental factors

A carelessly discarded cigarette is one of the most common reasons for 'paper bin' fires. The problem that occurs for hairdressers is that there are likely to be other types of waste in the bin. Cotton wool saturated with P.W. lotion or plastic gloves may give off toxic fumes on ignition; an empty aerosol of hairspray could explode.

Emergencies and evacuation procedures

Emergency situations arise from time to time and may be due to any of the following factors.

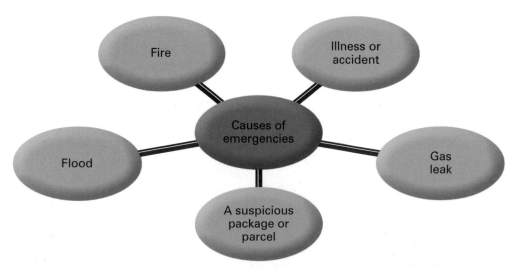

By now you should have identified those people in your salon who are responsible for first aid, health and safety and evacuating the premises.

Illness or accident

In the event of an accident or illness, you should report to the person responsible for first aid. Their responsibility is to take charge of the situation, assess the need for medical intervention and act accordingly. The appointed person should not give first aid unless they have been trained and hold a current first aid certificate. They may call an ambulance if they feel it is necessary.

Fire

In the event of a fire, you should follow the evacuation procedure laid down in policy within your salon. Do not take any unnecessary risks. You should:

- evacuate the premises by the nearest exit, taking your client/s with you
- close doors and windows en-route. A fire needs oxygen to continue burning; by reducing the amount of oxygen, it should contain the fire
- dial 999 for the fire brigade
- meet at the designated assembly point. The appointed person should now be checking to ensure that everyone has left the building.

When leaving the salon, you must not stop to collect your personal items as prolonging your stay in the salon could increase the risk of injury from the fire. Your evacuation policy should include provision for disabled people, as they may not be as mobile as you and should be classed as a higher risk. You should also be familiar with all evacuation routes. There may be instances where one fire exit is inaccessible due to the fire so you must know of other escape routes. Fire exits should be clearly identified and, in larger premises, green fire exit signs should indicate the way to safety.

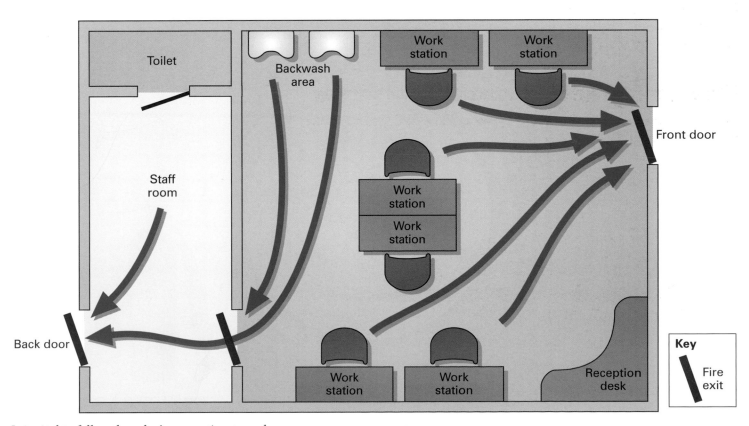

It is vital to follow the salon's evacuation procedure

Fire extinguishers

All new portable fire extinguishers are predominantly red with a zone of colour to indicate the contents of the extinguisher.

A **water** extinguisher should be used for fires involving wood, cloth, paper, plastics and coal.

A **foam** extinguisher should be used on liquid fires as it forms a blanket of foam over the surface of the burning liquid and smothers the fire.

A **dry powder** extinguisher is used for burning liquids such as oil, paint and grease. However, it MUST NOT be used on chip pan fires. The dry powder extinguisher does not cool the fire very well; care must be taken as the fire may re-ignite. A fire blanket will help to cool a fire and prevent re-ignition.

A **carbon dioxide (CO_2)** extinguisher may be used on burning liquids (except chip pan or fat pan fires) and electrical fires. Again, these extinguishers have limited cooling properties and a fire blanket may be used to prevent re-ignition.

A **wet chemical** extinguisher should be used to tackle fires involving deep fat fryers and chip pan fires. You may not come across this type of fire in the salon, however it is important to be aware of the different types of extinguishers available.

Water with additive

Foam

Wet chemical

Powder

CO_2 gas

Fire extinguishers

Identify the hazard	What is the risk?	What should I do?
Pouring water onto an electrical fire	Electrocution	• If in doubt, stay out and call the fire brigade. • Ask your employer to send you for training.

Suspicious parcels or packages

Suspicious parcels or packages should be considered high risk as they may endanger lives. Your salon should have a policy specifically for dealing with suspicious packages in a way that will reduce the risk to health and safety. It should include the following.

• Do not touch the package!
• Evacuate the salon.
• Call 999 for the police.
• Do not re-enter the salon until you have been authorised to do so by the police.

Flood

In the event of the salon being flooded due to a leak or burst pipes, it is necessary to follow your salon's procedures. In particular:

• the electricity must be turned off at the mains to prevent electrocution
• the water should be turned off at the mains supply to prevent further leakage
• call the plumber to fix the leak
• in extreme cases, it may be necessary to call the fire brigade to pump out the water.

Gas leak

In the event of a gas leak or if you suspect you can smell gas, procedures must be followed to prevent a gas explosion. You should evacuate clients and other staff not included in the salon's procedure for gas leaks.

Those remaining must ensure that:

- they do not turn electric switches on or off as they may 'spark' and ignite the gas
- they do not smoke or use naked flames
- they turn the gas supply off at the meter, to prevent any more gas escaping
- they open all doors and windows to get rid of the gas
- the appointed person will call the gas emergency number.

Check it out

If your salon does not have policies in place to cover the above emergencies, how would you rate the risk – high, medium or low?

Personal presentation

Hairdressing is a fashion industry and the way you look is important. Clients will judge you not only on your hairdressing skills but also on the way you look. Personal presentation also has important implications for health and safety, as outlined below.

Clothes

Your clothes should be regularly laundered and preferably made from cotton or a poly-cotton material, as these fabrics will allow your skin to breathe. Cotton fabrics also minimise perspiration and are easy to clean. Avoid wearing woollen clothes, as they may make you too hot; hair tends to stick into the weave and digs into the skin, which can be uncomfortable.

Shoes

Your shoes should have a low heel and a closed-in toe. Shoes with high heels throw your body out of alignment, which in time will lead to backache due to unnecessary stress put on the muscles and ligaments.

A closed in shoe will help to prevent hair cuttings from becoming stuck in the soles of your feet. This can be extremely painful as the hairs are not always easy to find and your skin may become infected. Hairdressers tend to stand for most of the day and your feet need to be comfortable. Leather shoes are best as they allow your feet to breathe.

Another potential problem is varicose veins which can develop as a result of standing for long periods of time. However, once they have developed, they are uncomfortable. Wearing 'support tights' may be helpful, especially if you are pregnant.

Personal health

Your own health, especially poor health, has serious implications for the people around you. If you have contracted an illness that is infectious or contagious, you run the risk of passing it on to your colleagues or clients. Ideally, you should not attend work if you know there is the possibility of you passing it on to another person. Remember, you have a duty of care towards your clients.

In the salon

Mr Lewis called into the salon for a beard trim with Shannon, the new stylist. Shannon had a small cut on her right hand from being careless with a bread knife. She didn't think she needed a plaster because the cut was quite small. As Shannon prepared to trim Mr Lewis's facial hair, she accidentally opened the wound on the edge of the workstation. The salon manager noticed what was going on and insisted that Shannon find a plaster in the First Aid box.

- What kind of risk did Shannon pose to her client?
- How could this situation have been avoided?

Knowledge check

1.   *Define the following terms:*
     - *a hazard*
     - *a risk*
     - *a control measure.*

2.   *List ten products used in the salon that are covered by COSHH regulations.*

3.   *Complete the gaps in the table below:*

Identify the hazard	What are the risks?	What should I do to prevent the hazard from becoming a risk?
Water on the floor		
Reaching for stock on a high shelf		
Trailing flexes		
Storing H_2O_2 near aerosols		
Running in the salon		

4.   *Name three methods of sterilization used in the salon.*

5.   *What are the potential risks of drinking alcohol in the salon?*

6.   *What should you do if you are ill at work?*

7.   *In the event of an evacuation, why is it important that you leave the salon as quickly as possible and do not stop to collect your personal belongings?*

8.   What type of fire extinguisher should be used for:
   • electrical fires?
   • non-electrical fires?

9.   When may it be necessary to use a fire blanket?

10. Why is it important to wear shoes with a closed-in toe when working in the salon?

Provide hairdressing consultation services

Unit G9

Introduction

The consultation is the most crucial part of any service offered in the salon. An effective and comprehensive consultation and advisory service will ensure the clients are satisfied with the service they receive and contribute to the overall professional image the salon is portraying. The consultation/advisory service should not finish when you start the required service, but continue for the duration of the client's visit.

In this unit you will learn the techniques needed to carry out an effective consultation and the importance of giving advice and guidance to your clients. This may include referring them to a specialist for further advice and/or treatment. You will also be encouraged to offer your support to colleagues who may be experiencing difficulties with their own consultations.

Effective consultation is the key to client satisfaction

What you will learn
• Identifying clients' needs and wishes
• Analysing the hair and scalp
• Making recommendations to your client
• Agreeing services with your client

You the stylist

As a stylist you must carry out thorough and effective consultations. You need to find out everything about your client's hair before starting work, as this will ensure you make the correct decisions regarding the services that are available to your client. This includes identifying the client's requirements using your communication skills, analysing the hair and scalp (including carrying out pre-service testing when necessary), and then making your recommendations. A good consultation instils confidence in the client and, as a result of this, you will build a good relationship with your client, based on trust. Your clients need to feel you have their best interests at heart, rather than being a means to boost your commission!

Once you have the trust of your clients, they will more readily accept your recommendations, as long as your recommendations are honest. It is not always easy to tell a client that their wishes are unachievable, but as long as you use tact and diplomacy, you will find that honesty is the best policy.

You should be able to participate in discussions with your clients regarding their needs and wishes as well as making general conversation. For many clients their visit to the salon incorporates the hair service and an element of socialising. A silent service can be uncomfortable for some clients as well as the stylist. You must learn to gauge the situation and make openings to encourage your clients to speak.

Hairdressers are renowned for discussing the weather and the client's last or forthcoming holiday, but this does not need to be the case. You should try to find out about your client's interests and bring these into the discussion. A quiet client may become quite animated when discussing an area they are interested in and the things you learn may surprise you! You will, however, come across the silent client, the one who shows no desire to speak once their needs and wishes have been established and the service is underway. You must respect their decision, as it may be the only time that day they have had the opportunity for peace and quiet.

Identifying clients' needs and wishes

Many clients find it difficult to express their requirements, as they do not always know how to explain what they want. As a professional hairdresser, you must be able to establish the exact nature of your clients' needs and wants. This requires you to have excellent interpersonal skills. You will need to use these skills to draw information from the client and also to make sure that both you and the client have a complete understanding before commencing any service.

Communication

Communication is a two-way process that involves both sending and receiving information. As a hairdresser, you are expected to be able to make conversation with your clients. However, good communication is not just about talking; it also involves listening, hearing and interpreting what the other person is saying in a positive manner.

We communicate in a number of ways, as shown below.

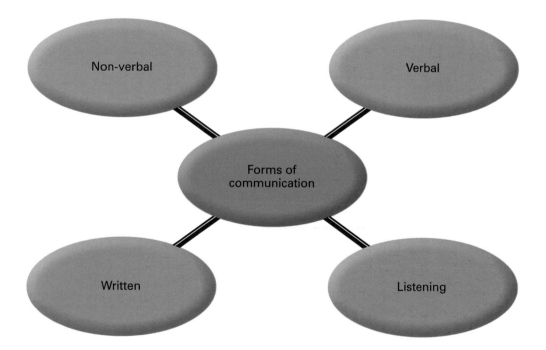

Verbal communication

When speaking to clients you must make sure the language you use is suitable for the recipient. You may need to simplify your language to ensure total understanding. Many clients are not familiar with hairdressing jargon and do not always understand what you are saying to them. For example, you might tell your client that you will taper the nape area, graduate the back and leave some weight on the top. Do you think your client really understands exactly what you mean or could this be better explained by using visual aids, for example, style books, colleagues in the salon, and so on? Many clients find it easier to relate to a picture than to words, as it conjures up a more realistic mental image and is easier for them to understand.

Some clients find it difficult to express their needs and wishes and require time and encouragement to put their point across. Your clients should never feel hurried as this may prevent them giving you essential information. At intervals you should stop and summarise the information the client has given you. This gives the client the opportunity to either confirm or refute your understanding of the conversation. For example, you could say, 'So do you want your hair to cover your ears?' or 'Do you want a heavy fringe?'

Using sign language can help you communicate with clients with a hearing impairment

Once you are both happy with the situation, you should move the conversation along to the next point of discussion. You should be able to initiate and focus on specific areas that need to be developed to ensure you have a total understanding. Remember to summarise when a new topic has been discussed. You may need to use explicit questioning to help draw the information from the client; this questioning should cover both 'factual' and 'feeling' questions.

Factual questions

You should use factual questions to find out relevant information about the client's hair such as home-care routine, previous chemical history, and so on. Many stylists like to use this type of question to open a conversation, as it is non-threatening to the client. For example, 'How often do you shampoo your hair? Which products do you use at home to style your hair?'

Feeling questions

Feeling questions should be used to establish the clients' fears, opinions, doubts or worries. These questions usually include words such as 'feel', 'think' or 'want', and are an excellent tool for finding out how the client really feels. For example, 'You feel a vibrant red colour isn't really you, but what do you think about this smoky, more subdued red?' You must treat your client's worries and doubts as important issues and readily accept their opinions. Ignoring their worries will lead to client dissatisfaction.

Remember

It is essential that you allow the client sufficient time to think and answer, as failure to do this could result in an unwanted outcome and a dissatisfied client.

Other types of questions

When trying to elicit information from your clients, the way you structure your questions is very important. You should try wherever possible to use **open questions**. These questions start with words such as 'what', 'why', 'when', 'how', 'where' and 'who', and will require the client to give a more detailed answer. For example, 'How did you feel about your last hair colour?' (This is an open and feeling question.)

Closed questions require either a 'yes' or 'no' answer and are not very good at drawing information from the client, for example, 'Same colour as last time?' This does not readily set the client up to express his or her wishes, but would be seen more as a lost opportunity to convey their views. However, you should use closed questions when closing the consultation or drawing a conversation to its end, for example, 'So you want a very soft curl, just to give the hair body and support the style?' This gives the client the opportunity to answer either yes or no.

When questioning the client, remember to give yourself sufficient time to reflect on what they have just told you. You should then summarise or re-phrase the information to ensure you have fully understood their requirements.

Non-verbal communication

Only a small percentage of the impression you create stems from what you say; the majority comes from your body language. It is very important that you are aware of your non-verbal communication skills.

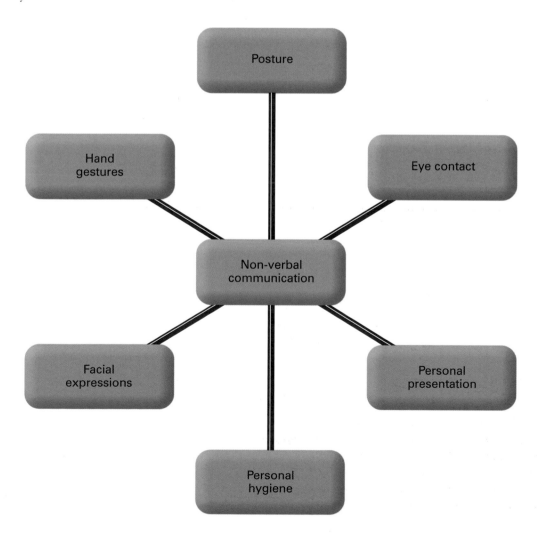

Posture

Try to maintain good posture. If you slouch around the salon, it gives the impression you do not particularly care and clients will assume this is reflected in the work you carry out in the salon.

Eye contact

You should make eye contact with your client frequently enough to show that you are responsive, but avoid staring at the client as this becomes intimidating.

Hand gestures

These are commonly used to convey feelings or to emphasise a point. However, overuse of hand gestures may appear ridiculous to onlookers.

Facial expressions

You should try to maintain positive facial expressions as these are seen as friendly and caring. Smiling at your client will make them feel more comfortable in your company. However, this does not mean walking around with a permanent grin on your face.

Your non-verbal communication should be positive at all times in the salon, for example, smiling, making eye contact, and so on. This will help to put others at ease, which includes both clients and other members of staff. When instructing junior members of staff, your body language should be open and unthreatening, as this will again be reflected in the salon's atmosphere and the willingness of others to help you. Other members of staff and clients may be easily offended by negative body language.

Personal presentation/personal hygiene

Personal hygiene is important to hairdressers as they work in such close proximity to clients. Your own hygiene should be excellent, as you do not wish to portray anything other than total professionalism to your clients. Stale breath and body odour will portray a negative impression of you.

Although hairdressing is a fashion industry, many salons now have quite strict dress codes for staff, for example, no sleeveless or cropped tops. It can be quite off-putting to have an armpit in your face or a large expanse of flesh showing. If you make the effort to look smart, clean and tidy, clients will assume you will take the same care and consideration over their hair.

Stylists should maintain a professional appearance at all times

---

Keys to good practice

- Keep in mind the phrase 'actions speak louder than words'. Your body language can tell someone far more about how you are feeling than what you may actually say.
- You may think you can cover up feeling hurt or angry, but those who can read body language will know exactly what you are saying without words!

Check it out

Ask a colleague or friend to watch you whilst you are working (or better still, make a video recording) and analyse your body language. Do you appear friendly and approachable? If you do not, now is the time to change!

Written communication

Some salons now use prescription pads to note a client's hair and home-care details. This then leads to a home-care maintenance programme that may be discussed with the client.

Aslone Kera-care
CONDITIONING HAIR CARE SYSTEM

Date: _____

Name: _____

Address: _____

City: _____ County: _____

Postcode: _____ Phone: _____

PLEASE TICK THE BEST RESPONSE TO EACH OF THE FOLLOWING

Scalp Condition:
☐ Dry/Itchy ☐ Normal ☐ Oily

Hair Condition:
☐ Virgin ☐ Relaxed
☐ Colour Treated ☐ Permanently Waved

Hair Texture:
☐ Fine ☐ Medium ☐ Coarse

Diagnosis:
☐ Weak ☐ Dry/Brittle ☐ Damaged
☐ Over processed ☐ Shedding ☐ Healthy
☐ Other

How often do you visit the salon for service?
☐ Every week ☐ Every Two Weeks
☐ Once a Month ☐ Every Two Months or longer

Do you shampoo at home between salon visits?
☐ Yes ☐ No

How do you usually have your hair styled?
☐ Blow Dry/Hot Curl ☐ Wrap Set ☐ Roller Set
☐ Rod Set ☐ Other _____

What is your daily active lifestyle?
☐ Aerobics ☐ Swimming
☐ Running/Jogging ☐ Other _____

How do you select products for home maintenance?
☐ Salon/Stylist ☐ Beauty Supply
☐ Other _____

Kera-care Hairscription

The following Aslone Hair Care Maintenance is suggested for your hair texture, conditioning, and daily styling needs. Follow this recommended hair care regime to restore and maintain healthy looking hair.

SHAMPOOS
☐ Dry & Itchy Scalp Moisturising Shampoo
☐ Hydrating Detangling Shampoo
☐ 1st Lather Shampoo

CONDITIONERS
☐ Leave-In Conditioner
☐ Humecto Cream Conditioner
☐ Dry & Itchy Scalp Moisturizing Conditioner

LIGHT OILS
☐ Oil Moisturizer with Jojoba Oil
☐ Conditioning Cream Hairdress
☐ Dry & Itchy Scalp Glossifer
☐ High Sheen Glossifer
☐ Essential Oils for the Hair

STYLING ESSENTIALS
☐ Protein Styling Gel
☐ Finishing Spritz
☐ Setting Lotion
☐ Silken Seal
☐ Silken Seal Liquid Sheen
☐ Foam Wrap-Set Lotion

Next Appointment: _____ Time: _____

Comments/Product Usage: _____
_____
_____

A hairscription

Completion of client record cards is essential to the smooth running of any salon. The information contained on a client record card should be legible, unambiguous and clear, and leave the reader in no doubt as to its meaning. Record cards that are filled in incorrectly or are incomplete may cause chaos in the salon, as mistakes can occur leaving the client dissatisfied with the service and the salon in breach of the Data Protection Act (see also page 78).

Listening

Listening plays a large part in any consultation as you need to listen to your client's requirements and act accordingly. Further questioning on your part to ascertain your client's wishes may follow this.

As a professional hairdresser, you should adopt an attitude of active participation when listening to your client's wishes. Maintaining positive body language and using words of encouragement may help you do this. You can show this by:

- facing the client
- maintaining eye contact
- leaning towards the client
- acknowledging what has been said.

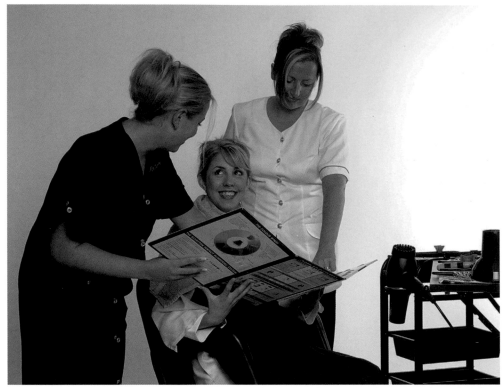

Use positive body language and active listening skills when discussing clients' needs and wishes

People are often heard saying, 'I know you're listening to me, but are you hearing what I'm saying?' meaning you are listening in a half-hearted manner and probably not trying to understand what is being said to you. This type of passive listening leads to mistakes and client dissatisfaction as the client's requests are often ignored.

You also need to learn the skill of listening to what your client is not saying! This involves learning to read the messages your clients are sending through spoken words, their facial expressions and body posture. You should pay particular attention to:

- what they say
- the way it is said
- what is not being said.

How often have you said something but not really meant it? A friend in an awful outfit asks if you like it and you agree so you do not hurt their feelings, but can you really lie that well? Most clients cannot. You need to take the time and effort to notice these things. You may also notice that the client's tone of voice alters. If the words become 'clipped', the client may not be happily accepting the information you are giving.

Keep a close check on your client's facial expressions. While you will hopefully have mastered the art of maintaining positive facial expressions, your client may not have and you should use this information to your advantage. This will obviously depend on the circumstances, but you may be required to ask further feeling questions to discover what the client is trying not to tell you. Have you ever taken the time to look for indicators such as these?

During your consultations you will be expected to adopt the techniques you have just learned and utilise them to the full. Your questioning and listening techniques, coupled with open and responsive body language, will ensure your client feels comfortable about asking you questions. You may be required to go over things several times to ensure the clients have a full understanding of the service they are to receive.

Check it out

If you have some spare time, study people's body language and their methods of communication. It is sometimes easier to do this when you are sitting on the outside looking in, for example, when the client belongs to another stylist.

Remember

Only when you are absolutely sure that you know what your client requires, should you begin to make your own service recommendations.

Keys to good practice

- Use all of your communication skills when identifying client's wishes.
- Use visual aids whenever possible.
- Thorough and effective consultations prevent mistakes and client dissatisfaction.

Analysing the hair and scalp

Before you are able to accurately analyse the hair and scalp, you should have a thorough understanding of the hair growth and the hair's characteristics, as this will have a considerable bearing on the outcome. To begin with, you should have a good understanding of the basic structure of the hair and skin and how they work.

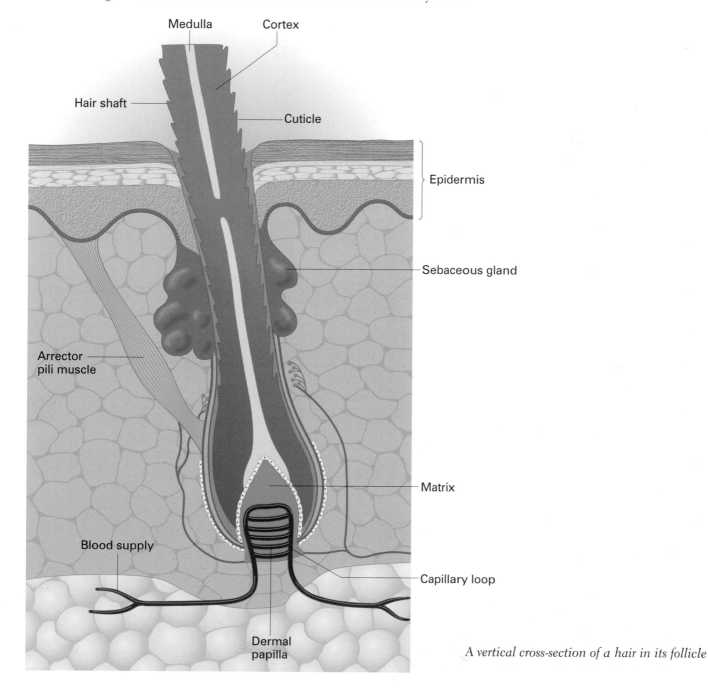

A vertical cross-section of a hair in its follicle

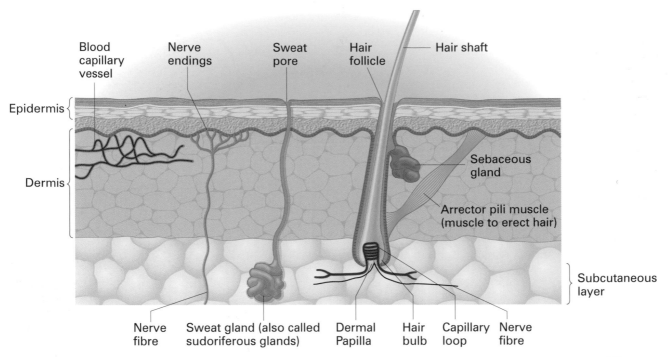

The structure of the skin

Parts of the hair

Cuticle

The cuticle is the outermost part of the hair and is made up from layers of overlapping scale-like bands. It acts as protection for the rest of the hair, but as keratin is brittle it may be damaged by harsh treatment and overuse of chemicals. The cuticle may not be present towards the ends of the hair, as it may have been damaged or destroyed completely; therefore the ends of the hair will be more porous.

The number of layers of cuticle scales varies depending on the type of hair. Coarse hair has the most layers of cuticle making it more resistant to chemicals. You may have discovered this already when perming or colouring coarse hair.

Cortex

The cortex makes up the bulk of the hair and gives the hair its strength and elasticity. The cortex is important, as this is where the changes occur during bleaching, perming, relaxing, colouring and styling. The cortex is made up from bundles of parallel fibres, which are in turn made up from smaller fibres.

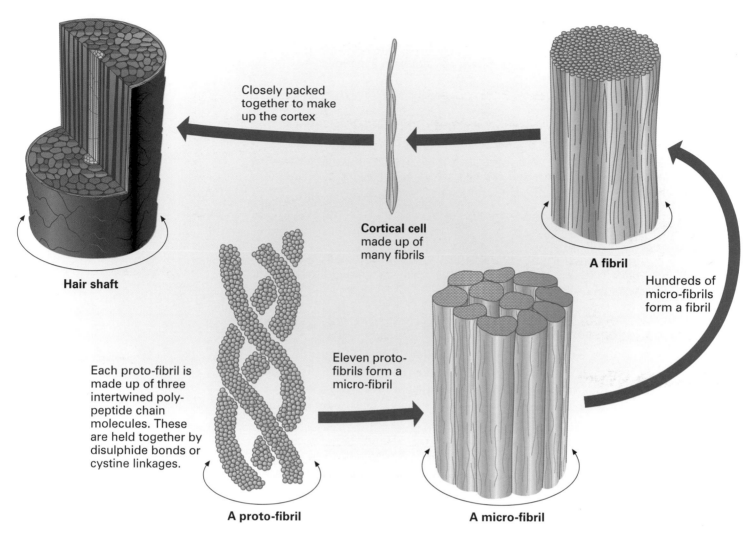

Closely packed together to make up the cortex

Cortical cell made up of many fibrils

Hair shaft

A fibril

Hundreds of micro-fibrils form a fibril

Each proto-fibril is made up of three intertwined poly-peptide chain molecules. These are held together by disulphide bonds or cystine linkages.

Eleven proto-fibrils form a micro-fibril

A proto-fibril

A micro-fibril

The cortex

Melanin and pheomelanin, the hair's natural colour pigment, is found in the cortex. African Caribbean hair has two different types of cortex, the ortho-cortex and the para-cortex. The ortho-cortex has a less crowded structure and always lies on the outer curve of a wave. It is less crowded as the hair is stretched at this point. It has a lower sulphur content than the para-cortex. The para-cortex is compressed on the inside of the wave, making this part of the cortex more crowded. When carrying out chemical treatments on curly hair, this must be taken into consideration, as the hair will absorb chemicals at different rates, giving an uneven result.

Para-cortex

Ortho-cortex

The para- and ortho-cortex

Medulla

The medulla is the central part of the hair and is made up from small soft cells with air spaces in between. People with very fine hair may not have a medulla.

Sebaceous glands

The sebaceous glands are sac-like structures attached to the hair follicles all over the body. They produce sebum, which is an oily substance used to lubricate and waterproof the hair and skin, and prevents them from drying out. If too little sebum is produced, the skin may become dry and cracked, which could lead to dermatitis. Sebaceous glands are plentiful on the face and scalp.

Arrector pili muscle

The arrector pili muscle is a small involuntary muscle that is attached to each hair follicle. When you are cold or frightened, the muscle contracts making the hair stand on end. It serves no purpose in hairdressing.

Sudoriferous (or sweat) glands

The sudoriferous glands are found in the dermis and look like coiled tubes that extend and lead to the surface of the skin to form a pore. The purpose of these glands is to regulate the body temperature through the excretion of sweat onto the skin surface. When sweat evaporates, it cools the skin and the body temperature becomes lower. Sweat is mainly composed of water, salts and waste products.

Hair follicle

The hair follicles are tiny indentations in the skin. The hair that is below the skin is contained within the follicle. The angle at which the follicle lies will determine the hair's natural fall.

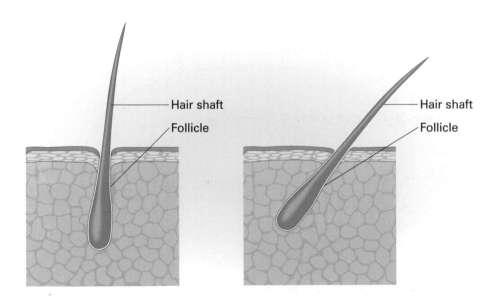

The angle of the follicle determines the natural fall of the hair

Dermal papilla

Often referred to as the growing factory. The base of the hair follicle is pushed upwards, like the bottom of a wine bottle. The papilla is situated in this space. The cells produced in the papilla are pushed upwards into the germinal matrix.

Hair bulb

The hair bulb has two distinctive parts – the upper bulb and the germinal matrix. In the germinal matrix all the cells look the same. In the upper bulb the hair starts to develop into its three layers.

Blood supply

The blood supply enters the papilla, bringing food and nourishment for healthy cell growth. It also takes away waste products.

Nerve supply

The nerve supply is also attached to the papilla. This supply is in addition to other nerves in the area, and it is what enables you to feel your hair being pulled.

Parts of the skin (see page 38)

Epidermis

The epidermis is the outermost layer of the skin. The part of the epidermis that we see is called the stratum corneum and this is made up of flat, horny cells. It is these cells that are constantly being shed and replaced. Skin problems associated with the production and shedding of these cells include dandruff and psoriasis.

Dermis

The dermis is situated below the epidermis and contains blood vessels, sweat and sebaceous glands, nerve endings and hair follicles. The dermis is made up from fibres of proteins.

Subcutaneous layer

The subcutaneous layer is situated below the dermis and contains fatty tissue, which acts as insulation (to prevent body heat from being lost), and acts as a defence to protect the internal organs.

The characteristics of different hair types and textures

Hair may be considered fine, medium or coarse in texture, but this may vary at different parts of the scalp and in the case of curly hair, along the hair shaft. The degree of curl in the hair may also vary. It is essential during your consultation that you consider all the hair you will be working with and not just the part that is easy to see.

Why do some people have straight hair and others curly?

There are currently three schools of thought surrounding this question but little solid evidence to support any particular theory.

1 The first theory suggests that the amount of curl in the hair is determined by the shape of the follicle, for example, a straight follicle will produce straight hair and a bent follicle will produce wavy or curly hair, depending on the degree of curvature.

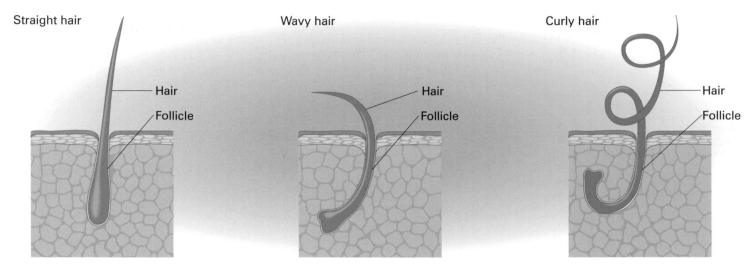

Straight hair   Wavy hair   Curly hair

— Hair   — Hair   — Hair
— Follicle   — Follicle   — Follicle

Different shaped follicles may produce straight, wavy or curly hair

2   The second theory suggests the amount of curl in the hair is due to an uneven rate of mitosis (cell division). Hair grows as a result of cell division in the germinal matrix. As the number of cells increase, they push the old cells upwards into the upper bulb. If the cells on one side of the hair are dividing more quickly than the other, this will make one side of the hair longer than the other, producing a bend in the hair. If the cell division alternates from one side to the other, the result will be curly hair.

Mitosis   Mitosis   Mitosis
faster here   `Papilla   faster here   faster here

To support this theory, think about a person who has undergone chemotherapy. The hair after treatment is often quite straight, whereas beforehand it was curly. The hair returns to being curly at a later date.

Curly hair resulting from an uneven rate of mitosis

During chemotherapy, the whole body's systems are disrupted and mitosis is suppressed. The body would naturally take quite a while to return to normal, even after the treatment has been completed, and this may include mitosis, hence the hair being initially straight but reverting to curly once the body's balance has been restored.

3   The third theory suggests that keratinisation occurs in the cortex asymmetrically. As the hair moves upwards in the follicle, the hair begins the process of keratinisation (where the living cells die and harden). By the time the hair is a third of the way up the follicle, the hair has been fully keratinised. On one side of

the cortex, keratinisation occurs early (and becomes the para-cortex) whilst on the other side, keratinisation is delayed (and this becomes the ortho-cortex). Until keratinisation takes place, the hair will continue to grow – so the ortho-cortex will be longer in length then the para-cortex, producing curl.

Check it out

Look at the above information and discuss the pros and cons of each theory with your tutor and group members. Then draw your own conclusions.

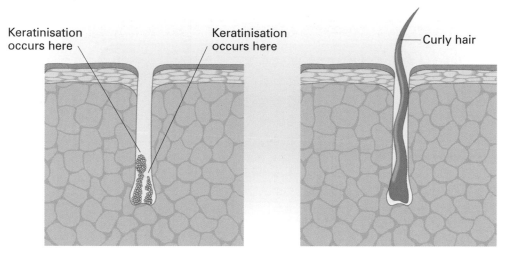

Curly hair resulting from uneven keratinisation

The hair growth cycle

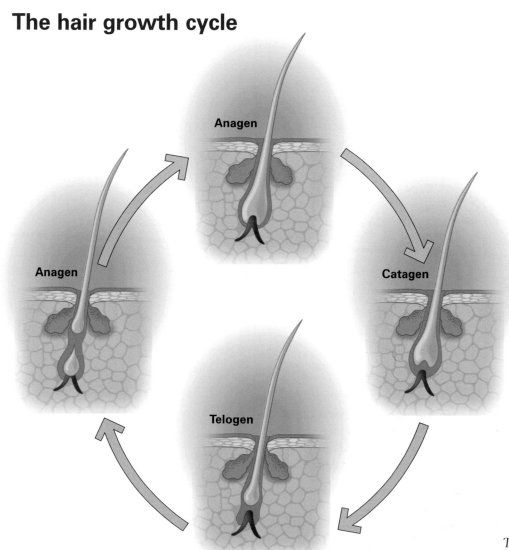

The hair growth cycle

At the base of the hair follicle lies the dermal papilla. The dermal papilla is fed by nourishment from the blood stream, which helps to produce new hair. Within each hair follicle there is a period of hair growth, followed by a resting phase. The total cycle goes through three separate phases, which are:

1 anagen – growth or active phase
2 catagen – transitional or changing phase
3 telogen – resting phase.

The hair growth cycle is repeated many times during a person's lifetime. Each hair grows then falls out and a new hair grows in its place.

Anagen

This is the growing or active phase of the growth cycle. There is plenty of activity taking place in the dermal papilla. This average phase lasts from one to six years, but some people have a short anagen cycle and regardless of what they may do, their hair will never grow long as it is predetermined to fall out after a specified time. Some people with very long hair have a much longer anagen cycle than average. The anagen phase is the longest with approximately 85 per cent of hair in this active state at any one time. Some areas of the body have a much shorter phase in the anagen cycle, for example, masculine facial hair.

Catagen

At the end of the anagen phase, hair growth stops and no new cells are produced in the dermal papilla. This phase lasts for approximately two weeks and during this time the follicle shrinks up to one sixth of its original length.

Telogen

This is a period of rest for both the follicle and the papilla and lasts between ten to twelve weeks. Approximately ten to fifteen per cent of the follicles are in this phase at any one time.

At the end of the telogen phase the hair follicle re-enters the anagen phase, the follicle lengthens downwards and the papilla becomes active again, ready for the growth of a new hair.

As each follicle across the scalp is at a slightly different point in the cycle at any given time, this explains why a client's haircut loses its shape after a few weeks. On a positive note, it keeps hairdressers in business!

During pregnancy, the hormonal changes in the body keep the hair in the anagen phase of the growth cycle for the length of the pregnancy and many women notice their hair becoming thicker during pregnancy. However, after giving birth, the hormone levels change yet again and all the hairs that should have been lost during the pregnancy are shed fairly quickly. This can be very distressing to a client who is not only contending with a new baby, but is also worried she is losing her hair. This condition does rectify itself eventually, but the client will require reassurance from you in the meantime.

Under normal circumstances, the hair growth cycle will continue for the duration of a person's life. However, there are factors that may influence hair growth or cause damage to the hair follicle. These factors include genetic influences (for example, male pattern baldness) or the results of scarring and radiation.

Reference to client records

Reference to client's previous records should be made whenever possible. This will give you a wealth of information the client may not know or understand, for example, allergic reactions to relaxing products previously used, type of colourants used, and so on.

Observation

An experienced stylist can tell a lot about a client's hair and scalp just by looking at it, for example, the texture, condition and any previous chemical treatments. Prior to questioning the client, you should have made an initial assessment of your client's hair and scalp and any potential problems that may arise from your observation.

Questioning

You should use questioning as a tool to find out as much as you can from your client, as this will enable you to make an accurate judgment regarding the most suitable service you can then carry out. You should use open questions whenever possible as you will gain more information from your client. However, not all clients are honest when giving information about their hair and the treatments that have been carried out on it, especially those done by a non-professional. If in doubt, carry out any necessary tests as this will save time in the long run and prevent client dissatisfaction.

Testing

Testing the hair prior to salon services is a practice that should be adopted by all professional hairdressers, especially as litigation is becoming more widespread. It only need take a few minutes to carry out some tests and could save you hours (not to mention money) if the service goes wrong and needs to be corrected, or the client sues the salon for negligence. If you have any worries or concerns regarding the suitability of a client's hair, carry out the necessary tests to eliminate the doubt and ensure the client's hair is suitable for the service they requested. All tests should be carried out following your salon's procedures and the manufacturer's instructions.

The kinds of tests you should be carrying out are shown in the table on pages 46-7.

Remember
All information contained on a client's record card should be accurate and up to date to comply with the Data Protection Act, even if the information is handwritten!

Test	When it should be carried out	Why it should be carried out	How it should be carried out	The expected outcome	The potential consequences if it is not carried out
Porosity (sometimes called a texture test)	Prior to colouring, perming and corrective relaxing.	To assess the amount of damage to the cuticle; to check the speed at which products will be absorbed into the hair.	It should be carried out on dry hair. Hold a few strands of hair, run your fingers from roots to points and then points to roots. This test cannot be carried out on wet hair as the hair swells when wet and will not give a true indication of the hair's porosity.	The hair should feel fairly smooth at the root area, becoming rougher towards the ends.	• The result may be uneven. • The hair will become more porous.
Elasticity	Prior to colouring, perming, corrective relaxing, thermal styling and styling hair.	To assess the degree of damage to the internal structure.	Hold a few strands of hair between the fingers and thumbs and pull gently. Best carried out when hair is wet.	The hair should stretch and return to its original length. If the hair stretches and does not return to its original length, this indicates the presence of internal damage.	The hair may overstretch and/or break.
Incompatibility	Prior to colouring and perming.	To test the hair for the presence of metallic salts or other incompatible substances.	Take a cutting of hair from the affected part of the head, secure with cotton or sellotape. Pour 20 mls of liquid 6% H_2O_2 into a non-metallic bowl. Add 5 drops of ammonium hydroxide. Leave for up to 30 minutes.	If there are no incompatible substances on the hair, there should be no reaction in the bowl. If the metallic salts are present, the liquid in the bowl will effervesce and become hot. The hair colour may change to green, purple or black.	The hair colour may change. Extreme heat will be given off causing the hair to disintegrate and cause scalp burns.

Test	When it should be carried out	Why it should be carried out	How it should be carried out	The expected outcome	The potential consequences if it is not carried out
Skin test	24–48 hours before each colour service.	To test for allergic reaction to the product.	Cleanse a small area of skin behind the ear. Mix a small amount of the darkest colour with 6% H_2O_2 and apply a small amount to the cleansed area.	**A negative reaction** There has been no reaction at all. The skin looks as it did before the skin test took place. **A positive reaction** This can vary from redness and mild irritation to severe swelling rendering the client unable to close their eyes, speak or breath properly.	The client may have a severe allergic reaction.
Skin test before perming	24–48 hours before a perming service, especially if the client has known sensitivity.	As above.	Cleanse a small area of skin behind the ear. Apply a small amount of perm lotion to the cleansed skin.	As above.	As above.
Test cuttings	Prior to a colouring service.	To ensure optimum colour result. It is also reassuring for the client to see the results.	Take a few cuttings from various parts of the head and secure with cotton or sellotape. Mix a small amount of the desired colour/s with the correct strength of H_2O_2 and place the cuttings into the colour. Process as normal. Rinse the hair and assess the results.	This test will clearly indicate whether it is safe to proceed with the service.	Client dissatisfaction due to an incorrect result or possible damage/breakage to the hair.

Remember

Always follow your salon's procedures when carrying out pre-service testing. Most of these will reflect the manufacturer's instructions. Remember, they have tried and tested all their products and know how to achieve the best results.

In the salon

Dave had been colouring his hair blue/black for years. He did not always stick to the same product manufacturer, as the colour was always great. He was modelling for Greta as she was entering a hairdressing competition. He was quite happy about this, as his hair was to stay blue/black, but would be coloured professionally, which would save him money. Two days before the competition, Dave went to the salon to have his hair coloured. He had used the product before and never had any type of reaction, so Greta coloured his hair. The result was fantastic. Later that evening, Dave's scalp started to itch and his throat became dry and he found it difficult to swallow. During the night the itch became unbearable and Dave was having trouble breathing, so he got up. As he walked past the mirror he was horrified by what he saw. His face was blue and so swollen that he did not recognise himself. He felt very ill and was really frightened. A friend took him straight to the accident and emergency department at the local hospital. He was admitted to hospital as he had had a severe allergic reaction to the colouring preparation that had been used on his hair. As his face and throat had swelled, this had caused Dave to have trouble breathing and he was placed on a ventilator and given a massive dose of antihistamine. It took a few days for the swelling to subside and he was unable to model for the competition. Although Dave had always coloured his hair and even used the same product before, he had become sensitised to the product and the result was a severe allergic reaction.

- Was Greta negligent for not carrying out a skin test?

Healthy hair

Healthy hair is recognised by its shiny appearance. This is because the cuticle scales are closed and the light reflects off the hair giving it lustre. Curly hair, even in good condition, does not always appear shiny, as the light rays hit an uneven surface causing the light rays to scatter. Consequently, shine products may be used to give the illusion of healthy hair.

Hair in good condition

Hair in poor condition

Hair in good condition

Light rays
hitting the hair

Light rays are
reflected

Flat cuticle scales

Hair in poor condition

Light rays
hitting the hair

Scattered rays

Roughened or
raised cuticle scales

To keep the hair in optimum condition requires good health, a good diet, exercise and a skilled hairdresser who will provide excellent services and advise the client on first-rate home-care routine. There are many things that may adversely affect the condition of the hair, such as:

- chemical damage caused by overuse of chemicals or poor application
- physical damage caused by over-brushing, blow-drying and overuse of heated styling appliances
- weather conditions, both very hot and very cold
- certain medication
- illness.

The factors above should be taken into consideration when carrying out consultations, as their effects will impact on the services and products that are suitable for the client.

When discussing client's health and/or medication, both of which are personal and may be highly sensitive, you should always follow the salon's code of ethics and maintain confidentiality. Failure to do so may result in disciplinary action against you and loss of trust and goodwill on the part of the client.

Check it out

Does your salon have a policy of confidentiality toward the clients? What should be covered within these rules?

Factors that may limit or affect services and products

There are several factors that may limit or affect the services and products you provide in the salon.

Adverse hair, skin and scalp conditions

It is essential that any adverse hair, skin and scalp conditions are identified and taken into consideration during the consultation. If the client has an infectious hair, skin or scalp condition, it needs to be recognised before the service commences to reduce the risk of cross-infection within the salon.

There are many different types of adverse hair, skin and scalp conditions and these usually fall into four main categories as follows:

- hair disorders
- infestations
- infectious or contagious skin or scalp conditions
- non-infectious skin or scalp conditions.

Hair disorders

Hair disorders are not usually infectious but may require special consideration when carrying out hairdressing services. The hair may be damaged or porous and be susceptible to breakage.

Infestations

Infestation is the name given to animal parasites that live on or in another living creature and have the potential to cause harm. The most common infestation seen by hairdressers is that of the head louse, although many hairdressers still do not recognise this condition or know how it should be treated. This infestation is becoming more prevalent and it is up to hairdressers to educate their clients as to the correct procedure to follow.

Most clients or parents are upset to discover they or their children have head lice and you must display tact and diplomacy when informing them. Salon services must not take place if a client has an infestation, but the client should be reassured that the problem is a common one and treatable. You should question the client/parent, as head lice are a common problem and are usually caught through close contact with children. You should refer the client to the pharmacist to purchase a suitable treatment and ensure the client checks through every member of the family, as they too will require treatment should they have head lice.

Once the client has left the salon, any tools and equipment that have been in contact with the client should be sterilised immediately to prevent the risk of cross infection.

Name	Recognised by	Caused by	Referral to	Infectious/ contagious
Scabies	A rash of red, raised spots and severe itching, especially at night. The burrows are sometimes visible, especially around the wrist.	The sarcoptes scabiei mite, which burrows under the skin. The mite may be passed easily through close contact and commonly starts at the wrists (maybe through holding hands with an infected person).	GP	Yes
Head lice (pediculosis capatis)	Intense itching and the presence of nits (the small eggs that are attached to the hair shaft close to the scalp). On closer examination, there may be lice present.	A parasitic infestation.	Pharmacist or GP	Yes

Infestations

Infectious skin and scalp conditions

Infectious skin and scalp conditions will obviously cause problems if you fail to recognise them, or more importantly, the risk of cross-infection. An infection can usually be recognised by redness, swelling, excessive warmth to the touch or the presence of pus. The affected area will be sore to the touch and possibly itchy. Infectious conditions of the skin and scalp should always be referred to a GP, as medical intervention is required (see page 64).

Name	Recognised by	Caused by	Referral to	Infectious/contagious
Ringworm	First appears as small, round, red spots. As the spots enlarge, the centre begins to clear forming a ring with a raised border that is red and scaly. Hair may become brittle and fall out leaving bald patches.	A fungal skin infection.	GP	Yes

Infectious conditions by classification: fungal conditions

Name	Recognised by	Caused by	Referral to	Infectious/contagious
Impetigo	Small blisters containing a pus-like substance that may break and form a flat, honey coloured crust. Most commonly seen on the face.	Streptococcal or staphylococcal bacteria. Impetigo may be present as a secondary infection, associated with head lice. The skin is broken through scratching and the bacteria enters the skin.	GP	Yes
Folliculitis	Small yellow spot with a hair growing through, found in the follicle opening.	A bacterial infection of the hair follicle.	GP	Yes
Sycosis barbae (barber's itch)	A form of folliculitis. Small, red spots, often with a yellow pustule, around the follicle opening. Found in the beard area.	Bacterial infection. May be transmitted by infected shaving brushes, razors, etc.	GP	Yes

Bacterial conditions

Non-infectious skin and scalp conditions

Non-infectious skin or scalp conditions should pose no problem unless the skin is broken. If this is so, any products used may enter the skin and cause discomfort to the client. Clients with known scalp conditions should be informed if there is any deterioration in their condition. This will enable them to seek intervention before the problem worsens.

Name	Recognised by	Caused by	Referral to
Alopecia areata	A small round bald patch on the scalp, with surrounding hairs being short and appearing 'frayed'. The skin in the patch is usually pale and glossy. The patch may appear overnight with the hairs being evident on the pillow the following morning.	The cause is not fully understood, as there seem to be a number of possible reasons for it occurring. In some cases it is thought to be genetic; however, stress and shock are also thought to be contributory factors. In some instances there is no explanation at all.	Trichologist
Traction alopecia	Hair loss at the point of tension, for example, tight plaiting or braiding can result in hair loss at the base of the plait.	The loosening of the hair in the follicle from constant pulling. Recommend all tension be removed until the hair grows back and then treat with extreme caution to prevent a recurrence.	Trichologist
Cicatricial alopecia	Loss of hair over an area of scarring.	Baldness due to scarring. The follicles are absent in scar tissue. Scars may be due to wounds, burns or infections. Take care when using chemical relaxers as they may burn and damage the skin.	Trichologist, although there is little that may be done.
Diffuse alopecia	A gradual loss of hair without any itching or scaling present. Affects females for a variety of reasons.	Following pregnancy (see hair growth cycle, page 44) changes in hormone levels, the contraceptive pill, thyroid problems, iron deficiency, illness or a side effect of certain medication.	GP/Trichologist
Androgenic alopecia (male pattern baldness)	Usually starts with a receding hairline, followed by loss at the crown area. Eventually the whole vertex is void of hair. The length of time the hair is in the anagen stage of the cycle reduces and the hair becomes gradually shorter and finer until the hairs do not re-grow.	A genetic condition affecting some men from late teens through to old age, and some females after the menopause.	GP/Trichologist

Non-infectious skin and scalp conditions

Name	Recognised by	Caused by	Referral
Trichotillomania	Areas of hair loss that are rarely complete patches and have irregular outlines. In right-handed people the hair loss is usually on the right-hand side.	Children twiddling hair as a form of comfort or habit. Obsessive hair pulling is usually associated with some psychiatric disorders.	GP/Trichologist
Psoriasis	Well-defined, red, thickened areas of skin covered with large, silvery scales.	May be caused by stress. Sometimes a genetic disorder. It is not infectious and normal salon services may be carried out. It is not advisable to carry out chemical treatments if the skin is broken.	GP/Trichologist
Eczema	Patches of dry skin, which can itch, become sore, inflamed and weep. Usually found in the creases of the body, for example, behind the knees, but may affect large areas of the body.	External or internal factors that give rise to an allergic response.	GP/Trichologist
Fragilitis crinium	Split ends.	Harsh physical or chemical treatment or clients who do not have their hair cut regularly.	The only real treatment for this is to cut them off.
Dandruff	Dry, flaky scalp, usually accompanied by itching.	Over production and shedding of epidermal cells.	Trichologist
Seborrhoeic dermatitis (greasy dandruff)	Yellowish, greasy scales that flake, causing redness and itching. In severe cases this can extend into the eyebrows, around the nose and ears and onto the cheeks.	Over production of sebum in conjunction with dandruff and an inflamed scalp.	Trichologist

Non-infectious skin and scalp conditions cont.

Name	Recognised by	Caused by	Referral
Sebaceous cyst	A dome-shaped lump under the skin. They are usually skin coloured unless infection is present. They may vary in size from 1–4 cms in diameter.	The hair follicle has a small duct opening onto the surface of the skin. This sebaceous duct becomes plugged with sebum and the cyst gradually becomes larger. Many people with small cysts choose to ignore them. However, if they are unsightly or large, they may be removed by their GP.	GP
Keloids	Scars that heal as a firm, smooth, hard growth. They have a 'ridged' appearance. Keloids may be uncomfortable and itchy.	An over production of healthy tissue. It is seen more often in African Caribbean skin.	Trichologist
Trichorrhexis nodosa	Small, split swellings appear on the hair shaft where the cortex has split.	Harsh physical and/or chemical damage. Incorrect use of heated electrical appliances. Perm rubbers incorrectly placed or twisted. Use of elastic bands to tie hair up.	Trichologist
In-growing hair	A hard lump with a dark patch in the middle, underneath the surface of the skin.	Short, curly hair that grows back on itself. It is quite often due to friction, for example, a shirt collar rubbing against the neck. Not infectious unless the in-growing hair has become infected.	GP/Trichologist
Monilethrix (beaded hair)	Along the hair shaft there are nodes and constrictions that make the hair look like a string of beads. This is caused by an uneven production of keratin. The hair must be handled with care, as it is liable to break where the hair constricts.	A rare hereditary condition.	There is no cure for this.

Non-infectious skin and scalp conditions cont.

Incompatibility of previous services or products used

Once you have identified your client's wishes and carried out an in-depth analysis of the client's hair and scalp, you may identify factors that will be incompatible with the requested service. For example, the client may have coloured their hair at home with a colourant that contains metallic salts and is therefore incompatible with any products that contain hydrogen peroxide.

Sometimes the condition of the client's hair means you will be unable to carry out the requested service, since the hair may become further damaged or break. This can prove to be very disappointing to the client, but the negative outcome that would undoubtedly occur could end up being far worse than any frustration felt by the client. When handling these situations, you must be sympathetic towards the client when you explain the problem but remain firm about your decision. This is the time when alternative services or products should be suggested and their outcomes explained to the client.

In the salon

Mrs Smith went into the salon to book an appointment for a permanent wave. Sonia, one of the stylists, was sitting at the reception desk covering for the receptionist whilst she had lunch. Sonia looked at Mrs Smith's very fine, highly bleached hair and suggested a consultation before the appointment to be sure of the most suitable course of action to take. Mrs Smith agreed and returned to the salon later that day for her consultation appointment.

Sonia carried out a number of tests on cuttings from Mrs Smith's hair. The hair was porous and had very poor elasticity and it was obvious to Sonia that a perm was not advisable as it would cause severe damage to the hair and it would break. She explained the situation to Mrs Smith and then suggested a course of intensive conditioning treatments. She explained that when the hair condition had improved sufficiently, she would be able to carry out the perming service. Mrs Smith was not very happy with the outcome and said she would take her business elsewhere. Sonia was quite upset to have lost a client, but she still stood by her decision.

Four days later Mrs Smith returned to the salon, looking very uncomfortable. She was wearing a scarf around her head and asked to speak to Sonia. As Sonia walked over to see her, she removed her headscarf, which revealed hair that looked like cotton wool balls all over her head. She had taken her custom elsewhere and the result was disastrous. The hair had been over processed, which was not difficult given its condition to begin with, and there were random areas of breakage all over the scalp. Having realised her mistake, Mrs Smith went back to the hairdresser that she knew she could trust and asked for help to put it right. It was a long, slow process to repair the damage to the hair and Mrs Smith's confidence in hairdressers. However, Mrs Smith is still a regular client of Sonia's ten years later and has brought a lot of custom to the salon as a result of her experience.

- Was Sonia right to stand by her original decision?
- What would your professional opinion be of the hairdresser who carried out the perming service?

Head and face shape

Being able to carry out excellent hairdressing is only a part of what makes a successful hairdresser. You also need to be able to identify your client's head and face shape and ensure the service you provide will enhance it (or reduce the appearance of anything less than perfect). The illustrations below show a range of different face shapes. The oval face shape is considered to be the 'perfect' face shape and can support most hairstyles.

The oval face

The round face

The round face

To turn into
an oval

The heart-shaped face

The heart shaped face

To turn into
an oval

The pear-shaped face

The pear-shaped face

To turn into
an oval

The oblong face

The oblong-shaped face

To turn into
an oval

The square face

The square face

To turn into
an oval

The position of a parting can alter the shape of the face quite significantly. A client with a long face should avoid a centre parting, as this will lengthen the face; instead move the parting to the side and the face will appear shorter.

The position of the parting can lenghten or shorten the face

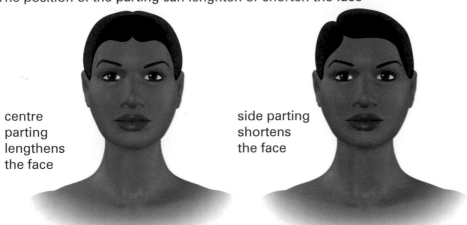

centre
parting
lengthens
the face

side parting
shortens
the face

A side parting suits longer face shapes

A client with a small face should avoid a hairstyle that involves a lot of hair on the face, as the face will appear smaller still. This is also true for a client with glasses, as the face becomes hidden behind the hair and glasses. The addition of a fringe can camouflage a high forehead or lines and wrinkles that are best left hidden. It also softens the facial features of a more mature client.

You should always check the shape of your client's head before starting any salon service. Not every client will have a perfect head!

The ideal head shape

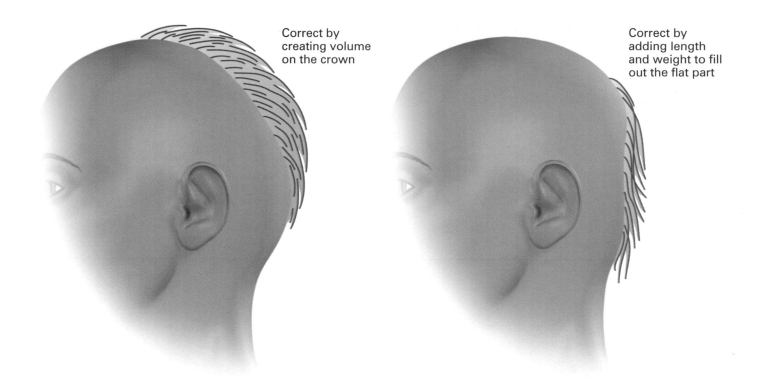

Correct by
creating volume
on the crown

Correct by
adding length
and weight to fill
out the flat part

Different head shapes and possible style solutions

Some salons now have a computer package that includes a digital camera that imposes different hairstyles and colours onto the client's face. This gives clients a visual impression of how they may look and removes the worry factor.

Lifestyle

Taking your client's lifestyle into consideration is vital. You must consider the following points:

*   what amount of time does he or she have to spend on their hair each day?
*   can he or she commit to the upkeep?
*   does the proposed service complement his or her occupation?
*   is it suitable for any leisure activities he or she may pursue?

All of the above should be addressed during the consultation to ensure the client will be able to manage their hair between visits. The style you would recommend for a busy working person may differ greatly from a style for a client with a lot of leisure time on their hands.

You must ensure the client can commit to the upkeep of the style or colouring services you propose. A full head bleach would not be practical for a client who visits the salon every four months, as the re-growth would be unsightly. It may be advantageous to suggest highlights, as the re-growth would not be as noticeable. Some occupations have quite stringent rules regarding the use of excessive styling and vibrant colours and this must be considered.

You should find out whether your client pursues any leisure activities that could impact on your decision. A client with long, thick hair who swims every morning before work should not have their hair bleached as it may discolour if incorrectly treated. Your client may ride a motorbike and need to wear a crash helmet and so a low maintenance style may be more suitable.

Remember

You should ensure you have all the necessary facts to hand before you make your recommendations, as this will prevent an inappropriate service taking place.

Hair growth patterns

Hair growth patterns may limit or affect some services in the salon. These must be taken into consideration to ensure a satisfactory result. It is always better to work with the natural fall of the hair rather than 'fight it' so that the hair lies another way. The styling will be more durable and therefore easier for the client to maintain. A soft perm can add movement to some strong growth patterns and make them more versatile.

Double crown

You should be careful not to cut the hair too short, as it will not lie properly. You should leave the hair longer in this area as the hair will lie better. The addition of a few perm rods in this area will create some movement and help prevent the hair from lying awkwardly. You should always try to work with the client's hair growth patterns wherever possible; for example, if the client requires a style that is short and spiky, utilise the double crown to help you to achieve this look.

Widow's peak

A widow's peak is a very strong growth pattern. Consideration must be taken when cutting hair, especially around this area. It can prove difficult when cutting a fine fringe, as the hair will easily lift and split. Again, work with the natural growth pattern whenever possible to ensure the best results.

Cowlick

A cowlick makes it difficult to cut a straight fringe, as the hair tends to grow strongly to one side. However, styling the hair and utilising the natural movement will make the style more durable.

Nape whorl

Nape whorls must be considered when cutting hair and dressing long hair. The hair may not lie flat in the nape area if the hair is cut too short. Analyse the nape whorls and check the direction in which the hair grows to try to incorporate it into your cutting or styling.

Examples of hair growth patterns

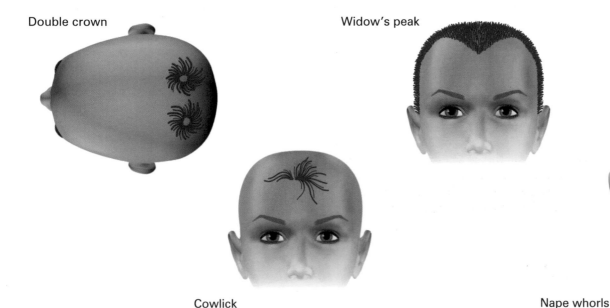

Double crown

Widow's peak

Cowlick

Nape whorls

Special occasions

If the client is having their hair styled for a special occasion, you must utilise the broad spectrum of skills you have and adapt them accordingly. For many clients, this type of occasion happens infrequently and therefore they will require something extraordinary. These occasions may include:

- bridal work
- fancy dress
- ball
- award ceremony
- milestone occasion (retirement, twenty-first birthday, and so on).

Once you become aware of the event the client will be attending, it should give you a clear indication of the type of service/styling the client may require. Remember to clarify the client's requirements as to whether they want something sexy and sophisticated, way out and funky, or modest but classy, but always ensure the service and styling will suit the occasion.

Some stylists like to carry out a trial run, as this helps to iron out any worries or anxieties the client may have. However, some stylists do not like to carry out trial runs as experience has taught them that it is not always possible to recreate the style so that it looks exactly as it did on the previous occasion. You should know your capabilities and use your own judgement as to whether the trial run is right for you.

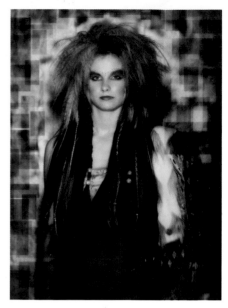

Your client may want a funky style for a special occasion

Keys to good practice

If carrying out trial runs, always take photographs of the final look the client decides on for the special occasion. This will help to refresh your memory on the day and ensure the client is satisfied.

Hair texture

The hair texture refers to the thickness of each individual hair. Fine hair is narrow in diameter, whereas coarse hair has a wider diameter. Fine hair is generally considered to be more receptive to perming and colouring services. However, you must remember there are exceptions to every rule, as some fine hair is known to be resistant to chemical processing. The hair may differ in texture across the head – it is usually finer at the front and this must be taken into consideration. It is essential that you know the texture of the client's hair prior to starting a service, as there are implications for most services carried out in the salon.

Hair density

The hair's density refers to the amount of hairs on the head. Many hairdressers confuse texture and density, as hair may be fine in texture but abundant in number. The average number of hairs on any head is said to be between 100,000–150,000, with blondes having the most and redheads having the least. However, blonde hair tends to be finer in texture than any of the other natural colours.

Providing analysis assistance to colleagues

There may be occasions in the salon when another member of staff is encountering difficulties with their own client analysis. This may be through lack of experience or lack of confidence. In either situation you should assist them promptly and effectively to enable them to continue with their work. This intervention should be carried out in an unthreatening manner to ensure you do not undermine their confidence.

Keys to good practice

- You should have a thorough knowledge of all aspects of the hair, skin and scalp.
- You should know how to gain information regarding the client's hair, skin and scalp.
- You should be aware of the importance of pre-service testing and examination.
- You should know about adverse hair, skin and scalp conditions and whether they may be treated in the salon.
- You should recognise the importance of identifying the incompatibility of previous services and products used.
- You should be able to identify head and face shapes and decide upon the most suitable style.
- You should consider the effects of the client's lifestyle regarding the suitability of services and products.
- You should be aware of hair growth patterns and how they affect your choice of styling.
- You should recognise the importance of getting it right for a special occasion.

Making recommendations to your client

Once your analysis is complete and you have identified your client's needs and wishes, you should then be able to make recommendations to your client as to the most suitable course of action. You must take into consideration the information you gained from your in-depth analysis, which includes the results of any tests you have undertaken. You must be aware of all the services and products that are available in the salon if you are to make an informed choice. This may include other parts of the salon that you are not familiar with. It would be advantageous for you to be aware of the beauty treatments that the salon offers so you can recommend a combined package to your client, for example, the bride or client about to take a holiday.

Keep abreast of current trends

Your knowledge of current fashion trends should be up to date so you can offer the widest range of services and products available to your clients. There are numerous ways of updating your skills and knowledge, including:

- referring to trade magazines, such as *International Hairdressers Journal*
- attending trade shows and exhibition
- attending courses run by product manufacturers
- watching television, for example, programmes about fashion
- accessing hair and fashion websites.

Remember

Under the Trade Descriptions Act 1968, any information you give to the client, including that of the features and benefits of a service or product, must be correct. You should be able to state the features and benefits of each service and product that is used or carried out in the salon. However, in reality, most clients are more interested in the benefits to themselves. Think about what the client has to gain from the service or product.

Check it out

Are you aware of all the services your salon offers to the clients? Can you state the features and benefits of each service and product used within the salon?

Keep abreast of current trends by visiting hair and fashion websites

You should be aware of current style icons and the impact they have on the general public and their concept of fashion. If you think back over the last few years, entertainers such as Madonna and Janet Jackson have re-invented themselves several times and on each occasion have helped to determine what becomes 'street fashion'. David Beckham's hairstyle became the ultimate fashion statement during the 2002 World Cup and was copied by many fashion conscious men, especially those in Japan. How many girls do you know who want to look like Beyoncé Knowles or Jennifer Lopez? You must keep abreast of these developments to ensure you can offer the requested service and know what the finished result should look like!

Some clients have aspirations regarding their hair that cannot be fulfilled. It is very disappointing for a client to be told the look they wish to achieve is not possible. There will always be a client with very fine, sparse hair who wants to look like Lily Savage! However, it is your job to explain the situation to the client using language the client can readily understand and offer alternatives. You may need to explore a number of different options until you find one that the client finds acceptable. You should display tact and diplomacy when dealing with this type of situation as the client's self-confidence may not withstand the brutal truth and you do not want to lose the client.

In some instances, the client's hair may not be able to withstand the preferred service and again you must explore all the options until you come up with a mutually agreeable alternative. You may wish to show the client evidence from any tests that you have carried out, especially those that clearly indicate deterioration in the hair's condition or unwanted colour. You should then make alternative suggestions regarding other services or products that may be used or given, which will give a positive outcome.

In the salon

A client comes into the salon for a re-growth application and has 25 per cent scattered white hair. However, since the last visit she has coloured her hair at home. An incompatibility test shows evidence of the presence of metallic salts, so you immediately know a permanent colour cannot be used. It may be possible to use a true semi-permanent colour (one that is not mixed with anything, but used directly from the bottle), as it does not contain hydrogen peroxide.

- What should you do next?

Referral

There are times when the client's preferred service is unavailable due to:

- the service not being offered in your salon
- adverse hair, skin and scalp conditions.

If a client requests a service that is not offered in your salon, rather than leave the client to find a salon that does offer the service, your salon should have a policy specifically for this purpose. If you refer the client to a specific salon, you must be sure the salon offers services to a good standard, as your reputation is at stake. If the service proves to be unsatisfactory, remember the client went there on your recommendation.

If your salon does not have a policy covering the referral of clients but intends to put a policy in place, make sure you do your homework and find the best place for your clients, as this will reflect on your judgement as a professional hairdresser. If the number of requests for a specific service becomes substantial, it may be in the interest of the salon to train one of their existing staff to fulfil this opportunity or employ somebody who can offer the service.

Check it out

Does your salon have a policy for referring clients to other salons?

Referring clients to specialists

Some hair and scalp disorders are treatable in the salon, for example, using special products or treatments manufactured for treating dandruff. However, some disorders will need to be referred to a trichologist for more specialist treatment. In some instances, clients with hair and scalp problems will go to their stylist as a first point of call. Many clients are unaware of the role of the trichologist or are unsure of how to access one. You should be encouraging and supportive towards these clients as they may find the situation quite distressing.

Keys to good practice

If you need to refer a client to see a registered trichologist and are not sure how to find one, the following website is very informative and user friendly: http://www.trichologists.org.uk

This website lists all the Institutes members from England, Scotland, Wales, the Channel Islands, Northern Ireland and the Republic of Ireland. Alternatively, you can call 08706 070602.

In the salon

Sally was a regular client. Every few months her mum Joan came to stay with her for a long weekend and as a treat she took her to the salon for a shampoo and blow-dry. Paul, the stylist, always did both Sally's and Joan's hair. One day, whilst blow-drying Joan's hair, Paul noticed a strange, dark brown, raised, unusual shape on the side of her face. He asked if it had been there long and Joan said she was not sure and asked him why. He made light of the situation but suggested she mention it to her GP when she was next there. During her next visit to the salon she told Paul that the doctor had 'burned the thing off her face'. He did not see Joan then for several months, but when she came to the salon, the brown, raised, unusual shape was back, but this time it was bigger. With each subsequent visit, Paul could see it getting bigger. He had no idea what it was, but felt it was not right and suggested again that she see her GP. He did not see Sally for ages and when she finally came into the salon she looked very worried. She told him that her Mum had been in hospital having the sinister shape removed and this necessitated her having facial surgery. She was very poorly.

Paul knew he had done as much as he could for Joan. He was not a doctor and he was not sure what the lump was, but at least he had suggested the initial visit to the GP.

- Could Paul have done anything more?

In these types of situations described above, it is important not to diagnose specific conditions to the client. Medical practitioners are the experts and although you may be right in your diagnosis, there is always the possibility that you are not. Firstly, you must consider the stress and worry the client will have to endure, especially if they have to wait several days for an appointment. Secondly, if you wrongly diagnose a client's condition, they may endure unnecessary stress and worry and inevitably blame you (even if you were trying to help!)

It is more professional to say to the client, 'I'm not sure what the problem is, but I would suggest you see your GP before returning to the salon.' This may offend the client, but if the client has a contagious or potentially serious condition, your actions will cause the condition to be treated more quickly, reducing the risk of it worsening and preventing possible cross-infection.

When referring a client with a suspected infectious condition, you should say as little as possible to get your point across effectively. In the event of a client with head lice, they do not need to know how many lice you have actually seen, but you should tell them there is evidence of the condition and refer them to a pharmacist. If you elaborate in these situations, you may find you are giving the client information that is not really your responsibility to give. You should speak quietly or move your client to a private area of the salon to maintain discretion and show that you are complying with the salon rules of confidentiality.

You must not show disgust or repulsion towards the client, but empathise with them instead and try to make them understand that these things are common within the salon environment (even if they are not). You should maintain a relaxed manner so you do not cause alarm and the tone of your voice should be authoritative to ensure the client takes your referral seriously.

In all instances, you must ensure your clients realise that you are a professional person and your recommendations are in their best interest. This will help to promote trust and goodwill between you and your clients.

Agreeing services with your client

When you are absolutely sure of your client's requirements, you should discuss what the service entails, the length of time the client can expect to be in the salon, and any special advice that may be necessary; for example, if you have a client having hair extensions, you must inform the client of the duration of the service, as they may not realise the length of time it takes, and the possibility that it may be uncomfortable. You must make sure the client has allowed sufficient time for the service to be carried out, as clients will quite often fit in a hairdressing appointment around other commitments.

It is frustrating for both the client and the stylist if the duration of the service takes longer than anticipated. This may involve the client having to leave the salon midway through the service or remaining in the salon but 'clock watching' the whole time. This leads to undue anxiety for the client and puts the stylist under unnecessary pressure. It shows a lack of professionalism and does not reflect well on the salon.

Check it out

How long does your salon allow for each service it offers? Make a comprehensive list.

Special requirements

Your clients should also be informed of any special requirements that may be needed for a specific service. It is very frustrating for a client to arrive at the salon for a service, only to be told the service cannot be carried out as something has been overlooked. Some examples of pre-service requirements include:

• the need for tests prior to the perming or colouring service – skin test, test cutting, and so on.
• special preparation requirements – a client having a relaxing service should not shampoo their hair for a least a week before the service as there should be a protective barrier on the scalp. They should be advised not to use excessive products on the hair during this time as it may prevent the relaxer from penetrating.
• special clothing that needs to be worn – if you are preparing a client's hair for a special occasion, you must ensure they are wearing clothing that may be removed easily without disturbing the finished styling. You may suggest the client wears a top that buttons or zips up the front rather than a jumper that will be dragged over the head.

Establishing the cost of the service

Your clients should also be informed as to the outcome of the service, the products you will use and the cost of the service. To do this you must be able to calculate the likely charge for the salon service, which means that you must be familiar with the pricing structure within the salon.

If your salon has staff with varying levels of competence, they may be allowed extra time to complete certain services; however, you need to be aware of this if you are to pass this information on to the clients. In some salons, the prices for certain services start from a specific price, for example, highlights from £30, in which case you must inform the client if his or her highlights are likely to cost them £30 or more.

Payment policies

Many salons have payment policies, which require clients to pay a deposit, or in some cases, pay for the whole service prior to their visit. Some salons maintain these policies at all times; others may implement the policies to cover:

* busy periods (for example, Christmas and New Year's Eve appointments)
* services that are time consuming (for example, extensions)
* clients who regularly default (do not turn up).

This is to ensure the salon receives an income even if the client has to cancel their appointment.

Record cards

Any information you have gained during your consultation that relates to the service your client will be having should be recorded on a client record card. Clients may not always have their requested service on the day of the consultation, therefore it is vital that you have the information to hand when the client comes in for the service.

A client record card

Check it out

To calculate the client's bill, you must ensure you have included all services the client has received, for example:

Cut	£14.50
Relaxing service and finish	£50.00
Semi-permanent colour	£15.75
Total	**£80.25**

Using your salon's price list, calculate the cost of:

1. a re-style, followed by a body perm and finish
2. colour polishing and cut and blow-dry
3. a man's re-style and re-design of facial hair.

You must include any additional products that may be used if these are charged separately.

Remember

Under the Sale and Supply of Goods Act 1994, there should be a reasonable charge for any service carried out unless a price was agreed prior to the service. As the client should be informed of the price prior to the service and their agreement sought, you should be fulfilling some of your responsibility under this piece of legislation.

To comply with the Data Protection Act 1998, all records should be accurate, up to date, legible and complete.

Once your client has agreed to the service, you are ready to commence. If the client has visited the salon for a consultation, you must ensure they make a suitable appointment prior to leaving the salon.

Keys to good practice

- Inform clients of the cost, duration and any special requirements that may be necessary.
- Know your responsibilities under the Sale and Supply of Goods Act 1994.
- Know how client record cards should comply with the Data Protection Act 1998.

Knowledge check

1. Why is it important to identify your client's needs and wishes during the consultation?

2. What are 'feeling' questions and why should they be used?

3. Name the two types of cortex found in African Caribbean hair.

4. Describe the hair growth cycle.

5. State the importance of carrying out pre-service testing.

6. Identify four factors that may adversely affect the condition of the hair.

7. How would you recognise the following conditions:
    *   psoriasis
    *   ingrowing hair
    *   keloid scarring
    *   alopecia areata
    *   sebaceous cyst

8. Describe the action you would take if a client with head lice enters the salon for a cut and blow-dry.

9. State three different types of poor hairdressing practice that may result in trichorrhexis nodosa.

10. You need to refer a client to a trichologist. How would you go about finding one in your area?

11. State four ways in which you can update your hairdressing skills and knowledge.

Promote additional products or services to clients

Unit G6

Introduction

The range of products and services available to promote within the salon is constantly changing, as you would expect from a fast-moving industry such as hairdressing. It is important for you to be aware of these changes in order to keep up with client's needs and expectations. This unit is primarily concerned with how you promote products or services to clients in order to extend their use of your salon. The benefits to the salon are increased revenue and, for the client, the improved condition of their hair and a manageable style.

What you will learn
• How to identify additional products or services that are available
• Informing clients about, and gaining client commitment to using, additional products or services, and salon promotions
• Salon and legal requirements
• Client rights

You, the stylist

As a stylist working in the salon, your job will involve promoting products and services to your clients. You will be required to keep abreast of changes and developments in the range of products and services that are available in order to maximise what you can offer your client. Excellent communication skills are essential in order to fully respond to the needs of your clients and present the products and services of your salon. You will need to be aware of each person's role within the salon and ensure that you are working as part of the team in promoting products and services.

Depending on your job role within the salon, the part you play in promotion may differ. For example, if you are responsible for stock ordering, you will need to be aware of which products or services are on offer to ensure you have enough of the items in stock. You may be responsible for organising the window display; therefore you need to be aware of what is on offer in order to change the window promotion. Staff meetings will play a vital role in ensuring that the correct information is shared and chairing these meetings may be your responsibility. If you are a senior member of staff in your salon, you will probably have a larger part to play in ensuring that the promotion of products and services takes place.

Keep abreast of the latest products so that you can advise your client on what is best for her hair

Remember

You may have productivity targets to reach on the promoting of additional products and services to clients. See pages 110-1 for information on productivity.

How to identify additional products or services that are available

In order to maximise the client's use of your salon, the whole team must play a role in making clients aware of what is available and encouraging them to return to the salon. There are many factors you should consider when promoting products and services. Both the salon and its employees have responsibilities to clients regarding legislation and regulations. The client also has rights as a consumer that you are legally bound to observe. These are covered in more depth later in this unit.

Products and services

The services that you offer in the salon are usually all the things that are listed on the salon's price list. However, there may be other services that on occasions you are asked for and will also provide, for example, special occasion styling or alternative colour techniques. The services you provide often change over time as your client's expectations and requirements change.

The products that you use and offer in your salon may be supplied from several different companies. This is often the best way to operate in a salon. Using only one product supplier can inhibit the services you offer, for example, your supplier may not produce a hair straightener.

Features and benefits

You will need to understand the features and benefits of the products and services before you can successfully promote them. Everything that you offer in the salon has a feature and a benefit. Features of a service or product are its attributes or characteristics, for example, using mousse will aid with the styling process. The benefits of a service or product are the advantages that it will give to the client. For example, styling mousse provides hold and volume to the finished look.

The products and services that you provide in your salon will differ from that of another salon and will depend upon the hairdressing abilities of your staff. For example, you may have a long hair expert working at your salon providing a lot of special occasion styles, or a nail technician, or even a trichologist with a specialist clinic. Whatever your salon set up, it is essential that you remain aware of the changes and developments to the products and services that you provide. There are several ways in which you can update your knowledge of products and services and each one may hold possible advantages and disadvantages for you.

Products have features and benefits – make sure you know what they are

Method of updating knowledge	Advantages	Disadvantages
College courses	Not linked to any one manufacturer and can gain further qualifications/certificates	May have to take time off work to attend
Reading trade publications or researching on the Internet	Contains lots of information regarding numerous products and services	Two dimensional; cannot try products and services yourself
Product manufacturer courses	Can gain further qualifications/certificates. Sometimes offer free courses as incentives	Can be the most expensive way of updating your knowledge
Trade events	Lots of companies to look at and can try products and services for yourself	May have to take time off work to attend

Informing clients about, and gaining client commitment to using, additional products and salon promotions

When supplying products and services to your clients you must also consider what you can promote outside of your salon. The term 'outside' does not have to mean exterior to the salon premises. It may just be a service that is outside of your hairdressing capabilities. Remember that you are trying to improve your clients' experience with you and this may require you to promote something that you do not necessarily provide yourself. There may be several other services that are linked to the salon, for example, a nail technician, beauty or holistic therapy services, or even a trichology clinic. It may even be something as remote as dog grooming or plumbing if the salon owner's partner also has a business. Through your communication with your client you will be able to determine their needs and advise accordingly. You must, however, take care not to offer the client something that is out of your reach as they may become disheartened. Ensure that if you are offering to supply your client with a product or service that you can fulfill their requirements.

In the salon

Joseph owns and works in a busy town centre salon. He has a varied client base but works predominantly as a colour technician in the salon. A regular client of his was going to a college ball and asked for her hair to be put up for this special occasion. Unfortunately, his long hair technician was away on holiday. Not wanting to lose the client or disappoint her, he agreed to put up the client's hair himself and booked the appointment. When the client came into the salon, she brought a picture of how she wanted her hair to look. Joseph took one look at the style and knew in his heart that he would not be able to achieve it; however he felt committed and did not want to let her down.

He tried to discourage her from the look and recommended something else but to no avail – the client had made her mind up. Joseph tried several times to achieve the look and the client was beginning to ask questions about whether he knew what he was doing. Eventually he admitted to the client that he could not achieve the look she wanted but could offer her an alternative style. The client had no choice but to agree in order to have her hair styled for the special occasion. However, she was very disappointed and, although a regular client at the salon, never returned again.

- Should Joseph have booked the appointment without letting her know that he was not a long hair expert?
- Do you think he lacked professionalism in his judgement of the situation?
- How could he have handled this situation differently without losing a client?
- Why do you think the client never came back to the salon again?

Salon promotions

There are various types of promotions that you will be involved in whilst working in the salon and you may even be responsible for running them. For example:

- promotional events at the salon
- advertising on radio or local newspapers
- using a website address
- advertising in trade magazines
- window display
- promotional leaflets or flyers.

Stages of a promotion

There are several stages to a promotion that must be considered. Initially, it should be well planned, looking at the budget and the resources available. The objectives must

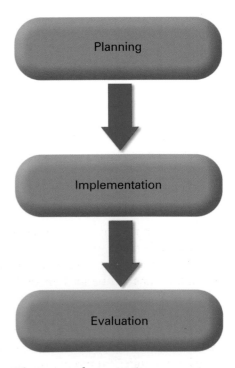

The stages of a promotion

be set to ensure each individual is aware of their responsibilities and what is expected of them. Next, implement the promotion, monitoring its effectiveness as it progresses. Every promotion reaches a saturation point when it is no longer commercially viable and should be brought to a close. This will become evident through careful monitoring. Then, finally, evaluate its effectiveness, again involving the people who took part to ensure all accurate information is gathered. The evaluation will provide crucial information on its effectiveness and whether or not it has achieved its objectives. This information can be used to assess the benefits of further promotions.

An attractive product display can catch the client's attention

You must be able to choose the most appropriate time and method of communication to introduce your client to additional products or services. Displaying the products for retail sale at reception is a subtle way of introducing your product range; you can then back this up by discussing their benefits whilst using them on your client. This type of promotion is commonly used; there are many ways of subtly bringing to your client's attention what you can offer, or alternatively, you may want to announce it in a loud and attention-grabbing way.

However you decide to carry it out, the timing and way you present a promotion is crucial. Clients can easily be put off by an attitude they find too brash. Alternatively, being quiet about it will not grab any attention. Think about what it is that you are trying to promote. If the product or service is new to the salon then you may want to make a big statement as it may attract new clientele to the salon. For example, if a new member of staff begins working at the salon, they may provide different services than previously offered or may want to inform their client base of where they are now working.

> ## Keys to good practice
>
> Take care when announcing a new member of staff that has previously worked locally. They may have a clause in their contract forbidding them from working within a specified area and you could end up being liable for poaching clients.

> ## Check it out
>
> Look at your contract. Are there any restrictions as to where you can work on leaving the salon? If you are the salon owner, is this something that you may consider introducing to your contracts with staff? It could save you money in the long term if an employee was to set up a business nearby.

Organise a launch party

If the salon is a new business then you may want to organise a launch party. This could be as small or large as you want it to be. Consider inviting local people to attend to have a look around without any obligation and even offer them discount vouchers for their first treatment with you. You may want to use a variety of sources to promote the event, but you should not restrict yourself to just using the salon facilities.

Set up a website

Many salons now have websites that tempt clients into the salon without them having to physically enter. You can use the website to promote all the services and products of the salon, the arrival of new staff, download discount vouchers, buy products, or even book appointments. One of the most important advantages of a website is that you can store lots of information about your salon and this should be as visually attractive as possible. You can also link to other websites, which is especially useful if the salon has a partner business, for example, a beauty salon. It has many uses and you cannot afford to overlook its numerous advantages. However, it should never be used as the sole medium of promoting, as you would be excluding a vast number of clients that are not computer literate. Using the local newspapers or radio station to

> ## Remember
>
>
>
> The cost of promoting should never exceed the financial gain of the promotion.

promote the salon can be an extremely good medium, as it goes out to a much wider audience. It can, however, be costly and this should be taken into consideration.

Window displays

The cheapest and most cost-effective way of promoting is using the salon window. You do not necessarily need to employ a professional window dresser – just use your imagination or there may be a member of staff with a flair for this. You can change the display according to the seasons or when sales are down in order to target certain services. The only disadvantage is that it will only reach a limited audience, especially if your salon is not in a busy main road position. However, if used in conjunction with other promotional media, then it can be extremely cost effective.

Promotional leaflets and flyers

If you have a particular announcement to make about the salon then promotional leaflets or flyers can be a successful way of getting the information across. You do, however, need to consider that they will have to be given out, which can take up a lot of working hours. Think about the amount of junk mail you receive yourself and what happens to it; this could be the money you have spent being thrown in the bin.

Magazine features

If you are a large salon with enough financial capital to spend then you may want to consider promoting your salon via a trade magazine. If you have recently undergone a makeover or are a newly opened salon, you could put yourself forward for a feature which would be a low cost option for the salon.

Whichever method of promotion you decide to use, choose the right kind of promotion for you and always follow the three key stages.

Promote your salon's makeover in a trade magazine feature

Communication

The way in which you communicate with your client will play a crucial part in the success of the promoting you do in the salon. Communication is the sending and receiving of information between persons by various methods. To make your communication effective you need to ensure that the information you are passing on is clear, legible (where necessary) and is fully understood by the receiver. In the salon you will communicate with your clients and staff in many different ways. The art of communication has greatly advanced due to the development of technology at such a fast pace. However, the basic methods of communication remain the same and these can be categorised into three areas: written, verbal and non-verbal.

Written communication

There are several forms of written communication that can be used effectively in the salon. Any written communication that takes place can be kept as proof of what has been said – for example, an invoice of outstanding payment or an enquiry about a product.

Possibly the two most important methods of written communication used in any salon are the appointment book and record cards. Firstly, the appointment book is essential in organising your working day. If the information stored in the appointment book is

> **Check it out**
>
> List all the types of written communication that are used in your salon and the advantages and disadvantages of each. This will help you to decide if you need to make any changes to the lines of communication that you are using.

incorrect, this will lead to major disruption in the salon. It is therefore essential that all the staff be fully conversant with how the appointment system works. Secondly, the record cards are a necessary requirement in order to retain information about the client's hair, the treatment received and his or her personal details. The information stored on the card must be accurate, legible and up to date: this is a requirement of law under the Data Protection Act (see page 78). For an example of a client's record card see page 67. Written communication for promotion may take the form of posters, flyers, salon websites or notices in the salon window, or reception area. Whatever form you use it should be clear, legible and stylish. This will also present a professional view of your salon.

Verbal communication

This type of communication applies to everything that is spoken in the salon. This includes both face to face and telephone conversations. In the salon you will have to deal with a variety of people, not all of them clients. Therefore, your communication skills will have to expand across many levels. You should pitch your conversation to the level of the client you are dealing with. Being versatile enough to recognise the level of language to use with different clients is essential. For example, the way you speak to a teenage client would be very different from the way you would talk to an elderly client. When speaking face to face and over the telephone, you need to be sure that you are clearly understood. The consultation process relies on good verbal communication, essentially to ensure you reach a positive end result for your client. Misunderstanding when communicating will lead to client dissatisfaction and lack of job satisfaction for you as a stylist. Therefore, maintain clear, concise and understandable communication at all times. When promoting verbally it is essential that you have a thorough and up-to-date knowledge of your products and services. You should be able to clearly explain the features and benefits of each product or service in order to sell it well.

Non-verbal communication

This type of communication covers everything that is expressed via your body language or facial expressions. It is the one type of communication that we often have little or no control over. It can be quite difficult to be continuously aware of what we are saying

> **Remember**
>
> A record card could be used as evidence in a court case if proceedings were to be brought against you. Therefore, it is crucial that the information stored on it is completely accurate.

> **Check it out**
>
> Ask someone you work with to look at your body language over a short period. Is it aggressive, intimidating or appropriate? Do you say one thing but convey something completely different with your body language?

Observe your client's facial expressions when discussing the service – she may not like what you have in mind!

eyes

tone of voice

hands and arms

gestures

angle of head

face

posture

muscle tension

Non-vebal communication is expressed through your body language and facial expressions

with our body language and facial expressions. However, it can be used to your advantage, as the stylist, when communicating with your client to try and determine their requirements. For example, if you spot a client's attention drifting over to the retail display, or reading promotional materials, then this would be a good opportunity to introduce the benefits of what they are looking at, which could result in a sale.

Keys to good practice

When you are in the salon, mirrors surround you. Even if you think no one can see what you are doing, it is likely that someone will notice your facial expression. A client may easily take offence at a frown from you, even if it was not aimed at them. You should make a conscious effort to look at your non-verbal communication and ensure that it is appropriate.

Making eye contact

Positive eye contact is essential. Have you ever noticed how difficult it is to talk to a person without looking at them? You must be sure to look at the client you are dealing with, as offence can easily be taken if it appears that you are not paying attention. However, too much eye contact can be a negative. For example, if the client is shy then trying to maintain eye contact can be an uncomfortable experience for him or her. The correct use of body language and facial expression can go a long way to impress the client and this should never be forgotten.

Whichever way you communicate with your client, it should always be clear, polite and confident. This is important to ensure that there is no misunderstanding between you and it will help to increase his or her confidence in your ability as a stylist. You should consider the manner with which you communicate; do you use a sympathetic tone or an empathetic tone? As an experienced hairdresser you will have come across many problems and crises that you have discussed with a client. Because of this vast experience it will be much easier to empathise with a client's needs based on the theory that you have dealt with this type of problem before. If you can only sympathise and not offer any real solutions then your client may feel disheartened and lose confidence in your ability.

The communication skills that you use when promoting additional products or services need to be appropriate and balanced. It is of little use explaining to the client all the features and benefits of something if it is not what he or she is interested in. It is likely the client will become bored by you and may not return to the salon. Your knowledge of what you are promoting will help to increase your confidence in the way you communicate. If you have a strong and thorough product and service knowledge, and are able to relay all the features and benefits to the client, then this will be reflected in how you communicate with him or her.

In the salon

Rosalyn had just started a new job at a local salon. Within the first few days she had been looking at the product range to familiarise herself with the features and benefits. On her third day she had a client booked with her for a re-style and from starting the consultation it was obvious to her that the client was open to using additional products and trying out new services. Rosalyn recognised a good promotional opportunity but felt that she did not yet have a thorough knowledge of all the products and services available at the salon.

Not wanting to miss out on the opportunity, she asked the client if she would mind if she consulted with a senior member of staff about her requirements. Rosalyn took care to explain to the client that it was not due to the fact that she did not know what she was doing, but just felt that because she was new to the salon she may miss telling her about something that would be of benefit to her. This reassured the client of her ability as a stylist. After the client agreed, Rosalyn asked her colleague, who was a senior staff member, to lend a hand. The situation was resolved in a satisfactory way for both the client and the salon. No promotional opportunities were missed out on and the client received the best advice possible.

- Do you think that Rosalyn showed professionalism in her approach to the situation?
- What might have been the outcome if she had not brought in a colleague to assist?
- Have you ever been in this situation yourself and felt that you were out of your depth and, if so, would you have the confidence to ask for help?

Salon and legal requirements

The products and services that you promote and provide in the salon are covered by many legal requirements. You should have a thorough understanding of what is expected of you if you are delivering products and services to clients. You must remember that any rules and regulations are set to protect all staff, your clients, and the environment that you work in. There are specific aspects of a salon's legal requirements that are very important and they are:

- health and safety
- data protection
- equal opportunities
- disability discrimination.

Health and safety

The laws and regulations relating to health and safety are extensively covered in Unit G1 (see pages 6–16).

Data protection

It is an essential requirement for you to keep records of client information; for example, the client's personal information and details of the chemical services that you have carried out in the salon. The Data Protection Act covers all the information that you store on your salon database. It requires you to take appropriate security measures to safeguard the information you keep from unauthorised or unlawful access or processing. Like many government written laws, it is very detailed and complex. Anyone processing personal data must be familiar and comply with the Data Protection Act (see also Unit G9). If you are holding data on anyone then you must register with the Information Commissioner. You will be given a certificate to display in the salon to inform clients of this fact.

The Data Protection Act contains eight enforceable principles of good practice. These state that all data must be:

- fairly and lawfully processed
- obtained and used only for specified and lawful purposes
- adequate, relevant and not excessive
- accurate where necessary
- kept up to date and for no longer than necessary
- processed in accordance with the person's rights
- kept secure
- transferred only to countries that offer adequate data protection.

With the introduction and widespread use of CCTV cameras, many small businesses, like hairdressing salons, are ignorant of the fact that you must register your usage with the Information Commissioner. Failure to do so could leave you liable for enforcement action and any recorded evidence you have may be inadmissible in court. Always be aware of the Data Protection Act when collecting information from clients regarding your promotional activities e.g. the personal information given on a survey evaluating a promotion.

Remember

Most salons do not let the client see information on a record card, as there are concerns that they may go to another salon. However, under the Data Protection Act, clients have a right to see all the information you store on them and you must comply with this. In the salon you will be held responsible for the processing of information on your clients. If your salon database is stored on a computer then you will have to comply with the Data Protection Act or you could face prosecution.

Check it out

Take time out in the salon to look over your client record card system and salon database. Is it up to date and accurate? If not, then you are failing to comply with the Data Protection Act. Update, and amend if necessary, the system that the salon uses.

Equal opportunities

The Sex Discrimination Acts of 1975 and 1986 are concerned with the equal treatment of men and women. They are written in terms of discrimination against women but apply equally to discrimination against men.

The Equal Opportunities Commission (EOC) is the leading agency working to eliminate sex discrimination in the UK. This commission was established in 1975 under the Sex Discrimination Act. The EOC is an independent statutory body with the following powers:

- To work towards the elimination of discrimination on the grounds of sex or marriage
- To promote equality of opportunity for women and men
- To keep under review the Sex Discrimination Act and Equal Pay Act
- To provide legal advice and assistance to individuals who have been discriminated against.

Both the employer and the employee have a responsibility to comply with equal opportunities.

Employers' responsibility

The employer must ensure that there is no unlawful discrimination. It is important, however, that measures to eliminate discrimination or promote equality of opportunity should be understood and supported by all employees. Employers are recommended to involve their employees in equal opportunities policies.

Individual employees' responsibilities

While the main responsibility for eliminating discrimination and providing equal opportunities is that of the employer, individual employees at all levels have responsibilities too. They must not discriminate or knowingly aid their employer to do so.

Keys to good practice

It is good practice to introduce equality into your salon procedures and practices even if the present law does not require it. This will include any promoting you do. For instance, a window display must not discriminate against the needs of men or women.

Check it out

Does your salon have an equal opportunities policy? Most small businesses will not have a written one. However, all the salon's written policies and procedures should have equal opportunities running through them. Review these and see if there is any discrimination that you feel should be eliminated. Advice on discrimination is available from both the Equal Opportunities Commission and the Commission for Racial Equality. Look up their websites.

Equal opportunities policies

The aim of a good policy is to ensure that everyone receives fair and equal treatment. Each individual company's policy will differ depending on the salon's size, its resources, the facilities and services it provides, and the industry's demands. According to the EOC, a policy should include five main points as shown below.

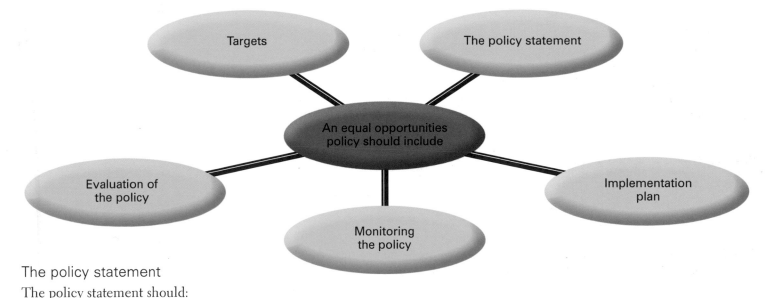

The policy statement

The policy statement should:

- explain who is covered by the policy
- explain what is meant by goods, facilities and services
- state the aims and outcomes of the policy
- link to the organisation's vision or mission statement and business plan
- make reference to the legal requirements
- indicate who has responsibility for its implementation.

The implementation plan

The implementation plan should include:

- commitment from senior management and staff
- consultation with customers, staff and the wider community
- the training of staff to promote ownership and good practice
- target setting with timescales
- establishing methods for monitoring and measuring progress
- communicating the policy to customers and staff.

Monitoring the policy

Monitoring should include the collection of data by gender for:

- applications for services
- those refused services
- customer retention
- complaints.

Evaluation of the policy

If the policy and implementation plan are successful, monitoring results will show:

- there is a fair representation of people from all groups in the community
- the levels of customer retention and customer satisfaction
- the reputation of the organisation in the local community.

Targets

After evaluation, targets can be set to improve future performance when needed. The laws regarding sexual discrimination are complex and very detailed, but in the salon you need to be sure you are not discriminating in any way. The fairest way to do this is to follow the salon's written Equal Opportunities Policy. If there is no written policy then you must ensure you understand the fundamental principles of the Sex Discrimination Act 1975 and that you are adhering to its rules.

> ### Remember
>
> Any promotional activity that you carry out in your salon should take into account equal opportunities. Discrimination can take many forms and your promotional activities should be designed in a way that takes everyone into account regardless of age, race or gender.

In the salon

Nubira was responsible for the window display at the salon. It was the beginning of summer and she was deciding what theme to use as their summer display. She came up with the idea of a beach/holiday theme and, as usual, had to present her idea to the salon owner before making the amendments. The salon was currently promoting a new range of shampoo and conditioning products and, as the hair can often feel dehydrated after a summer holiday, this was going to be her focal point.

When Nubira presented her ideas to the salon owner, she felt that the poster using an example of a man with dry hair was not necessary. The salon owner's argument was that it is predominantly women that suffer with dry hair and only a very small percentage of male clients ever buy the shampoo and conditioning product range. Nubira was quick to defend her decision and explained that it is a necessity of the Sex Discrimination Act that both the needs of men and women are catered for, but that was exactly her reason for using a male image in the window display. It would be a good opportunity to educate men that their hair also needs to be looked after in the sun. The salon owner thought about her argument and realised that Nubira was in fact right and that this was a market that needed to be explored. She changed her mind and asked Nubira to go ahead with the display, thanking her for her forward thinking.

- Was Nubira right to consider the needs of men and women?
- Has she covered her responsibilities under the Sex Discrimination Act?

Disability discrimination

Under the Disability Discrimination Act of 1995, you must not discriminate in any way against a person with a disability. In October 1997, the government made public its commitment to developing comprehensive and enforceable civil rights for disabled people. From this, the Disability Rights Commission (DRC) was formed in April 2000, its statutory duties being:

- to work to eliminate discrimination against disabled people
- to promote equal opportunities for disabled people
- to encourage good practice in the treatment of disabled people
- to advise the government on the working of disability legislation (the Disability Discrimination Act (DDA) 1995 and the Disability Rights Commission Act 1999).

The main function of the DRC is to assist disabled people to secure their rights. However, they will also provide information to employers and service providers, for example, salon owners, about their rights and duties under the DDA 1995. They can advise on good practice and help to ensure that you meet the obligations of the DDA within the salon.

You have a duty within the salon to promote equal opportunities for disabled people with those of non-disabled people. Your salon should be promoting good practice by widening its service provision depending on the needs of each individual.

Under the Disability Discrimination Act 1995, service providers (such as salon owners) must abide by the duties imposed. From 1 October 2004, service providers may have to make 'reasonable adjustments' to their premises so that there are no physical barriers stopping or making it unreasonably difficult for anyone with a disability to use their services. If you are refurbishing the salon, it would be a good opportunity to implement the changes to the physical features of the salon. If not, then you will need to consider a continuing access improvement programme. You have a responsibility to start preparing now for these changes in the law.

The salon you work in will have many rules and regulations regarding the promotion of products and services to clients. As a member of staff responsible for carrying out promotions, you must be fully conversant with all of these. Consider also that in the eyes of the law you are classed as a service provider and it is essential that you are familiar with the relevant laws that cover the promotion of that provision.

Check it out

Is your salon discriminating against disabled people in any way? Do you provide wheelchair access? Does anyone employed in the salon know basic sign language? Do you have a price list in Braille? Look at ways in which you could improve the service you provide by encompassing wider needs. If you are unsure then you can seek advice from the Disability Rights Commission.

Remember

Think about whether you are discriminating in any way against a person with a disability, for example, by not providing wheelchair access. Think about the large number of clients and revenue that you are losing.

Check it out

Look at any written rules and regulations in your salon and check to ensure that you are complying with the relevant laws that affect the promotion of products or services to clients. You may want to recommend some changes.

Clients' rights

If you are promoting services or products to a client then they will have their own rights as a consumer within the salon. As the stylist, you must be aware of and conform to these rights. You should think of your client as a consumer – any person who purchases goods or services for his or her own personal needs. There are several government acts that you must comply with that offer protection to the consumer.

The Sale of Goods Act 1979

The Sale of Goods Act 1979 (and amended in 1995) states that goods must be:

- of satisfactory quality – this means that products must last a reasonable time and not have any minor or cosmetic defects or substantial problems. However, if the fault was pointed out at time of sale, it does not give you any rights.

- sold as described – this means that the goods or products sold must match the description given, regardless of it being a verbal or written description.
- fit for purpose – this means not only the obvious function of the item but any queries that were made on its function and assurances given on its suitability.

Anything that you buy is protected under this law and you are entitled to your money back. Faulty goods must be returned immediately and as the supplier you must seek compensation from the manufacturer. This Act covers the rights of a consumer who buys from a trader, although not through a classified advertisement, for example, private sale.

The Supply of Goods and Services Act 1982

This Act covers all the work you do for a client as you are supplying a service that they pay you for. This law imposes a strict liability on any materials that you use. For example, if you put hair extensions into a client's hair and they loosen and come out within a couple of days, then you have a responsibility to replace them. You will also be liable for any damage that may be caused to the hair from the extensions being faulty. This Act clearly states that as a professional you have a 'duty of care' towards your clients and that any price or standard you agree must be honoured. Although there is no provision in the law for the time a job might take, it does require that any service carried out be done in a reasonable time.

Unfair Contract Terms Act 1977 and Unfair Terms in Consumer Contract Regulations 1994

These two Acts provide your client with the right to challenge any terms in a contract that they have signed with you if they seem unfair or unreasonable. There are very few examples of contracts drawn up between a hairdresser and a client, but be aware that there may be contracts between the salon and clients if you also offer beauty therapy services, for example, a course of treatments may be paid for in instalments.

Consumer Protection Act 1987

If a product the client uses turns out to be faulty then, as a consumer, they have a right to compensation for death, injury or damage to property (over £275). Although this action would be taken against the manufacturer, as the retailer, you have to state which manufacturer it is. This law also makes it an offence to display a misleading price. In summary, it provides protection from anything sold that is not safe.

This Act gives consumers protection against companies that provide credit, for example, the right to look at a credit file or the right to pay off credit early. You must clearly state the interest charges for credit. If your salon provides any services that you supply credit on then you must observe and comply with the conditions and procedures of this Act or face criminal prosecution.

There are many acts set out to assist us to run the everyday business of the salon in a legal and proper way. As the provider of a service or product, it is crucial that you have a thorough understanding of how these acts play a part in the way the salon runs. A good understanding of these will not only assist you in the salon but also in your own life as a consumer outside the salon.

Check it out

Do you have a returns policy at the salon? What is it and do you display this for customers to see?

Remember

If a client has particularly long, thick hair and you think this will increase the time of the service considerably, you should inform them of this fact. If you have discussed it then it prevents any misunderstanding between yourselves.

Check it out

Think about the promotion of additional products and services in your salon. Check to ensure that they comply with the relevant laws and if they take your clients' rights into account. You may want to recommend some changes.

Knowledge check

1. What are the benefits, to both the salon and clients, of your salon promoting additional services and products?

2. Why is clear and effective communication important in the salon?

3. What type of questions elicit your client's feelings?

4. List five methods of promoting the salon.

5. What are the three stages of a promotion?

Support customer service improvements

Unit G10

Introduction

This unit focuses on how you can improve the services you provide in the salon. Being aware of your clients' needs and making improvements that reflect those needs is essential. You should be prepared to keep an open mind and not allow yourself to be blinkered or narrow minded in your decision making, as this can adversely affect your judgement about the right way for your salon to move forward. Throughout this unit, you will become familiar with ways of determining what your clients' needs are and how improvements can be made to the services your salon provides.

Making your clients feel at ease is an important part of running a successful salon

What you will learn
• Using feedback to identify potential customer service improvements
• Contributing to the implementation of changes in customer services
• Assisting with the evaluation of changes in customer services
• Salon and legal requirements
• Clients' rights

You the stylist

As a stylist, your job involves delivering a service to clients. It is important for you to be fully aware of your responsibilities regarding customer services. There are several factors that you must consider.

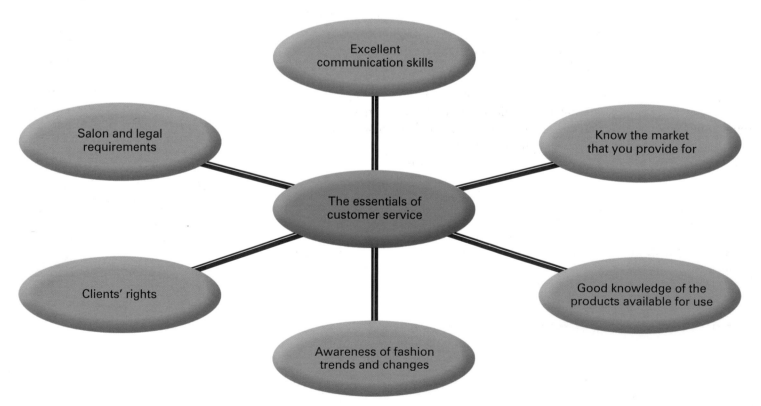

Salons change the way they deliver services to clients because clients demand change. You should, however, be aware that making changes for the sake of it will not always make good business sense. For example, if your client base is happy with the level of service you provide and your salon systems work well, why cause unnecessary disruption? You need to be aware of other salons and the services they provide in order to keep your eye on the competition. If your salon is implementing improvements then you must support them and present them positively to your clients. Listening to clients' comments and putting your own views forward is an essential part of your job role. As a stylist in the salon, your opinions will matter to the salon owner. It will be the salon owner's responsibility to judge if your ideas have possibilities for change and improvement.

Communication

Understanding the importance of effective communication is an essential part of working in the salon. But what is meant by 'effective communication'? This is a common term that you will have come across many times whilst completing your hairdressing training, but do you fully understand it? Communication is the sending and receiving of information between people using various methods. In the salon there are three methods that are relevant to you as a hairdresser. These are written, verbal and non-verbal communication. Refer to Unit G9 (pages 31–37) and Unit G6 (pages 74–77) for more information on and examples of methods of communication.

Products and services

The products and services that you offer in your salon will be similar to that of other salons but not exactly the same. The services you offer will be dependent on the ability of the staff that work in your salon and the needs of your clients. If your salon is located in an area where there is a large ethnic community then you will be looking to provide specialist hairdressing services in order to service your local community. If your salon is located in a rural village, you will not necessarily have the same demands for updating the services that you offer. You need to target the services you provide in relation to the client base you are providing for.

The services that you provide are enhanced by the products you offer. Again, your product range needs to be relevant to your clients' needs. It does not make good financial sense to buy products that your clients will never require or they would consider too expensive. Enhancing the services you provide with small but important features, for example, free refreshments or a discount for loyalty, will ensure your clients' satisfaction.

> ### Keys to good practice
>
> Word-of-mouth advertising is completely free to you. If a client leaves the salon with a fantastic hairstyle and feels you have treated them well, they are sure to tell their friends. However, you must not forget that clients will also be quick to tell their friends if the service was poor and this will harm the salon's reputation.

> ### Check it out
>
> Discuss with your clients if they are aware of your responsibility for implementing service improvements. Check that you are fulfilling your job role in this area – it is easy to become indifferent about what the salon has to offer.

> ### Check it out
>
> Think about the lines of communication that you use in the salon. It is easy to forget their importance when you are using them on a daily basis in your working life. List them all and then as you progress through this unit, check to see if there are any that you have forgotten.

The products you provide should be suited to your client base

Using feedback to identify potential customer service improvements

You need to look at ways of finding out how clients feel about the services you provide in the salon. There are various methods you can use to identify your clients' needs which can be labelled as either formal or informal.

Informal methods

Informal methods are probably the most commonly used. Each day, whilst dealing with your clients, you will question them and extract information about the products and services that you offer. Most of this information will never actually be recorded anywhere for future reference. Non-verbal communication is another form of informal feedback. For example, if a client is not happy with the service provision, although they may not say it directly, the look on their face can tell a different story. Perception of non-verbal communication, such as body language and facial expression, is crucial in order for it to be used as a means of identifying feedback. You may occasionally write a comment on a client record card regarding a product or service used, especially if a client had an allergy or dislike. At staff meetings, management may ask for client feedback, particularly if there have been any changes at the salon. This will be an opportunity to discuss and formalise (via the minutes of meetings) client feedback gained on a day-to-day basis.

Formal methods

It may, from time to time, be necessary to carry out a formal client feedback procedure to ensure that you are maintaining a high level of service provision for your clientele. The need to develop and enhance your service provision may have been highlighted by informal feedback given by clients. For example, if, during a discussion at a staff meeting, you uncover the same negative comments from several clients, then this should be recognised and acted upon.

There are a variety of methods that you can adopt in order to gain formal feedback from your client base including:

- a written survey
- a telephone survey
- an interview
- client suggestion box
- via the salon website.

Discussing different products with your client can help you to identify his needs

Written client survey

In order to improve services that you provide in the salon, you may consider using a client survey. This will be more effectively carried out in written form to enable you to collate all the information given. It is a valuable tool if used correctly. Consider keeping it anonymous to try to extract your client's true feelings. If not, then think of the implications of storing information under the Data Protection Act. You need to be clear about what you are trying to gain from the survey before you start. This will ensure you retrieve the information you require in order to make your improvements. You could post it on the website allowing clients to complete it in this way.

These are just a few of the many different facts and figures you may want to look at. How you deliver the survey is also an important factor. You also need to consider whether the survey caters for the needs of all your clients, for example, both men and women. If your client base is mainly one sex then you must ensure that if the survey is to be given out to both, that it will be fair. It would be beneficial to discuss this with all the staff and decide among yourselves how you will deliver it in the salon. This will ensure fairness and you will know that everyone is informed of his or her exact role.

You need to develop a plan for completion of the survey from start to finish, ensuring start and end dates are included. You will need to consider:

- where the survey is to be carried out, for example, in the salon or clients take it home
- at what time during the service will the client complete the survey, for example, whilst waiting at reception, during chemical processes or paying at the end
- how the survey is to be carried out, for example, client completes it anonymously or staff ask the questions
- who is responsible for ensuring its completion, for example, the receptionist or the stylist.

Types of questions

In the survey, there are specific ways in which you can question clients to determine the information you require.

Closed/open questions

Closed questions are more commonly used, as they make a survey quick and easy for a client to complete. You will ask a question and the client will only have to give a yes or no answer. This type of information is much easier to collate and analyse. However, you should consider that this could limit the amount of feedback you will gain. To overcome this, you may want to follow it with an open question. This type of question is much more difficult to collate and analyse, as it requires the client to put down their own thoughts and feelings. Open questions will generate a wider response and is particularly useful if you are not sure of the likely replies.

Leading questions

Leading questions are easy to devise, especially if you have a strong opinion on the questions you are asking. Be careful of using a leading question – if you are prompting a particular response to the question, would you be receiving the client's true feelings?

Personal information

A client may be put off completing the survey if you are asking personal questions, so only put them in if it is absolutely necessary. Make sure they are aware of why you are asking them to give reassurance, and put these types of questions towards the end, so as not to put them off. If you are trying to extract information from a client that is personal, such as age or income, then do not ask for specifics. It is much more likely that they will reply if they are offered a range. Look at the client survey for an example of this. When you have decided on the types of question you are going to ask, devise the survey in a logical order, for example, grouping the questions in sequential order so that one question leads to another.

Client Survey

As part of our ongoing commitment to the services we provide in the salon for you, we ask you to take a small amount of time to complete this short questionnaire. It is necessary to assist us with our improvements that we ask for a small amount of personal information. May all the staff at the salon thank you in anticipation of your completion of this survey, as it will greatly assist us to improve the services we offer you.

1. Do you feel the reception/waiting area is welcoming and comfortable?

    Yes/No

2. When you entered the salon were you greeted immediately and in a friendly manner?

    Yes/No

3. Do you feel the retail display looks inviting and attractive?

    Yes/No

4. How do you think the retail product range could be changed to encompass your needs?

    _____

    _____

    _____

5. Which age category do you fall into?

    Under 18   19–28   29–38   39–48   49–65   over 65

6. Are there any other comments that you would wish to make about the services, facilities or products used at the salon? If so, please write your comments on the next page.

    Many Thanks

Check it out

When did your salon last complete a formal client survey? Do you feel it would be beneficial to the salon's needs? Devise a survey that you could use in your salon depending on the information that you need to gain.

Remember

For any survey to be successful, you need to stay focused on its main objectives. Check it on an ongoing basis to see if it is achieving what you require. You can then implement any necessary changes as you go along.

Telephone survey

This type of survey can take up a lot of working hours, as staff would actually have to take the time to read out the questions and write out the client's response. The advantage is the immediate response you get from it. You would have to go through the same process of devising the questionnaire as you would for a written survey, looking at the types of questions and how it should be collated.

Interview

Interviewing a client to get responses will allow you to focus on an issue in more depth. As it involves speaking to the interviewee directly, it captures in greater detail personal views and experiences. Interviews can draw out feelings and reasons in a way that a questionnaire cannot. However, you should bear in mind that the interviewer may influence the answers given. Normal gestures shown by the interviewer, such as nodding or smiling, can lead the interviewee to give a false response. Using a tape recorder will allow you to replay the interview many times and extract the correct information.

Client suggestion box

Consider how many times you have taken the time to write down how good a product or service was compared with the amount of times you have taken the time to complain. Receiving constructive feedback from a suggestion box is unlikely and it also limits the type and amount of information you can get. However, if you actively encourage all clients to regularly complete the suggestion slips and use it as a tool to make improvements or stay up to date with your clients' needs, it can prove to be a useful resource.

Salon website

Using the salon website as a means of obtaining feedback is a good method. There are many uses of the website; in fact, all of the methods listed can be used successfully with the exception of an interview. If a client is looking at your website, they are more likely to take a minute or two more to complete a questionnaire or comment box. You can ask as much or as little as you like without the client feeling embarrassed or uncomfortable at not having enough time or not being interested.

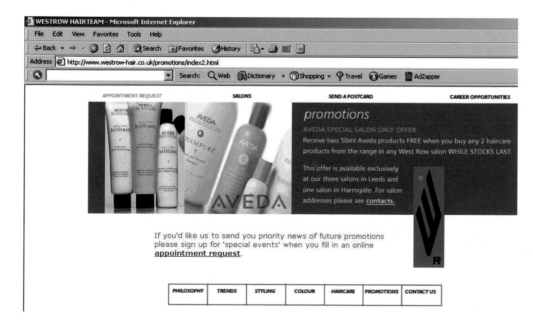

Websites can be used to inform and obtain feedback from clients

Identifying the improvements to be made

When the survey has been successfully completed, you must collate the information and decide how you will use it. It may be beneficial to share this information with staff and decide amongst you all what the best options for your salon would be. You will need to decide if the information gained from the survey should be made public to the staff. Sometimes it can contain comments that are not entirely complementary. You will need to deal with this as you see fit. For example, if a comment made about a receptionist states that his or her telephone manner is poor then you will need to raise this on an individual basis. An important question that you must ask is, did it achieve the objectives set? If not, do you need to revisit the survey and look at ways in which you can alter it to meet your requirements? The client survey should provide you with an opportunity to look at any improvements you need to make. It is important that, following its completion, you act upon this and implement the necessary changes. These changes may take many different forms. For example:

- re-pricing the product range
- re-pricing the service charges
- changing the product range
- introducing special offers
- staff training
- enhancements to the services offered
- updating facilities
- organising social events
- introducing new products and services.

If you show the clients that you have acted on the information given in the survey, you will be showing that you value their opinion.

Contributing to the implementation of changes in customer services

When working in the salon as part of a team, you will have to implement changes in the services you provide. It is important to work as a team and stay positive and focused whilst implementing any changes. Ensure that you all communicate and check the progress of the changes as you go along. This section covers:

- recognising the need for change
- presenting your ideas for change
- how to implement changes
- working as a team to implement changes.

Recognising the need for change

How will you know when your salon needs to implement changes? You are now familiar with the ways in which you can gain client feedback to help determine any changes required. You also have a responsibility to be alert to the changes that need to be made yourself. If you work in the same environment day in and day out, it is easy to become indifferent to your surroundings.

Updating the salon can be a small task or a major overhaul depending on your financial situation. A new coat of paint can dramatically change the appearance of your surroundings without costing a lot of money. If, however, you are in a position to redesign the salon then this would be a good time to ask your clients' opinions.

Check if your clients have any particular requirements that you may have overlooked. They may provide you with a wealth of good ideas. The changes that you feel need to be implemented may not even be on so grand a scale. For example, you may feel that the stock ordering system needs updating or a new method of distributing the tips given by clients is needed.

Presenting your ideas for change

Regardless of how trivial or crucial the change you feel is needed, it is important to bring it to the attention of the appropriate staff. How you do this is vital as to whether or not your suggestions are taken seriously. You need to be sure that you can justify why the changes are necessary, especially if you have to present your ideas to a manager or salon owner. Decide if you may need the other staff to support your idea and, if so, discuss it with them first. This option could be particularly useful if you need help on deciding how you will present your ideas. Alternatively, it may be a suggestion that you would like to discuss with management without the other staff knowing, for example, if you felt certain staff needed more training in a particular area. You will need to judge the delicacy of the situation and how others might feel about the proposed changes.

> ### Remember
>
> If you are redesigning or making any physical changes to the salon, check that these changes comply with the Disability Discrimination Act. See page 94.

In the salon

Following a recent client survey, Ali, the salon owner, decided to redecorate and modernise the salon. After a brief meeting with the staff, during which he informed them of his intentions, he set to work planning the improvements. Ali was very busy over the next few weeks with research and planning. Finally, he called another meeting to inform the staff of his ideas. The staff were already feeling concerned at not being involved in any of the planning and on seeing their boss' intentions they became alarmed at the changes he was proposing.

Firstly, the salon had a large storeroom upstairs that the staff also used as a staff room. Ali was proposing to change this into salon floor space and for all the chemical work to take place upstairs. The staff pointed out that not only would it limit access for clients with disabilities but that they would lose their recreational area. Secondly, the layout of the salon and the choice of decor would be very restrictive. The staff felt that putting in more salon stations would reduce each other's workspace and again limit access for clients with disabilities. They also felt that the blue colour scheme Ali was planning for the salon would adversely affect the colours reflected on clients' hair.

At first, Ali was hurt that all his hard work was being dismissed in this way, though he soon realised that he would have to listen to what his staff felt about the improvements. After much discussion, which at times became heated, Ali and the staff managed to make several compromises. He understood that the changes to the upper floor would be depriving the staff of their recreational area and decided to scale down the changes, allowing them to keep an area for themselves, but placing a couple of work stations upstairs for training purposes or when the salon was extremely busy. He allowed the staff to have input into the new colour scheme for the salon and to show him different ways of how it could be laid out utilising the space available to its best advantage. When all the staff had agreed as a team on the way to go forward with the improvements, Ali began to put them into place. Once finished, the team and clients were extremely happy with the outcome, feeling the improvements to the salon's surroundings and facilities were beneficial.

- Did Ali initially consider the needs of all his staff on making plans for improvements?
- Why do you think the staff was concerned when he did not involve them?
- Would you feel upset at not being consulted about major changes that affected your working conditions?
- Do you think his staff were justified in pointing out his discrimination to disabled clients?

Keys to good practice

To keep a successful and happy team, you must communicate openly and discuss ideas and changes freely.

How to implement changes

When you have decided what changes need to be implemented, you must then look at how this will be done. You need to be sure that all staff are made aware of how the improvements are to be carried out and that clients are also kept informed. You can use various methods to inform clients of the changes; however, you need to be sure you choose the right one. The table below indicates a few methods, with the advantages and disadvantages of each listed alongside.

Method	Advantage	Disadvantage
Poster	Good to inform of specific information, e.g. prices, dates or times	Clients will still ask and you will have to discuss it with each one
Inform each client on an individual basis	You can be sure you have told them exactly and explained the benefits fully	You may forget to tell someone and it could be particularly important
Leaflet distribution	A leaflet can contain lots of information about the salon, e.g. special offers, location	Time consuming and is easily dismissed as junk mail
Media advertising	Will reach a wider audience	Can be very expensive and not all your clients may see it
Internet via website	Can reach a much wider audience	Not all clients have access to the Internet

Working as a team to implement changes

As a team, all the staff need to present a positive approach to the improvements being made. If you or anyone else has any doubts about the changes then it will become difficult to remain enthusiastic. This will be reflected in your approach to the improvements and clients will become aware of it. If you display concerns then clients will lack confidence in the improvements being implemented and this can result in disaster for the salon. Alternatively, if you present a positive, united campaign then clients cannot fail to be impressed by the improvements made.

Assisting with the evaluation of changes in customer services

Evaluating the changes

Staff meetings are crucial at this stage to evaluate the improvements you have made. As a team, you will need to work flexibly. Ensure that each individual is fully aware of their responsibilities and is working towards achieving them. If problems do occur then they need to be addressed. A group discussion will help to formulate a plan of action and this is where flexibility is paramount. It may be that job roles have to change and as an individual you will have to adapt. You may also have to support other staff with this task, again showing your flexibility. Client feedback is very important at this stage. Each member of the team will have different comments to make known and it is important that they are considered no matter how trivial they appear.

Dealing with negative feedback

One problem that you may encounter is how to present negative feedback to staff, especially if the changes were their ideas. Any negativity needs to be handled with caution. It is easy to upset a person's feelings with a flippant comment and you need to be tactful in your approach. Be sure to deliver it with a positive comment, then the negative, and finish with a positive. This is sometimes called a 'feedback sandwich'. This will show that you have considered their feelings and that you are not totally disregarding their ideas. Alternatively, it may be your idea that is being presented with some negative feedback. You must be able to look at it with maturity and not take it personally, especially if the feedback is constructive. Constructive criticism should be used as a learning tool. However, blatant criticism can be both de-moralising and de-motivating. Being able to evaluate ideas and correct any problems as they occur will ensure continued success for the salon.

Supporting customer service improvements can prove to be a motivating factor within your job role. It is essential that you see it as a necessity in order to maintain a healthy salon. Any support that you give must be positive and assured. This will promote a healthy working environment in the salon and help to increase the financial effectiveness of the business.

Salon and legal requirements

In the salon there are many legal requirements that you must observe. If you look at Unit G1 on health and safety, most of the laws that you need to be familiar with are covered there. However, with regard to the laws that are important for customer services, you need to think about:

- data protection
- equal opportunities
- disability discrimination
- racial equality.

Data Protection Act 1998

The Data Protection Act has been extensively covered in Unit G6 – refer to page 78 for a reminder of the details of this Act. Below is a brief summary.

The Data Protection Act contains eight enforceable principles of good practice. These state that all data must be:

- fairly and lawfully processed
- obtained and used only for specified and lawful purposes
- adequate, relevant and not excessive
- accurate where necessary
- kept up to date and not kept longer than necessary
- processed in accordance with the persons rights
- kept secure
- transferred only to countries that offer adequate data protection.

You need to think about how this will affect your work in the salon and consider all the information that you may collate and store that is passed on from your clients. This includes not only all the information on a record card but also any feedback that you have gained whilst determining your clients' needs. If you have carried out a written survey or used a client suggestion box then all of the information you have gained from this will have to be used according to the rules of the Data Protection Act 1998.

Equal opportunities

At every stage of the customer service improvements you are carrying out, you should remain aware of your responsibilities to equal opportunities, not only towards your clients but also towards the staff that you work with. You must consider other people's needs and feelings and present a positive and unprejudiced view of the salon. Refer to pages 78–80 in Unit G6 for more information on equal opportunities legislation.

In your working life you have a duty to comply with equal opportunities. A written policy will serve to ease your understanding of how this can be done and the aim of a good policy is to ensure that everyone receives fair and equal treatment. Although your salon may not have a written equal opportunities policy, especially if it is a small business, all the salon's policies and procedures should have equal opportunities running through them.

In the salon

Elisha was working as a barber in a salon with a predominantly female clientele. She was self employed and rented a chair at the front of the salon, offering men's hairdressing services. The salon was running a data collection survey to help determine the needs of its clientele. Elisha's boss had made what she felt was a flippant comment to her that she need not bother with her clients as they only ever popped in for a haircut. Elisha was enraged; she felt that her clients' feelings were just as important and relevant to the salon, and any consequent improvements, as the rest of the clientele. She wasted no time in telling her employer that, under equal opportunities law, she was discriminating against her male clients. She explained that just because the majority of them only had a haircut, their feelings and needs were no less important to the success of the salon than the female clients. Her boss was unsure but, not wishing to upset

Elisha, agreed to let her carry out the survey with any of her clients that wanted to.

On completion, the results of the survey highlighted that Elisha's male clients were looking for a styling product range that they could buy whilst at the salon. Elisha was happy to see a retail opportunity opened up in this way, proving to the salon owner that the discrimination initially shown could have cost the salon money.

- Why do you think Elisha was initially unhappy with the salon owner?
- Do you think Elisha was justified in pointing out to the salon owner her responsibilities under equal opportunities?
- Why do you think the salon owner was negligent in this way?
- Do you think the outcome would make both Elisha and the salon owner happy? Why?

Disability discrimination

Under the Disability Discrimination Act 1995, you have a responsibility not to discriminate in any way against any person with a disability. Unit G6 covers this in much greater detail – refer to page 81 for a reminder of your responsibilities. Under the Disability Discrimination Act 1995, service providers (such as salon owners) must abide by the duties imposed. Anyone with a disability has a right to the services you provide and these duties have been introduced in three stages.

- Since 2 December 1996, it has been against the law for service providers to treat anyone with a disability less favourably.
- Since 1 October 1999, service providers have had to make 'reasonable

adjustments' for anyone with a disability, such as giving extra help or changing the way they provide their services.

- From 1 October 2004, service providers may have to make 'reasonable adjustments' to their premises so that there are no physical barriers stopping or making it unreasonably difficult for anyone with a disability to use their services.

Keys to good practice

You have a duty within the salon to promote equal opportunities for people with disabilities. Your salon should be promoting good practice by widening its service provisions depending on the needs of each individual.

In the salon

Peter had just moved into a new town and was looking for a local barber's shop for a haircut. As a wheelchair user, he had specific needs and knew that although he needed somewhere close to home, it would also have to provide easy access and usability for him as a client. This proved to be a difficult task; the nearest salon was unfortunately above another shop premises and provided no access for him at all. He could, however, use a salon a little further away but would have to get a friend to help him gain access, as the salon had quite a large step up into the premises.

When he visited the salon for a haircut, he was happy with the finished look but explained to the stylist that he had difficulty gaining access. The stylist told him that the salon had just appointed a new manager and that he had introduced a suggestion box and asked him to complete a comment card. Peter did this and was contacted by the salon manager requesting more feedback. The manager asked for suggestions on how they could adapt the salon to encompass the needs of clients with wheelchairs. Peter was more than happy to help and told the manager that although the floor

space of the salon allowed him easy movement in his wheelchair, he could not gain access without assistance. He also felt uncomfortable at reception when paying, as the desk was too high for him to see over, which also prevented him looking at any promotional material displayed there.

From their discussion, a ramp access was fitted, at very little cost to the salon, and the reception desk was lowered in order for a client in a wheelchair to see above it. Peter was very happy that his needs as a wheelchair user had been considered and, over time, the salon found several new clients that had previously felt the salon unusable. This example shows how a client suggestion box can provide vital feedback in order to make service improvements.

- Are there any small changes that you could make to your salon to make it more accessible for a person with a disability? Consider several factors like the layout of the salon or reception area. Is the floor space used cleverly or are there unnecessary objects littering and hindering access?

Racial equality

The Race Relations Act 1976 and the Race Relations (Amendment) Act 2000 make it unlawful to discriminate against a person, directly or indirectly, in the field of employment. Employees of all racial groups have a right to be treated fairly in line with equal opportunities. It is the responsibility of employers to provide this. You must develop coherent and effective policies in line with the requirements of the Race Relations Act 1976. This will ensure that the hairdressing industry is utilising all the abilities of the full workforce. It is both the employer's and employees' responsibility to adopt good practice and secure such equality.

The Commission for Racial Equality was set up under the Race Relations Act 1976 and is a publicly funded, non-governmental body. The Commission states that 'it works in both the public and private sectors to encourage fair treatment and to promote equal opportunities for everyone, regardless of their race, colour, nationality, or national or ethnic origin'. Its fundamental principles are that it:

- provides information and advice to people who think they have suffered racial discrimination or harassment
- works with public bodies, businesses and organisations from all sectors to promote policies and practices that will help to ensure equal treatment for all
- runs campaigns to raise awareness of race issues and encourages organisations and individuals to play their part in creating a fair society
- ensures that all new laws take full account of the Race Relations Act and the protection it gives against discrimination.

Since many hairdressing businesses are classed as small firms, you will be working in close contact with all the staff. Therefore, it is much easier to be aware of any types of discrimination taking place and the assessment of equal opportunities is much less formal. This does not mean that your responsibilities can be ignored – they are just as important. However, it does mean that the monitoring of equal opportunities will be less evident. You have a right to raise any feelings you may have about racial equality at the salon, whether it is regarding improvements to be made or the way the salon is run.

Clients' rights

Your client has rights as a consumer within your salon. A consumer is any person that purchases goods or services for their own personal needs. You must think of this as the hairdressing services and the products that you provide in the salon. You should re-read Unit G6 to remind yourself of the legislation that is relevant to clients' rights and the importance of each act and regulation. If you are to successfully implement any service-related improvements then being aware of you clients' rights as a consumer is crucial. If you are not complying with the laws set out to protect clients then you are not only negligent but could face prosecution.

There are four main acts that you should be fully familiar with and they are:

- **The Sale of Goods Act 1979 (amended in 1995)**
  This Act states that goods must be of satisfactory quality, sold as described and fit for purpose.
- **The Supply of Goods and Services Act 1994**
  As a hairdresser, this Act covers all the work you do for a client as you are supplying a service that they pay you for.
- **Unfair Contract Terms Act 1977 and Unfair Terms in Consumer Contracts Regulations 1994**
  These two Acts provide your client with the right to challenge any terms in a contract that they have signed with you if they seem unfair or unreasonable.
- **Consumer Protection Act 1987**
  This Act gives consumers protection against companies that provide credit, for example, the right to look at a credit file or the right to pay off credit early.

These acts and their amendments can assist you in the way in which your salon is run on a day-to-day basis. Consumers have these rights to protect them legally and you cannot afford to ignore their significance. Your thorough understanding of them may also be helpful to you as a consumer outside of the salon.

> **Remember**
>
> You can find out more about your clients' consumer rights from agencies such as the Citizens Advice Bureau or via the BBC's Watchdog website.

Knowledge check

1. List four of the laws set out to protect consumer rights.

2. List five methods of written communication that are important in the salon.

3. What method of communication is most commonly used in the salon?

4. How is the client's experience influenced by the way the service is delivered?

5. List four methods of how client feedback may be obtained.

Contribute to the financial effectiveness of the business

Unit G11

Introduction

The main aim of any business is to make a profit and the hairdressing business is no exception. However, this should not be at the expense of health and safety, client comfort, or staff welfare and career progression. In this unit, you will learn about the ways you can help the business become more profitable by monitoring the effective use of resources, and the impact of productivity and development targets as a means of generating income. You will also need to ensure any other staff for which you have responsibility are working effectively.

What you will learn
• Salon and legal requirements relating to the use of resources • Contribute to the effective use and monitoring of resources • Meeting productivity and development targets

You, the stylist

As a stylist, you need to understand the implications of using resources effectively. This is to ensure maximum profitability and minimise waste. You will need to monitor members of staff whose job role is to assist you in your work to ensure that they comply with the above aims.

Throughout your working life in the hairdressing industry, you will be required to meet monetary targets; this is to ensure the salon owner's business remains viable. Hairdressing is a fast-moving fashion industry with new products and services being introduced all the time. You need to keep abreast of these changes if you are to remain a productive member of the staff; therefore, further training and development will be necessary to achieve this.

Ensure that stock levels of all products are monitored effectively

Salon and legal requirements relating to the use of resources

There are numerous legal requirements relating to the use of resources that are relevant to the hairdressing business, many of which have been covered in Units G6 and G10. These include:

- Health and Safety at Work Act 1974
- Manual Handling Operations Regulations 1992
- Reporting of Injuries, Diseases and Dangerous Occurrences Regulations (RIDDOR) 1995
- Electricity at Work Regulations 1989
- Cosmetic Products (Safety) Regulations 1996; and
- Control of Substances Hazardous to Health (COSHH) Regulations 2003

However, there is additional legislation you should be aware of to enable you to contribute to the financial effectiveness of the business.

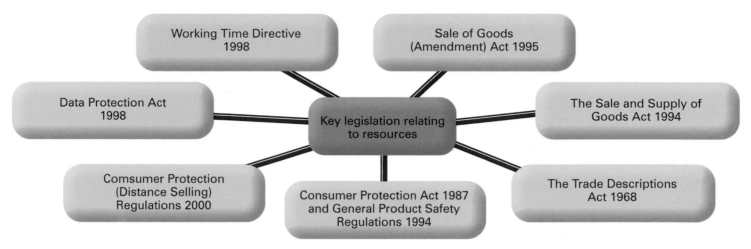

Much of this legislation is there to protect the salon from possible litigation. Any litigation against the business can prove to be costly in both time and money and the negative publicity will undoubtedly have an impact on the salon's financial security. Other pieces of legislation exist to ensure all members of staff are treated fairly and their working conditions are considered acceptable. Staff who consider their working conditions to be up to standard are more likely to co-operate with their employers and therefore the working environment will be conducive to good productivity.

Legislation and consumer rights

Sale of Goods (Amendment) Act 1995

When you sell goods or a service to your clients, you are entering into a legally binding contract. The contract may be written or verbal. The Sale of Goods Act states that goods must be:

- of satisfactory quality – this covers minor and cosmetic defects, as well as substantial problems. It also means that the products must last a reasonable length of time. It does not give the consumer any rights if a fault was obvious or pointed out at the time of purchase.
- sold as described – this refers to any verbal or written description made by the seller.
- fit for purpose – this means not only the obvious function of the item but any queries that were made on its function and given assurance on.

Anything that is bought is protected under this law and clients are entitled to their money back under certain circumstances. Faulty goods must be returned immediately and as the supplier you must seek compensation from the manufacturer. If the client feels the goods are not of a satisfactory quality, they have the right to return the goods and you must refund their money. In this instance, the client must return the goods within a reasonable time scale. Your salon should have a returns policy to ensure compliance with this Act.

The Sale and Supply of Goods Act 1994

This Act applies to the hairdressing industry, as it is a service provider. It has implications for both labour and the materials used during the service. The Act states that you must:

- carry out the service with reasonable skill and care
- complete the service within a reasonable time (unless a prior agreement was made specifying the time)

> **Remember**
>
> A business does not have to refund a client for a service that was badly done, unless:
>
> - the client can prove they have received no benefit at all from the work
> - the business is proved negligent
> - another salon has to repair the damage.

- make a reasonable charge for the service (unless a price was agreed prior to the service)
- use materials that are of a satisfactory quality and fit for the purpose.

It is also becoming a more recognised procedure within the hairdressing industry to make clients aware of the cost of the service beforehand. In the past, the hairdressing industry has gained a bad reputation for adding items onto a client's bill without their knowledge. This type of practice caused clients to mistrust hairdressers. With the heightened awareness of consumer rights, this type of poor practice will no longer be tolerated.

Check it out

Have you received sufficient training for the services you carry out in the salon, thus covering the 'reasonable skill' issue within this Act?

The Trade Descriptions Act 1968

This Act ensures that the description of goods, services and prices is accurate and not misleading in any way. The trade description may be given verbally, in writing, by photo, or by inference, but whichever way it is made, if the information is incorrect, it is an offence, even if it was made unintentionally. Therefore, it is important to think carefully before you unwittingly give out incorrect information, as you can still be penalised if you have acted without due diligence. Failure to comply with these regulations could result in lack of client confidence, negative publicity, and/or loss of clientele, not to mention the cost of litigation.

Consumer Protection Act 1987 and General Products Safety Regulations 1994

This Act is the main piece of legislation dealing with consumer safety. It is there to protect the consumer from defective products, that is, products that do not reach a reasonable level of safety. The Consumer Protection Act gives consumers the right to sue for damages if they have been injured or suffered damage to property (over a certain value).

The General Product Safety Regulations 1994 also deal with product safety and, in part, replaces the Consumer Protection Act 1987. It is the responsibility of all businesses to ensure that their products are safe. The responsibilities included within this piece of legislation are to provide relevant information to consumers regarding the risks of the products they are supplying.

Consumer Protection (Distance Selling) Regulations 2000

These regulations were introduced to increase consumer confidence. They will apply to you if the salon where you work sells goods or services via the Internet, by phone, by fax, or mail order. The key points of the regulations are:

- the consumer must be given clear information about the goods or services on offer. This information includes the price, delivery costs, arrangements for payment and delivery, and so on
- the consumer must be sent confirmation after making a purchase
- the consumer must have a seven-day cooling off period (this supposedly equates to the time the consumer would spend in the salon deciding whether to purchase).

It is likely that this regulation does not apply to your salon if you do not usually supply clients in this way, but you agree to as a one-off request. However, if the business regularly handles one-off requests, it is likely the salon should comply with these regulations. If this is the case, the salon should also ensure it has registered with and is fulfilling the requirements of the Data Protection Act 1998.

Data Protection Act 1998

The Data Protection Act is in place to protect the personal information you hold on individuals. You are required to ensure appropriate security measures are in place to prevent any unlawful or unauthorised access to data.

If your salon is holding personal data, you must be registered with the Information Commissioner. It is worth checking to find out if you should be registered, as failure to do so may result in prosecution.

Working Time Directive 1998

Up until the Working Time Directive was introduced in 1998, employers were free to set working times and holiday entitlements. Although many employers and employees negotiated terms and conditions, some employees were still treated badly by their employers. The general rule, which has been applicable since the introduction of this law, is that an employer must take reasonable steps that are in keeping with the need to protect the health and safety of their employees.

The main provision of the Working Time Directive relating to hairdressing salons includes:

- a limit on the average working week
- minimum daily and weekly rest breaks
- rest breaks at work
- paid holiday entitlement.

The law applies to full-time, part-time and casual workers, which is anyone with a contract of employment (whether written or not). These regulations do not cover the self-employed.

Key points of the Working Time Directive
- You should not be asked to work more than 48 hours a week, averaged over a seventeen-week period.
- You are entitled to a rest period of eleven consecutive hours between each working day.
- You are also entitled to a minimum of one day off per week.
- You are entitled to an uninterrupted break of twenty minutes if you work more than six hours per day. It should be a break in working time, not taken at the start or end of the working day.
- You are allowed at least four weeks paid holiday per year. This is calculated on your right to take a twelfth of your holiday entitlement for each month worked (rounded up to the nearest half day). One week's holiday is the equivalent to the time you would normally work per week, for example, if you work three days per week, your annual holiday entitlement would be twelve days. If your contract of employment is terminated before you have taken your leave entitlement, you have the right to payment in lieu.
- For staff aged over sixteen but under eighteen, the law is slightly different. The entitled rest period is increased to twelve consecutive hours rest in every twenty-four hours, and they are entitled to an uninterrupted break of 30 minutes if they have worked for more than four-and-a-half hours.

Your employer must keep records to show they are complying with this directive and they must keep them for two years from the date on which they were started.

Check it out

Can you remember the eight enforceable principles of good practice relating to data protection? If not, refer back to Unit G6, page 78.

Remember

It is not only client record cards that are covered by this Act. If your salon carries out distance selling, any information held on the client requires the salon to be registered. The salon may hold staff details, for example, salary, commission paid, working times, and so on, and these are covered by this Act. Some paper-based data is also included.

Contribute to the effective use and monitoring of resources

The resources covered within this part of the unit are:

- stock
- tools and equipment
- human resources (people)
- time.

Stock

Stock is a valuable commodity within any salon. A business may have large amounts of money tied up in stock and it is essential that the stock is used appropriately as misuse may cost the salon owner money.

Stock control

Stock control is an important aspect in any salon, as it is essential to the smooth running of the salon. If the salon were to run out of a specific item, it could lead to a disappointed client and give an unprofessional image of the salon, both of which may lead to negative publicity. There may also be seasonal changes that need to be considered, for example, more clients request blonde highlights during the summer months and warm/red colours in the winter. The salon may stock holiday hair products to retail during the summer and this should be well thought out when ordering stock. If the salon is running any promotional offers, it is essential that the stock be available.

Ensure that you stock holiday hair products during the summer

Stock includes items such as:

- products used for salon services
- retail items
- equipment used in the salon, for example, hairdryer, climazone, and so on
- consumable items, such as cotton wool and tissue
- semi-consumable items, for example, protective gloves and aprons.

Stock should be monitored following the procedures laid down by your employer who should set minimum stock levels for both products used in the salon and retail products. They should also set the frequency of the stock taking. Minimum stock levels are set to ensure the stock on the shelves does not exceed its shelf life. Items of stock that are used frequently or a good retail line may have a higher minimum stock level set than items that are seldom used. For example, you may retail more shampoos and conditioners for colour treated hair than dandruff control shampoo. Therefore, the minimum stock levels for the range of products for colour treated hair would be greater as you will use or sell more.

Stocktaking should be carried out on a regular basis and may be done in several different ways. Your salon may stock take manually, that is, to count each individual product and record your findings. You should then compare this against the minimum stock level set and this will tell you if the product needs re-ordering. Manufacturers will often provide stock sheets to record your stocktaking.

An example of a manufacturer's stock sheet

Styling Range		STOCK LEVEL		DATE													
		MIN	MAX	UNIT	STOCK	ORDER	STOCK	ORDER	STOCK	ORDER	STOCK	ORDER	STOCK	ORDER	STOCK	ORDER	STOCK
073000	Sleek Frizz Free Serum 50ml			6													
073001	Stretch Straightener 100ml			6													
073002	Pearl Strong Hold Gel 150ml			6													
073005	Shape Soft Wax 75ml			6													
073062	Control Wax Stick 75ml			6													
073007	Stay Strong Hold Hairspray 300ml			6													
073010	Stay Strong Hold Hairspray 500ml			1													
511552	Stay Strong Hold Hairspray 750ml			1													
073009	Free Flow Flex Hold H/spray 300ml			6													
073008	Free Flow Flex Hold H/spray 500ml			1													
511554	Free Flow Flex Hold H/spray 750ml			1													
073011	Lift Strong Hold Mousse 250ml			6													
073013	Lift Strong Hold Mousse 500ml			1													
073015	Move Medium Hold Mousse 250ml			6													
073014	Move Medium Hold Mousse 500ml			1													
073016	Animator Ex Strong Gel Spray 200ml			6													
073017	Massive Volume Pump Spray 200ml			6													
073018	Constructor Gum Paste 75ml			6													
073020	Definition Texuriser 150ml			6													
073061	Fizz Wax Spray 150ml			6													
073072	Create Styling Cream 150ml			6													
Style Active																	
070735	Hair & Body Shampoo 250ml			6													
070744	Hair & Body Shampoo 1 litre			1													
070753	Multi Care Conditioner 250ml			6													
070762	Mutil Care Conditioner 1 litre			1													

Many salons have computerised systems, which deduct the specific stock used during each transaction. The system is then able to identify products that need to be re-ordered. This will only work if accurate records are made of the products used within each service. This method readily shows any discrepancies in the stock and highlights, for example, any shortfalls in the stock.

STOCKINFO				Date: 25/05/03
Description	Product ref	Reorder level	Instock	Quantity required
Control Shampoo 250ml	8385	10	8	10
Control Conditioner 150 ml	8275	10	4	12
Control Shine Serum 50 ml	8573	10	5	8
Control Gel 30 ml	9835	10	6	8
Active Shampoo 250 ml	8935	10	9	12
Active Conditioner 150 ml	9275	10	5	10
Active Shine Serum 50 ml	4625	10	4	7
Active Gel 30 ml	3857	10	7	6
Style Shampoo 250 ml	2746	10	8	12
Style Conditioner 150 ml	6236	10	2	15
Style Shine Serum 50 ml	5254	10	5	6
Style Gel 30 ml	3646	10	3	4
Ordered by: Ros				

A computerised stock sheet

In the salon there should be one person responsible for stock control. Their responsibilities include:

- carrying out regular stock checks
- ordering stock
- checking the stock on arrival at the salon
- dealing with any discrepancies
- storing the stock, including stock rotation
- monitoring stock usage
- keeping the necessary records relating to the above.

Ideally, stocktaking is carried out at a set time each week and the subsequent order placed with the supplier. In a busy salon this is not always possible and stock control may become haphazard, which may lead to problems, as low levels of stock may not be noticed until it is too late. You should be aware of your salon's ordering system, as this will allow salon staff plenty of time to inform the person responsible for ordering stock if there are any shortages that may have been overlooked, or if they become aware that a large amount of a specific product be required the following week.

Check it out

- Does your salon have an appropriate system for stock control?
- Who is responsible for ordering stock in your salon?

Resource problem	Possible causes	Outcome	Solution
No base colours	• Poor stock control • Unexpected usage over a short period of time • Poor service from the supplier	Client dissatisfaction	• Implement a good stock control system • Inform staff of the procedures if and when they notice low levels of stock • Try to come to an agreement with the supplier or shop around for a more reliable one

Ordering stock

There are several different methods that may be used when ordering stock. Whichever method your salon employs, records must be kept to show this. This is to make sure the order is correct on its arrival.

Stock may be ordered by:

- sending your order by post
- telephone
- fax
- e-mail
- in person.

The method your salon uses should be reliable, ensuring the required stock arrives on time. Your employer may need to shop around to find the most competitive prices and a supplier who can guarantee efficient service.

Checking the stock on arrival

When the stock arrives, it should be accompanied by a delivery note that states the contents of the package. This should be checked against the original order to make sure the delivery matches and the correct goods have been received. The delivery should then be checked to make sure the order is complete and undamaged.

Dealing with any discrepancies

Any shortfalls, discrepancies or breakages, should be reported to the salon owner (if applicable) and the supplier immediately. Damaged, substandard or unrequested goods should be returned to the supplier with a returns note, stating the problem.

Storing the stock, including stock rotation

All stock should be stored in the correct place in the stock room. Large or heavy items should be stored at ground level; this is to safeguard against it falling and injuring someone. Frequently used stock should be stored at eye level to ensure it is easily accessible. All products covered by COSHH should be stored according to the regulations. This is to maintain health and safety within the salon and to prolong the shelf life of the products. For example, aerosols should be stored in a cool place away from direct sunlight and other sources of heat.

Stock rotation is an integral part of the stock control system. All new stock should be placed at the back of the shelf and the old stock brought forward. This will ensure that the stock is used in the order in which it was purchased and should guarantee it is in optimum condition. Some salons find it advantageous to date all stock as it arrives, allowing them immediate information regarding the age of the product.

> **Check it out**
>
> How do the Manual Handling Operations Regulations relate to your work role and that of others when receiving and storing stock?

Monitoring stock usage

You are responsible for estimating the amount of stock you require for each service. Although you must make sure you are using sufficient products to carry out the service effectively, you should also try to eliminate any waste. Any leftover products that have to be disposed of equate to money down the drain for your employer. You should be able to estimate the quantities of each product you will use and prepare them accordingly to minimise wastage.

Keys to good practice

If you find it difficult to estimate the quantity of product to mix, it is more cost effective to mix more as and when it is needed.

If you are responsible for other members of staff, for example, juniors, you are also accountable for their product usage. It may be that you are required to train your staff to use all resources effectively to minimise waste. This may include turning off the taps whilst shampooing to save money on heating the water or using the telephone for business calls only, as using the telephone for personal calls will run up unnecessary phone bills and also prevent clients getting through to make appointments. If it is not within your job specification to deal with resource problems such as this then you should notify the person responsible as soon as possible. Your salon should actively encourage you to put forward any recommendations for improving the use of resources.

When making recommendations, you must be able to justify them and state the reasons why they will benefit the salon. In the instance above, you may suggest a pay phone is installed for staff to use, reducing the telephone bill and not tying up the line for incoming calls. If the salon is to carry out training in the effective use of resources, it is more cost effective to carry out this type of training with several staff members at a time. This will also ensure that the information they receive is identical, which will ensure consistency within the staff.

In the salon

Shabir was a colour technician in a busy salon. To save time he always asked the junior stylists to mix the tint for him, as they had been trained to mix colour products and knew which ratios of colour to oxidant to use. Some of Shabir's clients had up to four different colours on their hair. He always noticed that when Michael mixed the colour there seemed to be a lot left in the tint bowl at the end of the service. After several weeks, Shabir asked Michael how much tint he was mixing. Michael replied, 'Oh, a whole tube. It's easier to work out how much oxidant to use.'

- How do you think this affected the salon's finances?
- What should Shabir do now he has identified a problem?

Keeping the necessary records

All records or documentary evidence relating to the salon's stock control systems must be accurate and up to date. There are two main reasons for this.

1   To check the stock levels are accurate at any given time.
2   These records will also be used by the salon's accountant when drawing up the end-of-year accounts.

Consumable and semi-consumable items should be checked and ordered following the same procedure. It would not be safe, practical, or professional, for the salon to run out of essential items such as cotton wool or protective gloves.

Keys to good practice

If items such as cotton wool and protective gloves do not appear on your stock sheet, suggest to the member of staff responsible for stock to add them on at the bottom to ensure they are not overlooked.

Check it out

To whom would you go when suggesting recommendations for improving the use of salon resources?

Tools and equipment

Salon tools and equipment are monitored in the same way as salon and retail products; the main difference is that stocktaking of tools and equipment is carried out more infrequently, as tools and equipment should last longer provided they are properly maintained and only used for business purposes. To ensure the optimum life expectancy of electrical equipment, you should make sure you are complying with the Electricity at Work Regulations (refer to Unit G1 if you are unsure).

It is important to monitor the levels of tools and equipment in the salon for several reasons, which are:

* to ensure the correct number of working items that are needed to ensure the smooth running of the salon (some may be out of use, either broken or awaiting repair)
* to calculate if the levels need to be increased to meet the demands of the salon (if there are more stylists employed, more equipment will be needed)
* to make sure the end-of-year audit is correct with regard to items that may be offset against tax due from the business.

All salon equipment should be regularly checked and maintained

If you are aware of any shortages of tools and equipment, you should report them immediately to the designated person within your salon. This will ensure the smooth running of the salon, avoiding unnecessary problems such as clients being kept waiting whilst another stylist finishes their client.

Resource problem	Possible causes	Outcome	Solution
Five hairdryers broken within the last few weeks	• Misuse • Accidental damage • Unauthorised use for out of salon work	• Clients kept waiting until resources become available • Client dissatisfaction	Ensure resources are repaired or replaced in sufficient time to ensure smooth running of the salon

Human resources

The people that work in the salon should be a valuable asset to any business. However, for the salon to remain profitable, this should mean employing the right people for the right job; for example, your colour technician should have received proper training in this area and have the expertise to carry out the role. If they do not, this may lead to client dissatisfaction, resulting in loss of clientele, negative publicity, and/or litigation (see the Sale and Supply of Goods Act 1994, page 99). A stylist carrying out the duties of a junior (on a stylist's pay) would not be cost effective, as the stylist would not be bringing sufficient revenue into the salon to cover their wages.

Remember

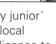

If you employ a 'Saturday junior' you need to check your local by-laws. Do you need a licence to employ people under 16?

Resource problem	Outcome	Solution
Stylist phones in sick	A whole column of clients have no stylist	• Try to share out the work amongst the other staff (with similar levels of competency) • Telephone clients, explain the situation, then reschedule where possible • Cancelling appointments should be a last resort

All staff should have good working conditions as laid down in law, examples of which are the Working Time Directive and The Health and Safety at Work Act.

Time

Time is another valuable resource in the salon environment. It is essential that all staff make good use of their time at work, as time is money! All the services carried out in the salon are priced to include the cost of materials (products, electricity, water, etc.) and the time it takes to complete the service. It is essential that you are able to carry out all salon services in a commercially viable time and, by doing so, you are fulfilling part of your obligations under the Sale and Supply of Goods Act 1994.

Some services allow time for other services to be carried out whilst the stylist is not needed, for example, the stylist should be able to carry out an additional client while another client's hair colour is developing. All appointments should be booked in this way to allow optimum use of time. This will benefit both the business and the stylist, as it will bring more money into the salon and increase the amount of commission the stylist earns each week.

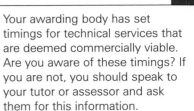

Check it out

Your awarding body has set timings for technical services that are deemed commercially viable. Are you aware of these timings? If you are not, you should speak to your tutor or assessor and ask them for this information.

A page from an appointments book

Date:	Thursday August 16th				
	Tracey	Aleisha	Katie		
AM 9.00	Sprott	Michaela			9.00
9.15	cut &	relaxer			9.15
9.30	colour	semi-colour	Suzanne		9.30
9.45	Laura		full head		9.45
10.00	c/blow (long)		foils		10.00
10.15					10.15
10.30	Reynolds	Joanne	Alison		10.30
10.45	c/blow	foils & c/b	semi-colour		10.45
11.00			(foils along parting)		11.00
11.15	Elsie		Suzanne		11.15
11.30	sh/blow	Tim	c/blow		11.30
11.45	Tim	(child cut)	Alison		11.45
12.00	gents cut	Lucy	c/blow		12.00
12.15	LUNCH	(child cut)	Mrs Robertson		12.15
12.30		LUNCH	c/blow (long)		12.30
12.45	Debbie				12.45
PM 1.00	cut & foils	Tina	LUNCH		1.00 PM
1.15		spiral			1.15
1.30		perm	Mrs Williams		1.30
1.45	Sue		s/s		1.45
2.00	cut &		Jane		2.00
2.15	colour		c/blow		2.15
2.30			James		2.30
2.45	Elaine c/blow		(child cut)		2.45
3.00		Syra	Finish		3.00
3.15		sh/blow			3.15
3.30	Jim				3.30
3.45	cut & colour				3.45
4.00	(polish)	Mrs Simms			4.00
4.15		cut & set			4.15
4.30	Mary				4.30
4.45	c/blow				4.45
5.00					5.00

In the salon

Sylvie worked as a stylist in a busy salon. Each Friday she carried out a full column of cut and blow-dries. The salon allocated 45 minutes per cut and blow-dry client. Despite the amount of work she carried out, she still needed to earn more commission each week (as her expenses were more than her income). On looking through the appointment book, she noticed that the way her appointments had been booked, she sometimes had an hour to complete each client. She then realised that if her clients were rescheduled, she could actually do another three clients each Friday and still have a lunch break! Sylvie explained this to the salon receptionist and asked her to reschedule all her clients (as far as she was able) and to then make sure she booked all her cut and blow-dry clients at 45 minute intervals so she could maximise her opportunities to meet her targets and increase her commission.

In the future, it may be necessary to allow the stylist more time per client when booking appointments and/or the stylist may need retraining in certain areas to enable them to get up to speed.

- Was this Sylvie's responsibility?
- Whose responsibility is it to ensure that all working time is utilized to the full?

Resource problem	Possible causes	Outcome	Solution
Stylist is continually running behind schedule	• Stylist is not up to speed • Junior member of staff is not fulfilling their own job role effectively causing unnecessary problems for the salon • Instructions from the stylist are unclear or poorly timed	• All other clients kept waiting, leading to client dissatisfaction • May cause unnecessary friction between the stylist and the junior • Stylist may not meet productivity targets	• Enlist the help of other members of staff to either take over one of the clients or assist the stylist in order to help to catch up • Junior needs retraining

Meeting productivity and development targets

Hairdressing is a fast-moving industry. In order to keep abreast or ahead of any competitors, it is essential that you continually update your existing skills and learn new ones. To maintain your client base and generate income for the salon, it is important that you do not allow yourself to stagnate professionally. Change can sometimes be viewed as threatening; however, if it enables you to remain in employment it must be looked upon in a positive manner. To enable you to fulfil the requirements of this outcome, you should have regular meetings with your employer/salon owner to discuss, negotiate, and review your productivity and development targets.

Your employer should have quite clear objectives regarding the salon's business and ways of keeping up with or ahead of the competition. This is a necessary skill for any employer who wishes to maximise the potential of their business. You may also be able to identify gaps in the market or areas you feel could be developed within the salon. You may get ideas from reading trade journals such as *International Hairdressers Journal*, as these contain information relating to all areas of the industry. You should also be expected to analyse your own performance in the salon and identify any areas of weakness you may have that you can then work to improve. This will have a positive impact on the salon and your productivity levels should improve accordingly.

Productivity

Within a business context, the salon's income comes from your ability to produce work of a good standard (in other words, you continue to bring money into the salon). Your employer needs to make sure you are able to maintain the required level of productivity to ensure both his/her and your income. If your wages cost your employer more than you bring into the salon, the business may not remain viable. Many employers offer incentive schemes or productivity bonuses to ensure their staff remain motivated and enthusiastic. You may already work in a salon that offers commission or other bonus schemes if you meet or exceed your targets.

Productivity targets cover retail sales and technical services. Retail sales are an excellent source of income for a salon, as any profit made does not need to be offset against the service. All members of staff may have productivity targets for retailing. To succeed in selling retail products, you must have excellent product knowledge to ensure you are selling the correct product for the client's requirements.

Knowing your product range well will help you to achieve your productivity targets

Any productivity targets should be negotiated and agreed by both you and your manager then recorded for future reference. The information may be recorded manually or the data may be entered onto the computer (if this is the case, the information held is covered by the Data Protection Act). Any targets set should be short term, for example, four to six weeks, and reviewed on a regular basis. The monetary targets that are set will vary depending on your capabilities and the prices charged in your salon. Any targets that are set should be achievable; there is nothing more de-motivating and de-moralising than failing to achieve your targets week after week. If you meet your targets easily, your employer may increase them to make sure you are working to full capacity and maintaining the challenge. However, if you fail to meet your targets, it may identify areas of weakness, for example, poor knowledge of retail products and their uses. This will necessitate additional training to improve your knowledge.

There are many different types of opportunities within the salon that you may use to help you achieve your productivity targets.

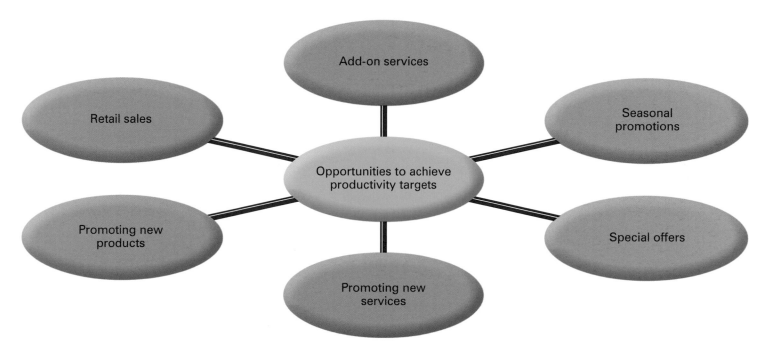

However, to carry these out effectively, you must have excellent product knowledge and a good awareness of other services that are offered within the salon.

Developing targets for personal learning and improvement

In addition to your productivity targets, you should also be encouraged to develop new skills and improve your existing skills. In this way you will continue to be an asset to the salon.

Before meeting with your employer to negotiate targets for your personal learning and development, it is a good idea to analyse your own performance in the salon and identify any areas of weakness you may have. You may also find it useful to gain feedback on your work from other members of staff. This information will enable you to put forward your own suggestions at the meeting. This should be looked upon in a positive way, as it shows you are able to be objective about your capabilities and limitations.

You may have your own thoughts regarding ways in which the salon can improve its financial effectiveness, for example, by introducing new services or products. However, when presenting this information, you must make sure you have given adequate thought to your suggestions, any potential problems that may arise, and how the problems may be overcome. This should enable you to present the benefits of your recommendations in a positive way. The way should then be open for you and your employer to discuss your suggestions objectively.

Any developmental targets set by your employer should have been negotiated and agreed by you both, with the necessary documentation completed. If you do not feel the targets your employer suggests are achievable, you should discuss this with them, using sound reasoning. Your targets may then be adjusted accordingly. Your employer may want to introduce new services into the salon, in which case you may be required to undergo training. It can be very difficult for a salon to progress if the staff are resistant to change and the atmosphere in the salon becomes tense. This does not reflect well on the salon, as the clients will pick up on the negativity. This will have an adverse effect on the business, therefore you should take up the challenge to progress and help the business and yourself whilst doing so. You may also be required to develop and improve your existing skills, as this may improve your productivity within the salon.

The timescale for developing new skills should be longer (than for productivity) and reflect the amount of time needed to perfect the skill. However, it is important that you meet your targets within the allocated timescale, as your employer may have included the potential income in the salon's business plan.

If you become aware that you are not going to achieve your developmental targets, you must inform your employer as soon as possible and give reasons as to why this is so. It is better if your employer hears this from you, rather than from another member of staff, as this can cause friction between the staff and create an unpleasant working environment. Your employer may ask you to explain the reasons why you are unable to meet your targets and if your reasons are justifiable, your employer may reconsider the original timescale, providing it is within the salon's budget.

Communication

Communication is an all-important part of salon life. Effective communication ensures total understanding between all the people involved. It will promote a professional image to both clients and junior members of staff (remember, they learn

---

In the salon

Salman was a junior in a busy salon assisting several of the stylists with their work. Mercedes, one of the stylists, had a habit of barking orders at Salman, whereas Natalie, another stylist, always asked him nicely if she required assistance. Salman liked to work with Natalie, as she did not make him feel insignificant or stupid in front of the clients. Salman began to hate working with Mercedes and avoided her whenever he could. Consequently, Mercedes found it difficult at work, as she did not receive the support she ought to. This had an impact on her ability to achieve her productivity targets.

- What should Mercedes do to improve the situation?
- If you were a junior member of staff, which of the stylists would you want to work with?

by example). It also sends a good message out to the clients, which will gain their trust and goodwill. Refer to Unit G9 (pages 31–37) and Unit G6 (pages 74–77) for more information on and examples of methods of communication.

You may be required to order stock by telephone, in which case you must make sure your requirements are made quite clear. It is good practice to have your order repeated back to you. This way you can check there have been no misunderstandings. You will also need to communicate effectively with your employer during reviews or appraisals to negotiate productivity levels or development targets.

Keys to good practice

'Actions speak louder than words.' Your body language can tell someone far more about how you are feeling than you may actually say. You may think you can cover up feeling hurt or angry, but those who can read body language will know exactly what you are saying without words.

Written communication

Although the majority of your job role involves verbal and non-verbal communication, there are certain times when written communication needs to be used. This may be when compiling an order form for stock purchasing, completing stock records, or filling in target sheets with your employer.

It may be necessary to use written communication on the staff notice board when notifying staff of your intention to send an order for stock and asking if they have any suggestions. This is especially effective if the salon has part-time staff and you do not always see them. It allows these staff to feel valued members of the team. Client record cards must be completed accurately, as the information contained on a client record card communicates to other members of staff the exact nature of the service. A badly filled in record card may be misinterpreted by another member of staff and cause client dissatisfaction if the end result is not as expected. It will also cost the salon money to fix the client's hair in terms of time and products.

Receiving and dealing with negative feedback

It is not always easy to deal with criticism or negative feedback; however, provided the criticism is constructive, you should use this as a tool for improvement. When responding to suggestions made for your self-improvement, these should be seen in a positive way and any constructive criticism accepted readily and acted upon. It is not always easy to respond in a positive manner, especially when you have received negative feedback and your immediate instinct is to feel hurt. However, it is important that you try and remain positive and look upon this as a learning tool, that is, something that is there to help you. This will lead to a more pleasant working environment for all the staff, which will be reflected in the salon atmosphere.

When receiving negative feedback, you must also remember your non-verbal communication skills are sending a message back to the sender and although you may be saying all the right things, your non-verbal communication may be sending out a different message.

Knowledge check

1. Which consumer legislation applies to you when you are providing services to clients?

2. Explain the importance of a good stock control system.

3. Why is important to check all stock deliveries when they arrive?

4. Why is it important that all records relating to the salon's stock control systems are accurate and up to date?

5. Why is it essential to your employer that you utilise all your working time effectively?

6. Why should you continually update your skills and learn new ones?

7. Why is it important to have excellent knowledge of the salon's retail range of products?

8. What action should you take if you know you are unable meet your productivity targets and why?

9. Name four different types of opportunities in the salon that you may use to help you to achieve your productivity targets.

10. List the ways you contribute to the financial effectiveness of the business and consider how you can improve on these.

professional SKILLS

Develop and enhance your creative hairdressing skills

Unit H24

Introduction

To create exciting new styles you will need creative hairdressing skills

This unit is about developing your creative hairdressing skills in a way that enhances your own professional profile. You will need to carry out research and planning, while exploring a variety of different hairdressing techniques, in order to create a range of images that demonstrate the diversity of your skills. You will also need to be able to work as part of a team as you will be working in conjunction with others. Once you have created the images, you must carry out an evaluation of your results. Finally, you will be expected to look at ways that your images may be adapted or modified for commercial use.

What you will learn

- Plan and design a range of images
- Produce a range of creative images
- Evaluate your results against the design plan

You the stylist

To succeed in developing and enhancing your creative skills, you need to have belief in your own ability, as well as having confidence in exploring new techniques. Think about the opportunities that you may have for this in the salon. For example, many salons carry out activities on a regular basis, which enable the staff to develop and enhance their creative skills. This may be an annual hair show, which seeks to raise the profile of the salon and increase salon business. The salon may also choose to use this type of activity to launch the season's new look or introduce the salon's new collection. This may be carried out in conjunction with photographic work, e.g. the collection is then photographed and displayed in trade magazines such as the *International Hairdressing Journal*.

Other salons use competition work to encourage the staff to show off their creative talents. There are competitions to suit all levels of hairdressers, from trainees through to very experienced stylists.

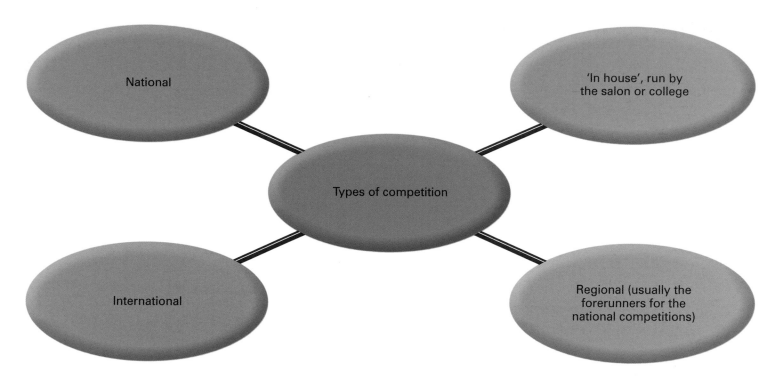

Plan and design a range of images

You must first decide which of the activities you intend to carry out. This will be dependent on your level of ability, the support networks within the salon, the resources available to you and the financial assistance that you will be given. The activities you may choose from are:

- Photographic work
- Hair shows
- Competition work

Whichever activity you choose to undertake, planning has to be the key factor. Detailed and accurate planning will ensure everything runs smoothly. Without meticulous planning and attention to detail, the activity may prove to be disappointing. You should leave nothing to chance and work on the principle of good time management, which means that nothing is left until the last minute.

Keys to good practice

Think carefully about your level of ability and that of others involved. Planning to the best of everyone's ability will help to guarantee success.

Design principles and presentation

When creating your image, you should be aware of the basic principles of design as this will enable you to produce images that are aesthetically pleasing, well balanced and express your visual ideas. You need to think about a number of basic elements including colour, shape and texture.

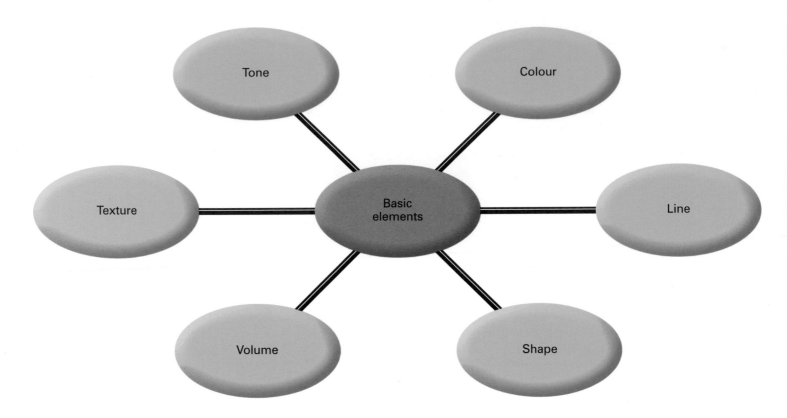

All of the above elements relate not only to the hair you are working with, but also the fabrics, make-up, etc.

You should now consider the design principles and how you can achieve the best effects possible. The following principle should be considered: emphasis, harmony, unity, opposition and balance.

Emphasis may also be described as the centre of interest. It relates to dominance and influence. Do you want to have one major focal point of interest, or do you hope that all parts of the work will be equally exciting? One major focal point could be used for competition or photographic work; however, for a hair show, all the work should be equally exciting to hold the audience's attention.

Harmony describes complex but pleasing visual combinations. This should apply to any work you perform.

Unity could best describe a whole image with no distractions. Again, in relation to competition or photographic work, unity is ideal, as it does not detract from the main point. However, unity without any variation can be uninteresting especially within the realms of a hair show.

Opposition is based on contrasting visual concepts, e.g. rough and smooth, dark and light, curved and straight etc. – any may be applied to any of the activities in this unit.

Balance refers to the consideration of visual weight and importance on both sides of the image. Asymmetrical balance is usually more interesting and dynamic. All images should have good balance (but not necessarily symmetry) to be aesthetically pleasing.

Once you have been given information regarding the theme for the activity, you may need to carry out some research, especially if your creative styling is based on historical or cultural influences, to ensure accuracy in your design. This information may be sought from the library, trade journals, magazines, television or the internet.

When you have several ideas, discuss them with friends and colleagues in order to gauge the opinion of others. Remember to use open questions if you require a full answer to any questions you may ask. You may be required to use a varied vocabulary when discussing ideas with friends, especially those who do not have a hairdressing background, as you must ensure your ideas are fully understood by all involved. Your friends may be able to give you additional ideas or information that you may not have thought of, and this may include your interpretation of the theme.

When receiving information you should actively listen to the speaker and ask relevant questions to show that you value his or her thoughts and ideas. When you feel you are in possession of all the necessary facts, you should summarize the key points to clarify your understanding, with a view to developing these areas more fully, but always making sure you remain focused on the purpose of the conversation. This will enable you to develop your ideas further. (See Unit G9 for further information on communication.)

Keys to good practice

Keep notes and sketches of all your ideas, as it is easy to go off at a tangent and forget what you should actually be doing! This evidence may be used as a record of your planning. If you are good at graphic design, a computer-generated image is an excellent medium for you to work from. You may modify and adapt your original ideas, while keeping an overview of your intended image.

You will be required to create a design plan that should contain sufficient information and be explicit in its content. Your design plan must include:

- Your intended activity
- Your objectives (what you want to achieve)
- Images that are suitable for the activity
- The roles and responsibilities of the people involved
- The budget you have to work with
- A comprehensive list of the resources you will require
- Ways in which health and safety risks may be reduced
- Any foreseeable problems and a contingency plan where possible
- The venue requirements, if applicable.

The objective of the activity

The objective of any activity is what you hope to achieve as a result of undertaking the task. There may be many reasons for carrying out this type of activity, including:

- Positive advertising for the salon, thus increasing revenue
- To increase your personal profile
- To improve your employability
- Self-fulfilment.

Whatever your desired outcome, it must be quantifiable in some way. Therefore when planning your objectives, consideration must be given to the way it can be measured after the event.

Suitable images for the activity

There are two types of images that must be covered:

- Thematic, e.g. based on a theme
- Avant-garde.

You should have explicit guidelines that indicate which of the above you are expected to cover. An avant-garde image is a look that is a forerunner of fashion or a style beyond what would be commercially expected.

An avant-garde style

However, you may create an avant-garde style that is based on a theme, thus covering both of the images together. The theme you may be working towards can be virtually anything, e.g. bridal work, historical figures, moods and/or emotions. Some are more prescriptive than others, so you may need to use your own interpretation of the theme.

There are many options for you to explore, depending on the objectives you are planning to achieve.

A look based on the theme of 'Hippy Chic' from John Carne's collection

---

Keys to good practice

If you opt for competition work, it is essential that you thoroughly understand the rules of the competition. Many competitors are taken aback on reaching the competition floor, only to find their design doesn't abide by the rules. This is very disappointing when you have spent many hours practising and preparing for the event.

The roles and responsibilities of others

You will need to enlist the help of others to enable you to carry out your work effectively. Each member of the team should know their own roles and responsibilities and those of the others involved. Whilst working with others it is essential that you communicate effectively to ensure the complete understanding of all of the people involved. Effective communication should ensure mistakes are avoided and nothing is overlooked as being somebody else's responsibility.

When giving instructions to other members of the team, you should ensure their understanding by asking them to confirm what you have said to them. Remember this if you are asked to carry out a task; you should confirm your own understanding of the task in hand. You will need to have regular meetings with the people involved in the activity to discuss the progress each person is making and to ensure there are no problems. The meetings may be informal or formal (with an agenda of items to be discussed). Remember, if a member of your team is having difficulties regarding their specific duties, you should offer support and advise them how to resolve their difficulties. This may be indicated to you by their manner and tone of voice, e.g. they may appear quite forlorn and speak quietly. You, in turn, should think carefully before you speak to ensure you don't turn the situation into a huge problem! For each problem encountered, there should be a number of solutions. Your role may be to find the most appropriate and workable solution to the problem.

Check it out

Write a list of all the people involved with your activity and note their roles and responsibilities. Distribute a copy to everyone involved and include a copy on the wall in the staff room. This will help to ensure that nothing is forgotten.

The importance of working to a budget

Once the budget has been set it is important that you keep your outgoings within the budget. Any activity must be cost effective for the salon, i.e. it will not cost more to carry out than the expected long-term revenue the salon can expect to receive. The amount of money you have to spend will vary depending on the budgetary constraints of the salon. Within your plan, you should be able to get a good idea of the amount of money you will need to cover your expenditure. You must be realistic and able to keep your expenditure to a minimum (unless of course the salon has an unlimited budget for this kind of activity). Failure to produce a plan containing sufficient details of possible expenditure will undoubtedly lead to you exceeding your budget. All those little things that spring to mind at the last minute will undoubtedly end up sending your expenditure soaring.

Resource requirements

In your design plan you must state all the resources that you will require. The budget that you are set will impact on the resources that you are able to purchase. Therefore you may need to look at other ways to obtain the necessary resources that you require. Make-up artists should provide their own make-up, although you may wish to obtain specific items the make-up artist does not carry. This must be checked and confirmed prior to the activity, to ensure that you have all the necessary items on the day.

You must remember to include any hair products that you may need to use, both prior to and during the activity. Your salon will most probably provide these; however, it may be useful to contact a product manufacturer or other large business to enquire about sponsorship. Additional media, such as clothing and accessories, may be acquired from other people or hired for the purpose. Your local theatre company may lend you costumes and accessories, although there may be a nominal charge. Check with designer retailers to see if they would be willing to supply you with clothing and accessories for the activity (with a little publicity for them of course!).

If you require props for the activity, these must be included in your plan, but consideration must be given to the health and safety implications of any such items being used.

Health and safety requirements

When carrying out any type of creative activity, health and safety must not be forgotten just because you are not in the normal salon environment. You must still abide by:

- The Health and Safety at Work Act
- COSHH (when dealing with products covered by this legislation)
- Electricity at Work Act (when using electrical equipment)
- Manual Handling Operations Regulations (when moving equipment and props around, etc.)
- Personal Protective Equipment Regulations.

You must remain alert to the presence of hazards while working in other venues, in order to avoid accidents. This may necessitate you carrying out a risk assessment. It is likely that the venue will have a designated person responsible for health and safety. However, this does not mean that you can afford to be unaware of any potential hazards, just because the responsibility lies with someone else. You should clarify with the venue manager the areas they are responsible for and those for which you are responsible.

> ### Keys to good practice
>
> Even if the venue assumes responsibility for health and safety, the salon should carry out its own risk assessment and implement steps to reduce any identified. This shows a professional attitude towards health and safety. You must not overlook your duty of care towards others for whom you have responsibility.

Some possible hazards may include unstable equipment, trailing wires, or stairs the models and stylists need to use to gain access to the stage area, all of which should be considered prior to the event and control measures put into place to reduce the risk (as far as is practicable).

When using any additional media such as props, you should identify any potential hazards that may occur, e.g. if using props, are they likely to fall and injure someone, or are they highly flammable? Wherever possible you should try to use alternative media that are less hazardous or ensure that any props used are sturdy in design. This will necessitate you carrying out a risk assessment of each additional piece of media used.

As stated above, most venues have their own health and safety procedures, which cover fire and first aid. You must ensure that you are familiar with these procedures when working in any venue, so that you are able to act safely in the event of an accident or emergency.

Insurance must also be given consideration. In the event of an accident occurring you must be confident that your insurance will cover any eventuality. You must have public liability insurance and possibly an entertainment licence, but check with the venue and your insurance company to ensure no other insurance is required.

Problems and ways to resolve them

Problems may occur in even the best-planned events; however, being aware of some of the more common faults and ways in which they may be resolved should help to prevent problems from occurring during your activity.

> ### Check it out
>
> Are you aware of your responsibilities under the legislation listed here? If not, see Unit G1.

> ### Check it out
>
> List the potential hazards you would need to consider when carrying out:
>
> - A competition
> - A photoshoot
> - A hair show

> ### Check it out
>
> Are there any local bylaws, or other legislation, that may limit your use of tools and equipment that you should be aware of when working in venues other than your salon?

Photographic shoots

Common problems	How to resolve them
Model doesn't turn up for the shoot	Have a stand-in model/s.
Model is pretty but not suitable for the look	See photographs of all models beforehand. Have a stand-in model/s.
Weather	Arrange suitable alternatives if the photoshoot is to be held outdoors.
Equipment breakdown	Always carry spares.
Running out of film	Always carry spares.
Time overruns	Stick to the agreed plan.
Clothes do not fit the model	Ask the models to bring their own clothes, but make sure they are in keeping with the finished look. Have fittings beforehand to make sure the clothes fit properly. Ask the models to send you details of their measurements.

Clothes are an important part of the finished look

Hair shows

Common problems	How to resolve them
Model doesn't turn up for the show	Make sure you have sufficient 'back-up' models.
Model is late	Within your preparation time, you must allow much more time than you anticipate you will need. You should still have time to prepare your model.
Models not ready on time, e.g. hair still wet, run out of hair grips, etc.	Ensure plenty of time for preparing models.
Equipment breakdowns	Always carry spare hairdryers, etc.
Show overruns	The show should be rehearsed until it is 'time perfect'.
Pauses in the show	Rehearse everything until the show is 'time perfect'.
Electrical problems, e.g. lighting too low, microphone distortion	Ensure everything is thoroughly checked before the show.
Poor seating, audience not able to see the show	Make sure you check there are no blind areas – prior to the show.
One of the make-up artists doesn't turn up	Re-allocate the work amongst the other make-up artists.
Poor choreography	Make sure there have been sufficient rehearsals.
Hair and make-up don't look as good under the stage lighting as they did when done in the make-up room	Check hair and make-up under show lighting.
Model/s are allergic to false eyelash glue	Carry out sensitivity testing (glue) 24 – 48 hours before the show.

Thoroughly check everything, including ornaments and hairpieces, before the show

Competitions

Common problems	How to resolve them
Model doesn't turn up for the competition	Ensure there are suitable stand-in models.
Not adhered to the competition rules	Ensure you have read the rules thoroughly. If there are any areas you do not understand, ask for clarification from either an experienced colleague or contact the competition organizers.
Left some equipment or products behind	Ask other competitors for help.
Run out of time	Practice until you are 'time perfect'.
Equipment breakdowns	Always carry spares / ask other competitors for help.

Competition work

Venue requirements

During your planning, you should check the venue to ensure there will be no foreseeable complications on the day. This may include the use of basins for shampooing models, sufficient plug sockets in the correct place and whether the venue's electricity supply can accommodate the possible surge of electricity. If you require refreshments for your audience, does the venue have a licence or the facility to provide food? You must also consider public liability insurance when presenting a show. Are you responsible for this, or is it the responsibility of the venue?

You may need to set up the venue prior to the activity; check whether you can have access to the venue beforehand. If planning a hair show, do you require staging for the models to use as a catwalk? If so, can the venue provide suitable staging for your requirements? Will the staging be large enough to fulfil your requirements?

Remember

You must always remember the 5 Ps:

Poor **p**lanning **p**roduces **p**oor **p**erformance

Keys to good practice

You should test and evaluate your ideas now and ask yourself three basic questions:

- Does it work?
- Does it meet the design brief?
- Does it need to be modified in any way?

When you are happy with the outcome, all your planning has been carried out, and you are sure you have covered every eventuality, you should take your design plan to your line manager for approval. Any modifications or alterations must be carried out and shown as amended on your design plan. Only when you have your line manager's consent should you go ahead and produce your range of creative images.

Produce a range of creative images

When carrying out this type of work it is essential that you communicate effectively with all the people you are working with. This will ensure that there are no mis-understandings which could lead to problems later on. It is essential that all the people involved maintain confidentiality regarding the activity. This will help to prevent plagiarism by competing salons. If staging a show, it will heighten the impact of the show by adding an air of mystery.

Keys to good practice

Lighting and music play an important part in any show. The lighting must be bright enough to clearly show your creative work, but must not dazzle the audience. The music used to accompany your work should be in keeping with the image you are trying to portray.

Additional media

Your use of appropriate additional media can add dynamic emphasis to the work you create. The clothing you use must complement the image you wish to portray.

The make-up used should be in keeping with the overall image and should be used to enhance and complement the total look. When choosing a make-up artist, ask to see their portfolio of work, as this will give you a good indication of the type of work they have previously carried out and the quality of work you can expect.

Use a qualified make-up artist to ensure the best results

Bold jewellery can add emphasis to your creative style

If different models require identical make-up, use several make-up artists who can work on a conveyor belt system; e.g. the first make-up artist applies the base to all the models, the second applies the eye make-up, and another applies the lip colour. As the same make-up artist is responsible for a specific part of the whole look, it should be much easier to recreate an identical image. Accessories may be anything that you would use to complement the image you are creating e.g. added hair, jewellery, etc.

Whatever image you want to create, you must consider the most suitable techniques to use to achieve the desired effect. You will probably use several of the techniques listed below.

How you choose to apply the techniques will be dependent on the results you wish to achieve.

Check it out

Make a list of all the products, tools and equipment available for the techniques you plan to use and the effects they can create. (This may help you choose the most appropriate ones to achieve your intended look.)

Keys to good practice

Remember to follow the manufacturer's instructions when using any products, tools and equipment.

The use of added hair

Added hair has become very popular again over the last few years. However, for the type of work you will be carrying out, it has never really lost its appeal!

The main reasons for using added hair are:

- To add volume to fine hair
- To add length to the hair
- To add colour to the hair
- To blend or contrast giving maximum impact.

You should give considerable thought to the positioning of the added hair and how it may be incorporated most effectively into your styling. You also need to ensure that it blends effectively with the natural hair. The base or fixing of the added hair must be well hidden.

Most of the hairpieces available are made from synthetic fibres. The quality of these pieces is improving all the time. They come in a variety of colours and may be used to match your client's natural hair colour or add contrast. However, although acrylic pieces come in a variety of colours and styles, there are limitations to their use.

Great care must be taken when using heated styling equipment on synthetic hairpieces, as they will melt. Some heated styling equipment has a very cool setting, which may be used on synthetic hair; however, you should test it first on an inconspicuous part of the piece. Specialist products are required for styling and finishing, therefore you must adhere to the manufacturer's instructions. Hairpieces made from real hair are more versatile as they may be styled and dressed in the conventional way using normal salon products. However, they are more expensive to buy.

As with any hairstyling, the limitations of the piece will control your choice of styling; e.g. if your chosen image necessitates a long pony-tail, the hairpiece you use must be long enough to create such an image. When using hairpieces, it is essential that they are properly secured. Your catwalk models must feel confident that the hairpieces are secure when showing your creative styling. If the models don't feel confident, this will be reflected in the way they walk and carry themselves.

Hairpieces are available in a variety of different forms, from a traditional postiche e.g. a chignon, to fun-coloured slices attached to small combs or pins. Hair extensions are a good idea as they add length and volume to the model's hair, thereby allowing a wider variety of images to be created. Natural or synthetic hair extensions are available depending on the look you wish to create.

When styling hair there are numerous non-conventional items that may be used to give a variety of different effects, e.g. rolled or folded foil; etc. African Caribbean hair may also be styled using alternative or unconventional items such as drinking straws and rolled up brown paper.

> **Check it out**
>
> Discuss with colleagues/your tutor any non-conventional items that may be used when styling hair to give a variety of effects.

You must ensure that the final image meets your agreed design plan and any innovative features are clearly shown within the presentation of your work. Any work you produce should be of the highest standard if you wish to accurately reflect your creativity. The most effective way to do this is to practise your techniques until you are sure you could recreate the image under any circumstances and in any situation. Failure to do this may jeopardize your success.

Evaluate your results against the design plan

Once you have carried out your activity, you should be actively seeking feedback from a number of people on the impact of your image/s. This is essential if you are to evaluate your design plan effectively and make it better next time. An evaluation should be carried out both during and after any of the activities. During the activity, an evaluation should be carried out to consider the effectiveness of your proposed image/s and seek ways to improve them. You should have this type of discussion with your colleagues and others who may be involved.

After the activity, an evaluation should be carried out for a number of reasons:

- To ascertain whether you have met the objectives stated in your design plan
- To gain constructive advice on your finished look/s
- To obtain advice on how to improve your creative skills
- To gather any information as to how you can improve in any of the above areas
- To assess the profitability of the event.

Feedback may be gathered from a number of different people including:

You should evaluate your own performance and try to be objective; in fact, you will probably be your own harshest critic, and therefore feedback should be sought from other sources.

You should try to gain feedback from as many different sources as possible. This will give you an insight into other people's perspectives. Most of the above are professional people who have great expertise in their own field of work and you should accept any criticism they give, so long as it is constructive. Any feedback given should be used as a learning tool that will enable you to develop and progress further in your chosen career. There are several areas on which you should actively seek feedback; most importantly, how your look was received. This should include information regarding:

- Your interpretation of the image
- The overall look you achieved
- The artistic quality of your work
- Your technical expertise.

Most of the feedback you receive will be verbal. However, when putting on a show, you may wish to ask the audience for feedback. This would usually be in the form of an evaluation questionnaire, whereby several well-thought-out questions are asked to the audience to gauge their responses, e.g. questions relating to the length and pace of the show, appropriateness of the music, suitability of the venue, communication prior to the show, etc. This will also give you documentary evidence to use when assimilating your feedback and looking for ways to improve.

It is also useful to be able to read an audience by their body language. If they are bored, they will usually shuffle around in their seats. This can give you a good indication of whether things require speeding up, etc. If they are maintaining an interest and appear quite relaxed, this would indicate that they are enjoying the show.

You should look to evaluate your activity as soon as possible after the event while it is still fresh in your mind. In addition to the feedback received from other professionals, you should also evaluate your own performance against your objectives to enable you to identify how and where your design could be improved.

In addition, if the image/s you created was avant-garde, you should evaluate the design image to see if it is possible for it to be adapted to make it more commercially viable.

Knowledge check

1.   What are the five basic principles of design?

2.   List all the information that should be detailed on your design plan.

3.   State the potential commercial benefits that can arise from creative hair design work.

4.   Why is it important to work within your budget when undertaking any of the activities listed in this unit?

5.   If you are working with a limited budget, state the ways you can obtain additional resources without overspending.

6.   State the potential consequences of failing to consider the 5 Ps when carrying out your activity.

7.   State the importance of using additional media within the image/s you create.

8.   State the 4 main reasons for using added hair.

9.   Once a photoshoot has been completed who should you get feedback from?

10. Why is it important to carry out an evaluation of your activity?

Contribute to the planning and implementation of promotional activities

Unit H32

Introduction

Promotional activities in the salon should serve to increase revenue, motivate staff and demonstrate your professionalism to clients. This unit is concerned with your contributions towards the salon's promotional activities. You will need to work with other people and be an active member of a team. You will work with others to plan, implement and evaluate hairdressing-related activities. You must be able to present information and interact with the public whilst competently demonstrating your hairdressing skills.

What you will learn	

- Contribute to the planning and preparation of promotional activities
- Implement promotional activities
- Participate in the evaluation of promotional activities

You the stylist

You will need to have a thorough knowledge of the range of services and products offered in your salon in order to fully sell their benefits. Recognising selling opportunities is important and in order to do this you will have to fine-tune your communication skills. Ensuring that you are always aware of your clients' needs and being able to advise them accordingly will also serve to assist you when carrying out a promotional event. You may need to support junior staff in their role, as you will have the benefit of experience when it comes to recognising client needs.

Contribute to the planning and preparation of promotional material

The promotional activities you must consider are:

- Demonstrations (both in the salon and at other premises)
- Displays (window displays/retail)
- Advertising campaigns (media, newspaper, website, trade publications, leaflets and/or fliers, etc.)

In order to make an informed choice regarding the promotional activity you wish to undertake, there are several questions you should consider:

- How much money do you have to spend?
- What type of activity do you wish to undertake?
- How do you think it should be done?
- Who will you be aiming the activity at?
- What do you hope to achieve?
- Will you need the help of others?

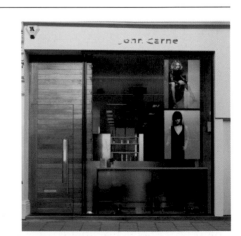

Your salon window is the ideal place to set up displays or advertising

- What resources will you need?
- When is the promotional activity to take place?
- Where will the promotional activity take place?
- How much time do you need to prepare for the event?
- What type of advertising are you thinking of using?
- How will you evaluate the activity?

Each of the above questions should be thoroughly thought out and your answers will enable you to produce an outline plan, highlighting your ideas. In addition to the above questions, it may be wise to check through the salon's past promotional events and their evaluations. This may prevent you from making mistakes or, better still, you may learn from other people's mistakes instead of your own!

The most important aspect of any promotional activity has to be the planning and preparation. These activities do not happen on their own; they require thorough planning followed by meticulous preparation.

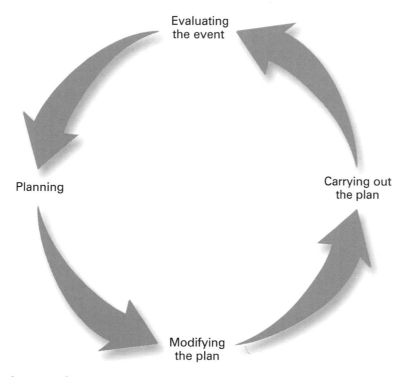

The cyclical nature of a promotion

Make your initial recommendations/proposal

You should make an appointment with the relevant person, e.g. the salon owner or manager, to discuss your ideas and recommendations for a promotional activity.

The meeting you have may be informal, where you can put forward several suggestions and discuss them on an unofficial basis. However, you will then need to prepare a more formal proposal which states the type of promotional activity you wish to carry out, your ideas as to how this may be done and the potential benefits for the salon. The most obvious benefit is to make money for the salon; therefore your ideas must be cost-effective; that is, they will make more money in the long term than the initial cost of the activity.

> **Remember**
>
> You must be prepared to justify your recommendations for promotional activities, as the salon will undoubtedly be paying for them and will expect a guaranteed return on their money!

The importance of working to a budget

You should be mindful that you will have a budget to adhere to and overspending may result in failure. Initially, when you are deciding on the budget for the promotion, and in order to safeguard your plan, you should allow for a pot of money to be put aside for emergency use. This will ensure that if problems are encountered you will have the money to provide a solution. Consider not only the money you will need to carry out the promotional activity but also the money you may need for your contingency plans. If several people are involved in the financial side of the promotion, regular reports on spending will be needed to ensure no overspending in any areas. Remember that your main objectives are to increase revenue and to raise the salon's profile. If the promotion fails through overspending then neither objective will be met.

Setting your objectives

There are many reasons for carrying out promotional activities, but the first questions you need to ask yourself are (a) what do you want to achieve?; and (b) what are your objectives for carrying out the activity?

Your main objectives should be to:

- increase the salon business
- enhance the salon's image.

There are many ways that these objectives can be met; for example, launching the new season's looks should increase business and enhance the salon's image. You may want to promote new product lines or services, or your activity may be a means to shifting stock that is lying dormant in the stock room.

Whatever your reasons, they should be thought through and then discussed and negotiated with your manager/salon owner. Any targets or objectives that are set should be mutually agreed.

When setting objectives for your promotional activity, you should ensure you follow the SMART principle; that is, you should make your objectives:

Specific – have you stated clearly what you intend to do?
Measurable – can you prove you have done it?
Achievable – do you have the potential to meet your target?
Realistic – are you planning something that is realistic?
Time bound – will you meet your target by a certain time or date?

You must also consider the target group at whom you are aiming your promotional activity, as this will undoubtedly have an impact on the type of activity you choose to undertake.

Selecting the target group

You may decide to aim your promotional activity at a specific age group that reflects the type of clientele you are looking to attract, e.g. 20 – 35 years. Alternatively, you may wish to open a section of the salon for men's hairdressing services if the salon doesn't already have one.

Once you have decided what you want to do, you need to think about how you are going to achieve it and which promotional activities will be best suited to your objectives and target group. You would not necessarily use the same activity aimed at a group of 16 – 20 year olds as perhaps the 50-plus age range as their preferences may be very different. Time and consideration must be given to these factors if you wish your promotional activity to succeed.

Demonstrations

There are various ways of demonstrating the work of the salon. You may want to offer the public the chance to see your work at a showcase event in the salon. Alternatively, you might be involved in a large event where you carry out various hairdressing techniques on a stage to promote the salon's range of skills.

When carrying out any demonstration, consideration should be given to people's attention span. Most people have an attention span of only 20 minutes and if you are demonstrating something for longer, you need to think about whether it will be exciting enough to maintain interest. Demonstrations are an excellent way of advertising the talent of your salon. Remember, any stylist showcasing his or her work in this way must have the confidence and hairdressing experience to carry it off. If you can wow the crowd with your hairdressing ability and charm them with your line of banter, then you are likely to be successful. On the other hand, if you lack the skills and confidence to perform in front of a crowd then it will not only be torture for you the stylist but it will also be professional suicide for the salon's reputation.

Displays

Displaying products at reception is a good way of attracting you clients' attention

Displaying products for retail sale at reception is a subtle way of introducing your product range. You can then substantiate this by discussing the benefits of the products whilst using them on your client. This type of promotion is commonly used; indeed, there are many ways of bringing products to your client's attention, be they subtle or attention grabbing in their approach.

The cheapest and most cost effective way of promoting products and services is to use the salon window. You don't necessarily need to employ a professional window dresser; use your imagination or find out if any members of staff have a flair for window dressing. You can change the display according to the seasons or when sales are down in order to target certain services. The only disadvantage is that it will reach only a limited audience, especially if your salon is not on a busy main road position. However, if used in conjunction with other promotional mediums, it can be extremely cost effective.

> **Check it out**
>
> Make a list of the different target groups you could aim a promotional activity at. Which type of promotional activity would be best suited to each of the target groups?

Your display may be at a larger promotional event, in which case consideration must be given to the audience it is designed for. You must decide the main objective of your display and ensure that you do not stray from this at any point. The design should be pleasing to the eye and not too fussy. The audience will be drawn to a focal point and this is where your main objective should be showcased. Unless you have an experienced designer on board, seek help from all the staff with themes and ideas. Bear in mind that different people have different concepts of what is and what is not attractive. To overcome this, seek advice and feedback from a wide range of people to enable you to produce a display that most people will appreciate.

Advertising campaigns

An example of salon advertising

Most salons use advertising in some form; however, for an advertising campaign to be successful you must have clearly defined objectives. Your objectives may be to:

- Increase the clientele
- Introduce new products or services
- Increase retail sales
- Promote a forthcoming event.

Whatever you decide, your objectives must be quantifiable and SMART.

There are many different forms of advertising and the one you choose will be largely dependent on your budget, as some forms of advertising are more expensive than others. Some examples are shown below.

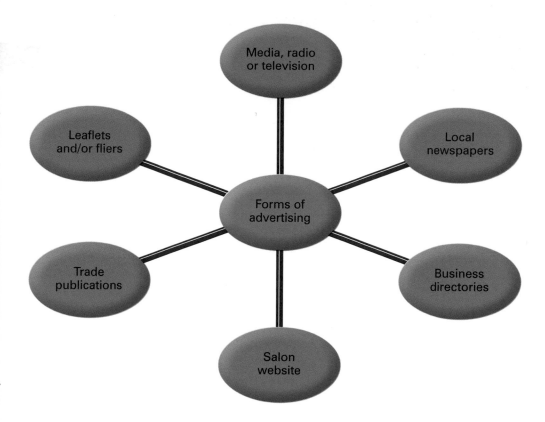

Media, radio and television can be used to reach potential clients throughout the day. However it can be expensive and often broadcast out of the vicinity of the salon. Using a local radio station may prove to be more successful, unless you are part of a nationwide chain and the advert can direct the audience to a salon in their area. You must consider this option very carefully as the high cost may outweigh the potential revenue gained.

Local newspapers may be a good medium for advertising, especially as most areas receive a free paper each week. The salon will have to pay for this type of advertising, so it is essential that the advert is both eye-catching and easily understood for the message to be successful. Newspapers like to run interesting stories, so if the salon is planning to carry out something 'newsworthy', e.g. a percentage of the salon's takings is being donated to a charity, the paper may well send a photographer and run a story on the salon. This type of advertising is free, but it must impact on the audience.

Business directories such as *Yellow Pages* are good for long-term advertising, as they are usually distributed to every household in the area. An advertisement in such a directory must be carefully worded, as it will be listed alongside all the other salons in the area.

Salon websites are becoming more widespread as the internet becomes more accessible to the general population. A salon website should be visually attractive to capture the eye of the user but easy to navigate with accessible information. The website may include photos of the salon and additional information regarding the services and products that are available. Websites are also a good medium to display this season's looks and update clients on current staff and the opening times of the salon.

Keys to good practice

If you are developing your own website, it is recommended that the home page be fairly simple with few or no pictures. A potential user is likely to become bored if they have to wait more than a few seconds for a heavily image-based website to open. Keep the design of the home page to a minimum with links to the more detailed pages.

A trade publication is a good place to advertise because you know the people seeing your advertisement will be interested in hairdressing. This will help to enhance the image of the salon. However, if your objective is to increase the salon's business, this type of advertising may not be the most suitable method.

Leaflets and/or fliers

Leaflets and fliers are a good way to advertise, especially if you do not have a substantial budget for promotional activities. The leaflet must be eye catching and the information easy to understand if your promotion is to impact on the public. Think about the amount of junk mail that you receive and never even read. If the leaflets/fliers are being hand delivered, you must ensure they are delivered to homes within the local vicinity of the salon. If you distribute the leaflets too far away from the salon then the chance of anyone responding to the leaflet/flier is far less. You should also consider the person-hours required to carry out a leaflet drop and if the person responsible is trustworthy. How will you know if they have been delivered or not? Many beauty or nail salons will display leaflets for hairdressing salons, as long as the favour is reciprocated.

The team

For most promotional activities you will need the assistance of others. This may be to exchange thoughts and ideas that will enable you to gain another person's perspective. If your proposed activity is large, you will undoubtedly need the assistance of others to enable you to realise your goals.

It is very important that you consider who you will need to help you and what you want them to do. Allocate responsibilities according to individual's talents, e.g. a good hairdresser should be given the role of demonstrator, or a good negotiator given the role of negotiating prices. They must be competent to carry out the roles you require. Failure to obtain competent assistance may lead to chaos. You should ensure that every member of the team wants to take part, as an unwilling member may cause problems later. If you suspect someone is losing interest or not fulfilling his or her role then this must be challenged and not left to create a problem for you.

Regular meetings of the team will ensure that each individual is maintaining their role and not failing. It will also serve to communicate any changes if they arise and ensure that each person is coping with the workload.

Check it out

Make a list of all the roles that need to be covered, outlining the responsibilities connected to each role. Allocate members of the team to cover each role.

Produce a detailed plan

By now you should have a clear idea of the exact requirements for the promotional activity. You will now need to produce a detailed plan.

The type of activity you choose to promote your salon will be the one that allows you to best achieve your objectives. Also consider any constraints such as the budget and resources. You must be sure the activity you choose is realistically achievable and thoroughly planned.

The objectives of the activity must be made known to everyone involved to ensure that each person is working towards the same goals. You must ensure that the objectives remain the main focus – do not allow the activity to be sidetracked from their importance.

The roles and responsibilities of others involved should be clearly defined from the start. Make sure that everyone is sure of their role and is comfortable with what is expected of them. Each person must be informed of whom to go to when there is a problem. If problems do arise it is important that they are dealt with quickly to prevent a more serious situation developing.

Resource requirements will need to be given careful consideration. It is crucial that detailed planning is carried out to ensure that no requirement is overlooked. Serious problems may arise if something of great importance is forgotten for the event. When making lists of what is required, involve all the team and brainstorm ideas to prevent any detail being missed.

Preparation and implementation activities will need to be attended by everyone concerned. If a member of the team does not attend at this stage then something of importance may be overlooked, thereby creating a problem at a later stage. If the promotion is well planned then implementation should run smoothly. However, if the planning stage is not given the serious consideration it deserves, problems will ensue.

Timescales need to be set to ensure that nothing is left to the last minute. A promotion should not be thrown together in a hurry. Each person involved must be aware of the timescales and the importance of working to them, otherwise problems will arise.

The budget will be set and agreed at the start and money put aside for any emergencies. If you feel at any time that the budgetary constraints are failing then this must be discussed and a solution found to ensure the success of the promotion. The budget is set at the outset to guarantee there will be enough money for everything needed to implement the promotion. Therefore, careful consideration must be given to this initially, in order to achieve the objectives.

Methods of evaluation should be considered during the planning stages in order to allow you to prepare materials required in advance, for example, feedback questionnaires or business reply questionnaires. If your evaluation requires you to carry out some activity at the end of the event then you must have materials ready for this. The methods of evaluation should gauge the effectiveness of the event and must therefore be suited to the purpose. For example, if your promotion is an advertising campaign, then checking for increased revenue would be required; alternatively, if you give demonstrations at an event, a short questionnaire may be more successful.

Venue and legal requirements

The requirements and restrictions of any venue will differ depending upon many factors such as the size of the event, the location, and the need for electricity and water. The venue will need to be carefully considered, as there will be health and safety implications and other legal requirements that will be of great importance.

You have the responsibility to think about the requirements and restrictions of the venue.

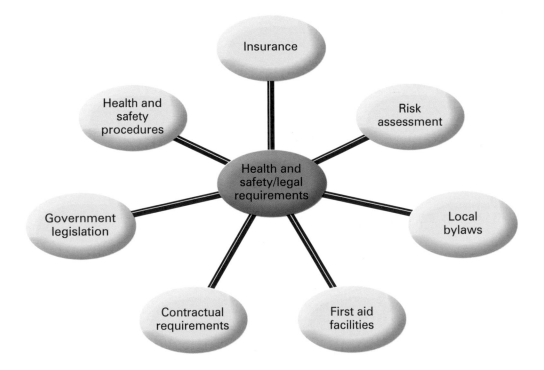

Insurance is an absolute must! You should look at the various types of insurance policies and check to be sure you are adequately covered. Most insurance companies will offer you free advice. Public liability insurance will most definitely be for a six-figure sum and, if you are using an external venue, you should check that the level of cover is adequate. You should also consider if an entertainment licence is required as your insurance could be void without one.

A risk assessment should be carried out prior to the event, in order to assess the steps needed to minimize any risk. All potential hazards will need to be considered and plans put into place to reduce exposure to these. Your risk assessment must take into account the safe use of utilities, e.g. electricity, equipment, chemicals, exposure to extremes of temperature or risk to health from vibration, noise or radiation. In your assessment you must take into account whether staff are properly trained to fulfil their role and plan for any restrictions that need to be imposed due to lack of training.

CONTROL OF SUBSTANCES HAZARDOUS TO HEALTH ASSESSMENT OF RISK

Expt. Title/No		Year	
Substance		Course	
Process			

Substance(s) used

Hazard(s) Please tick:

| Irritant | | Corrosive | | Harmful | | Very Toxic | |
| Oxidising | | Explosive | | Flammable | | | |

Where used pleas tick:

| Laboratory | Preparation Room | Chemical Store | Workshop | Other (specify) |

By whom please tick

| Lecturer | Technician | Student | Other (specify) |

Document(s) outlining working method(s) e.g. Safety & Science Lecturers Guide etc.

Expected Hazardous By-Product(s)

	Tick	Irritant
		Corrosive
		Harmful
		(Very) Toxic
		Oxidising
		Explosive
		Flammable

Likely route(s) of entry

| Inhalation | Mouth | Skin contact | Eyes | |

Specified safety measures to be taken

| Goggles | Fume cupboard | Apron/coat | Eye-wash bottle | Good ventilation | Safety screen | Wash hands | Gloves | Respirator | Dust mask |

Specified procedures for dealing with:

| First Aid ST or PH | Emergency Spillage SP | Fire | |

Assessor_____ Date of Assessment _____
Head of Department_____ Date of Authorisation _____

A risk assessment sheet

Local bylaws are specific laws written by your local authority. These laws may vary depending upon your locality. Therefore, it is a good idea to be aware of which area the venue for your promotional activity falls under. It is important that you are familiar with any restrictions under these laws and that you abide by them, not only to prevent the risk of prosecution but also to ensure that your insurance cover is valid.

First aid facilities are required by law. You must provide adequate first aid provision and it is important to check the facilities at any venue to ensure that you are fully prepared. You also need to be sure that you have designated personnel for the administering of first aid provision. It is crucial to check that these people have a current First Aid qualification or else you are leaving yourself open to possible prosecution or litigation if a situation was to arise.

Contractual requirements are the terms of any contract that you have entered into. It is essential that you are fully aware of the specifics of the contract to prevent any misunderstanding, which could result in an incident or accident; for example, checking to see who provides first aid provision. All aspects of the contract between yourself and another party must be thoroughly explored and, unless you are familiar with business law, you may want to consider employing the services of a business lawyer to check it over for you.

In the salon

Lisa and Claire were joint owners of a large city centre salon and were planning a promotional event to launch the salon's opening. After planning to showcase the work of the staff at a hair show event, they found a venue and signed a contract with the company, which required them to pay a substantial deposit upfront. As time went by, Lisa and Claire realised that the venue they had originally booked would not be suitable to meet their requirements and they made a decision to change the venue. When they contacted the company to let them know, they were told that their deposit was not refundable after thirty days. Claire and Lisa were both surprised and disappointed to discover they had lost a substantial amount of their budget. On checking the specifics of the contract they had signed, they discovered that these details were stated in print. They realised that they were unable to protest at the company's decision.

- In what area do you think Claire and Lisa were negligent?
- How could they have avoided being in this situation?
- Do you think it would have been beneficial to seek legal advice before signing the contract?

Government legislation relating to your promotional activity should be given careful consideration. You need to be sure that you are familiar with all the laws affecting the activity and that you abide by these. This is to prevent the risk of exposure to litigation, prosecution or rendering your insurance invalid.

Unless you have been involved in the management of a business or promotional event previously, you will need to extend your knowledge of the laws that affect your activity. You should seek advice from government websites or your local business advice centre. However, the laws that are relevant to your needs will depend upon the activity you are undertaking. For example, if you are retailing, you will need to consider such legislation as the Sale of Goods Act 1994, The Supply of Goods and Services Act 1982, and the Consumer Protection Act 1987. Information regarding each of these laws can be found in Unit G6.

Health and safety procedures such as fire evacuation must be explored thoroughly to ensure that everything is safe. The health and safety procedures applicable to your event will become apparent once you have planned the activity and booked the venue. Once you are aware of the use of electricity, gas, water, products, equipment and the size of the event, you can put into place any procedures to ensure safety. You should check that the venue has suitable fire fighting equipment and that the utilities you propose to use at the venue have been deemed suitable for purpose. All of this should be included during your risk assessment.

Check it out

In your work in the salon you will have become familiar with legislation that encompasses the needs of the hairdressing industry. Make a list of the relevant acts and regulations and decide which will need to be given consideration for your promotional activity. (See also Unit G1.)

Resources

All the resources required need to be listed and given careful consideration. Planning should be about not only how much is needed but also how to obtain back-up if required. The type of resources you may need include:

The resources you use should be both accessible and affordable. Your promotional activity relies upon the resources needed to produce the results. During the planning stage, you must consider what will be required and ensure that you have enough of what is needed. Poor planning may lead to disappointment for all concerned if you run out of resources. Alternatively, it may be costly to be left with unused resources, which might render your promotion a financial failure.

Implement promotional activities

This section is concerned with the practicalities of the promotional activity. In order to carry out the promotion successfully, all of the hard work completed in the planning stages must come to fruition. At this stage each person involved will be busy fulfilling their role but may still need a point of contact to discuss any problems as they arise. By maintaining communication throughout, not only will everyone be able to see how it is developing but if there is a problem, you can be united in putting into place any contingency plans.

Effective use of resources

As the event organiser you have the responsibility of making certain that the resources required are available for use. This is a very important task and should be given your full attention. Monitoring resource use is essential to prevent misuse and waste. You should also consider that the resources you are using might be governed by health and safety regulations. You must therefore ensure that everyone is aware of his or her responsibilities regarding safe use. You must also bear in mind any contractual agreement and whether or not there are any restrictions that prohibit use of certain equipment or materials. It is essential that any information regarding the use of resources be disseminated to each individual, to prevent problems arising later.

Features and benefits

Everyone involved in the promotional activity must understand the features and benefits of whatever you are promoting. These are your selling points and must reflect the best elements of the promotion. Features of a service or product are its attributes or characteristics, for example, using mousse will aid the styling process. The benefits of a service or product are the advantages that it will give to the client, for example, adding a colour to his or her hair to enhance the haircut. Whatever the objectives of your promotion, the products and services will have features and benefits, and a sound awareness of these is required in order to clearly understand the objectives of the exercise.

Selling skills

If you are to develop and use your selling skills to their best advantage, then it is important for you to recognise buying signals. A client will demonstrate buying signals if he or she is interested in your product or service. Failure to recognise these may lead to a missed selling opportunity.

Once you have established an interest, you must tailor your presentation of the benefits of the product and/or service to meet the individual's needs. In order to carry this out successfully, you will need to have excellent communication skills. These will have been developed over time during your hairdressing career. It may, however, be required of you to support junior members of the team in their role, in order to enhance their selling and communication skills. You should already be aware of how to communicate effectively with people of various age groups and social and ethnic backgrounds. You must now use these skills to present your promotion at a level that is most suited to the audience.

Communication

The way in which you communicate with clients will play a crucial part in the success of the promotional activity. To make your communication effective you need to ensure that the information you are passing on is clear, legible (where necessary) and is fully understood by the receiver. In your promotional work you will communicate with your clients and staff in many different ways.

Methods of communication

The methods of communication you choose to use must suit the type of promotional event that you are undertaking. For example, if you are showcasing your hairdressing work, invitations will need to be sent out, or if you are promoting a new product range then a salon display may suffice. Remember that you also want to create a visual impact and this should substantiate the objectives of your promotion. It is of little use having your best stylist demonstrating his or her skills if you are in drab surroundings and the promotional materials you use are of a poor quality.

If you are conveying information via a presentation, it is important to remember that most people have an attention span of only 20 minutes, so keep it short. Make sure that you have planned the timing and pace and that your methods of presenting information suit the purpose. For example, if you are using presentation software such as Microsoft PowerPoint, are you fully conversant with how to use it and will it fully showcase what you want to demonstrate? You should judge how best to get the information across, for example, using pictures, graphics, music and varying your tone of voice.

You will also need to consider how information will be disseminated among the team. To ensure success, each person must be fully informed at every stage. You must decide how best to update the team, for example, via regular meetings, memos/bulletins or e-mail. Ask the team how they would like to be updated – they may be able to offer alternative ideas.

Presenting and demonstrating

During the event, you need to look at which method of communication is likely to have the most impact on both the team and the target audience. Presenting information in logical steps will assist the listener in grasping the concept of what you are communicating. For example, if you are demonstrating a skill, carry out a skill analysis beforehand as this will allow you to break it down into easy-to-follow steps. Alternatively, if you are advertising, your advert needs to follow a step-by-step progression in order to help the reader/listener to understand your main selling points. You should encourage the target group to ask questions about the services and products you are promoting. This will not only give you an opportunity to sell the features and benefits, but it will enthuse the audience and help them to understand why they need your product or services.

When you are presenting or demonstrating, ensure that you have informed the audience of when to ask questions, as interruptions during your presentation may be off-putting. As you begin discussing the products and services on offer, you must be able to respond to questions in a way that promotes goodwill and enhances the salon's image. It is of little use having an audience sending out buying signals if you proceed to put them off with your replies to their queries. Your manner should be confident and assertive; let them know you completely understand what you are offering. This is where your knowledge of the products and services on offer must be thorough and exact. If they are looking for an answer to their problems then empathise by offering advice based on your experiences.

Problems and how to rectify them

During your planning of the promotional activity you should have set up contingency plans in case of problems arising. Although you can never plan for every eventuality, it will help if you have considered what might go wrong in order to pre-empt a situation with possible solutions.

Problem	Possible solution
Supplier lets you down	Have an alternative supplier ready and waiting
Venue is double booked	Have an alternative venue planned
Models don't arrive	Have alternative models planned
Change of details, e.g. date of event	Set up viable methods of communicating changes to both staff and audience
Staff are off sick	Ensure that staff are trained to cover other roles if required
Show/event is running over time	Plan for shortening demonstrations/ presentation if needed
Show/event is running under time	Plan for extra activities if needed
Sound system malfunctions	Have a back-up system
Laptop crashes during PowerPoint presentation	Have a spare laptop available

After the event

When you have completed the promotional event, you must be sure to leave the venue as requested. All the products and equipment must be cleared away following both health and safety requirements and at the request of the venue. This will serve to prove your professionalism and assist you when negotiating future events. You should remember to include the clearing away in your initial plan. You must also allocate responsibilities for all resources used and the cleaning. This will not only prevent anything from being left behind or misplaced but will also look professional when you leave everything clean and tidy.

Participate in the evaluation of promotional activities

This section is concerned with the evaluation that takes place at the end of the promotional activity. When the promotional activity is over, you should collect all the evidence for your evaluation to enable you to gauge its effectiveness and success. This is the evidence you specified in your promotional plan. Once you have all the evidence, this should be collated and recorded in an easy-to-understand format. Charts and graphs are a good way to record the results, and may be used in conjunction with your evaluation presentation.

Methods of evaluation

The methods used to evaluate the promotion must suit the purpose. You will need to look at the elements that made up the event and decide what was promoted and how effective it was. It is of little use carrying out an evaluation if it does not give you the information you require. For example, asking for feedback on a questionnaire will be more successful if used immediately after the event. Not all evaluations can be carried out immediately. If your objective is to increase your client base then this may have to be assessed over a period of time. You may have to complete several different methods at a time to ensure it suits the target group. For example, a telephone survey to the suppliers may be more appropriate, as it can be seen as a courtesy call.

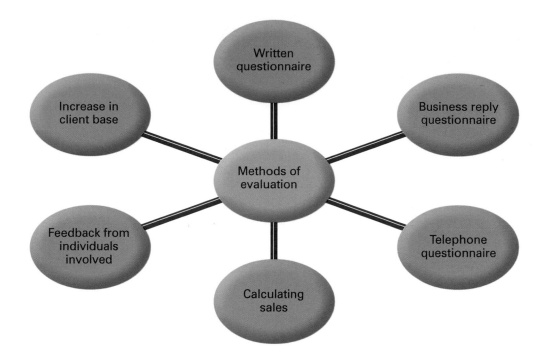

A written questionnaire should ideally be given out at the end of an event. This will ensure that a person's perception of the event is still fresh in their minds and will give you a truer insight into their feelings. It is a valuable tool if used correctly. Consider keeping it anonymous to try to extract people's true feelings. If this is not possible, think of the implications of storing information under the Data Protection Act. You need to be clear about what you are trying to gain from the survey before you start. This will ensure you retrieve the information you require in order to make your evaluations. For anyone leaving the event early or forgetting to complete a survey, you could post it on the salon website allowing them to complete it at their leisure.

Business reply questionnaires are sent out along with a reply paid envelope or on a reply paid postcard. This will help to retrieve the same information as a written survey given out at the event, but there is more incentive to return it if the postage is free. However, you must consider that a couple of days later the audience may have forgotten some vital points they would have brought to your attention on the day. Consider also the need to pay for the postage to send and receive the questionnaires – this could prove to be a costly option.

Telephone questionnaires can be quick and easy to carry out but do you have the person-hours available to administer them? If people are busy at work in the day and do not have time to talk to you then you might have to consider carrying it out in the evening. You will need to be sure that you have contact numbers for all the people you need to speak to.

Calculating sales may have to be done over a period of time, especially if your objective was to increase salon revenue. However, if the event was a one-off promotion, then this can be carried out immediately after the event. You must remember when calculating sales to deduct any VAT if necessary to give you a true figure.

Feedback from individuals involved can be gained in a number of ways, e.g. a written survey or staff meeting. Whichever way you choose, it must suit the purpose and gain the most effective feedback. If you are chairing a staff meeting then ensure your agenda reflects the feedback you wish to receive. You will need to produce a structured discussion plan and ensure you control it well, to prevent the discussion from straying off the track.

Increasing the client base will become evident over a period of time and you will have to structure a timetable of how and when the information will be collated. You will not only have to look at the number of clients coming into the salon but also the amount of money they are spending, particularly if the promotional event has targeted specific hairdressing services.

Collate, analyse and summarise feedback

You should next collate and analyse all the feedback from the activity and put it into an acceptable format. When collating your findings it will make the process much easier if you store the information on a computer, especially if you have access to a spreadsheet and database programme. This will allow you to manipulate the information and present it in different formats. Graphs and charts can be both colourful and interesting and are an excellent visual aid. You may also want to consider presenting your results in a PowerPoint presentation.

Keys to good practice
If you are storing information on a computer, you must keep back-up copies on disk. This will prevent you losing the information if you develop a system failure.

When analysing the information, you must check whether or not you have met the stated objectives. You will need to look at the elements that made up your promotional activity and decide which you are to assess. You must also consider if it was approached in the correct way and whether it could have been carried out differently. Finally, you should decide the best method to present your findings – this must be given careful consideration to ensure that the information is clear and concise.

Check it out

Extend your computer skills by inputting information into a spreadsheet and then trying to present the information in different formats, for example, using pie, bar or flow charts. If you are unfamiliar with spreadsheet programmes, seek advice from someone else, e.g. tutor, ICT technician at college, or a friend.

Presenting the evaluation report

When you have completed your evaluation you may have to present your findings to other people. This may be your employer, business partner or other individuals that were involved with the event. Your results need to be clear and easy to understand; do not use too complex a method to present your findings or else the group may lose interest.

The evaluation report should contain all the important information you gleaned from the evaluation methods used. The report will need to contain information to prove or disprove that you have met the objectives. You should consider including the following information:

- How much revenue has been gained or lost?
- Has the client base expanded?
- Was the venue suitable?
- What problems arose and how were they overcome?
- Did individuals fulfil their role?
- Were the timescales set appropriate?

This list is not exhaustive and could be expanded depending on the particular areas you were promoting.

Once completed, discussing your evaluation report will allow you to present your summary in a clear and structured way. It will also allow the group to clarify any areas that they do not understand. You must be prepared for questions and be sure that you fully understand the information you are presenting, to allow you to elaborate if needed.

Finally, consideration should be given to how improvements could be made. This should be discussed with everyone involved. You will need to look at how the activity can be made better in the future, and ensure that you learn from any mistakes made. All your records should be kept for future reference, as they will be extremely helpful when you are planning a promotional activity event in the future.

Knowledge check

1. Describe the cyclical nature of a promotional activity.

2. Why is it important to work within the constraints of a budget?

3. What are the two main objectives of a promotional activity?

4. What does the acronym SMART stand for?

5. How would you identify potential risks when working at an external venue?

6. What are the differences between the features of a service or product and the benefits of a service or product?

7. Why is it important to evaluate a promotional event?

8. List five methods of gaining feedback after a promotional activity.

Create a variety of looks using a combination of cutting techniques

Unit H27

Introduction

Cutting techniques can be used to create varied and contrasting looks

Throughout this unit we will be looking at how to use a variety of cutting techniques to create classic, current and emerging looks. You will see step-by-step examples of each of these three looks. There are many different techniques involved in cutting, all of which can be developed and applied in innovative and creative ways to produce varied and contrasting looks. You will use all of the basic principles that you learnt whilst completing your initial hairdressing training, but will now need to develop and apply those skills with greater accuracy and invention. The demands that a client will put on you for a total re-style or emerging look will require you to have a higher skill level and a broader use of imagination.

What you will learn
• Preparing the client
• Creating the look
• After the service

You the stylist

This is the point at which you will need to have self-belief in your ability and commitment in the work you produce. Free your mind, find your creative flair, and, most importantly, enjoy it.

Preparing the client

This section highlights all the things that are important when preparing your client for the cutting service, for example, using the correct personal protective equipment and ensuring you have ready the relevant tools that are appropriate for the task. As always, there are several health and safety regulations that you need to be fully aware of before you begin the cutting service.

Check it out

Re-read Unit G1 and make a list of all the acts and regulations that you think might be relevant to cutting a client's hair. Then, as you progress through this unit, check that you have remembered them all.

What you will learn

- Thorough consultation
- Use of visual aids
- Checking for contra-indications
- Personal hygiene
- Personal protective equipment
- Preparing your work area

Thorough consultation

When a client comes into the salon for a cut, it is important for you, the stylist, to conduct a thorough consultation with him or her. You must note what the client is wearing (ensure your assistant does not put a gown on until you have seen him or her). Ask about his or her job and lifestyle, for example, does he/she go to the gym regularly? Look at the client's hair as they enter the salon and before it is shampooed, just in case he or she asks for it to be styled in the same way. At this stage, find out as much background information as you can, as this will help you make an informed decision on the choices available to your client. Do not skimp on the detail and take the time to find out about them now, so that you can be sure to advise them on the best possible options that are available to them.

Use of visual aids

You will need to use sound communication skills to extract the right information from your client (see Units G9 and G10 for more information on communication skills). Your aim is to build up a picture in your mind of what exactly the client requires of you and you need to make sure that you are both thinking along the same lines. You must ensure that you fully understand your client's requirements; one method of doing this is to use stylebooks or magazines to illustrate the proposed look. It will be much easier for both you and your client if you have a firm idea of the look he or she is seeking to achieve.

In the salon

Shabia was cutting a client's hair in the salon. She asked her client, 'Would you like your hair cutting over the ear?' The client said 'Yes', so she proceeded to cut the hair off, leaving the entire ear exposed. She then noticed the look of horror on her client's face. When she asked her what was wrong, the client told her that what she had meant was over the ear, but still covering the top of the ear. What could Shabia do? She had already cut the hair off so she had to cut the other side to balance the look. The client was very upset about her new 'short' look. She explained to Shabia that she did not like her ears exposed as she felt that they were too big. Shabia apologised but the client left the salon and never came back.

- What should Shabia have done differently during the consultation?
- How could she have tried to retain this client and build her trust again?

An important factor that you must consider during a consultation is whether the client's hair has the potential to achieve the look that you both may want. A ten-minute consultation will be wasted time if the hair texture, length, or amount of movement is not suitable to achieve or maintain the look. During the consultation, it is good practice to push the client's hair back off the face so that you can look at his or her head and face shape. Keep a close eye on your client's facial expressions as these can reveal whether he or she is happy with your suggestions or not.

Checking for contra-indications

When you are looking at your client's hair, remember to check the scalp for infections and infestations. You should also be checking the hair's texture and density, as this can be a critical factor in determining the right style for the client. For example, if the hair is very coarse and abundant, and the client has chosen a look that is best suited to finer hair, you may have to advise him or her against it or adapt your cutting technique to take this into account. It may be necessary to use a razor or thinning scissors to remove some bulk.

You may need to ask your client when he or she last had his or her hair cut, as this will give you a good indication of how much to cut off, bearing in mind that most people's hair grows about one centimetre a month. Another good indicator is the demarcation line of a colour growing out, as this gives you an idea of your client's hair growth rate.

Once your client has been shampooed and has returned to you, look at the hair again and check the growth patterns. The client may have disguised these by styling the hair but shampooing the hair will allow it to lie back in its natural fall. Also, while the hair is wet, it is important to check the hair's elasticity: if it is poor and stretches considerably, this must be taken into account during cutting to prevent taking off too much.

Personal hygiene

During the time you spend with your client, you must consider your own personal hygiene. You will be in close contact with your client as you talk to them and lean over them. You should have fresh breath and a clean smell about you. Strong smells such as nicotine can be very off-putting for the client, particularly if they are a non-smoker. For this reason, it is good practice to appoint a rule of no smoking in the salon. Not only are there the risks associated with passive smoking, but there is also the risk associated with smoking near flammable products. You should ensure that your hands and fingernails are clean and presentable – this will instill confidence in both you and your client regarding your personal standards and professionalism.

Personal protective equipment

Once you have fully explored every option with your client and you have agreed on the end result, you must prepare the hair for cutting. Gowning the client and using the correct protective equipment is essential. For example, a cutting collar or towel will not only prevent hair from falling onto the client's clothing, which causes uncomfortable itching, but it is also cleaner and creates a professional appearance. Attention to little details like this is what distinguishes you from being a 'run-of-the-mill' hairdresser to being a specialist. Using a good shampoo and conditioner relevant to your client's hair type is essential. The hair must be thoroughly cleansed to aid with combing during cutting and also to prevent damage to your cutting tools. You will find the hair easier to handle if it is thoroughly detangled; this will ensure you take clean sectioning lines and keep good tension during cutting.

Preparing your work area

While your assistant is shampooing your client, you have a few minutes to prepare your work area. Utilise this time wisely to ensure that you get all the tools and equipment ready that you think you will need. Once you get into the routine of doing this, it will become natural good practice. You cannot always rely on your assistant to know which tools you are planning to use. However, you should be able to rely on the junior staff to ensure that all tools and equipment are clean and sterilised (see Unit G1). This will prevent any risk of cross-infection, infestation, or damage to tools due to them being unclean or unfit for purpose. Scissors and combs can be sterilised by placing them in an ultra-violet cabinet, but remember, they must be turned over to ensure both sides have been done. It is also good practice to keep combs in a chemical jar and replace the solution frequently to ensure its effectiveness.

Creating the look

You need to be skilled in creating three types of look: classic, current and emerging. We will look at each of these now, and then later in this unit you can refer to the step-by-step guide on how to achieve each look.

Classic

Current

Emerging

What is a classic look? A classic look is a hairstyle that has a timeless quality, for instance, a bob. This look has been around, in one form or another, for several decades and, although it has countless variations, it is a look that you will see on women of all ages.

A current look is the type of look that is very popular at any particular time, for example, the 'Rachel' cut (modelled on Jennifer Aniston's hairstyle in the television series *Friends*). These types of style change quickly and would suit a client who likes to change their hairstyle regularly.

Finally, there are emerging looks. These are looks that are about to come into fashion, for example, a look described in a magazine as next season's 'must-have' style. These types of styles are good for clients who like to look different.

Cutting tools and their uses

There are many cutting tools available for use. You need to be familiar with each one and the effects you can achieve by using them.

Scissors

Scissors come in many different designs and several lengths of blades. They are used for a variety of cutting techniques such as club cutting, slicing, texturising or thinning. It is very important to find the right pair; remember that they need to feel comfortable to use, as they are really just an extension to your hand. Be familiar with all the working parts of your scissors. It will help you to use them if you know how they work. Below is a diagram of a pair of scissors with all the parts labelled.

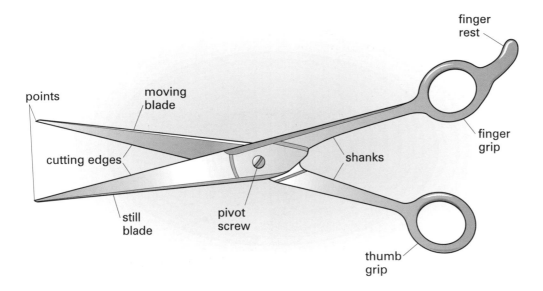

Thinning scissors

As well as straight-edged scissors, there are also thinning scissors with serrated edges. These can also be called aesculaps or texturising scissors. They have one or more edges with serration. It is also possible to buy scissors with varying degrees of serration, which allow the stylist to produce much more imaginative styles. Thinning scissors are used to remove bulk, not length, and must be used only on dry hair.

Thinning scissors

Clippers

Clippers are used for club cutting and are extremely good to use on very short styles. Clippers have two blades with serrated edges, one of which moves and the other stays still. Because of the type of edge, it is essential that you have them sharpened by the manufacturer or a specialist sharpening service. You can use small clippers for tapering and outlining as they cut much closer and finer. They are especially good for removing any hair outside of the hairline after cutting. Outlining is particularly important when providing a very short cut close to the skin as it can be used to neaten off a finished style. However, even when outlining, you can use ordinary-size clippers, but be sure to close the blades by using the lever on the sides, as this will give a much closer cut.

Clippers

Check it out

Look at the clippers that you use in your salon. Find out how they should be maintained and stored following the manufacturer's instructions.

Attachments for clippers

Clippers come with different-size attachments. These are usually numbered and, depending on their thickness, will cut the hair shorter or leave it longer. They are mainly used for club cutting, but if you are confident in their use then they can be used to create various effects, such as scooping out at the root area to thin the hair. Clippers must be maintained by removing the hair around the blades with a clipper brush with stiff bristles, often provided by the manufacturer. Use clipper oil on the blades regularly but ensure they do not have oil on them whilst cutting or else this will hinder their performance during the cut. In recent years, cordless clippers have become more popular and this type of clipper has the advantage of causing less of a hazard due to trailing wires. They are recharged when placed back in the base unit after use.

Cordless clippers with attachments

Clippers are now available with a pivot head, which makes them easier to use. They also come in various colours which appeal to our fashion-conscious industry. Hairdressers are often nervous of using clippers, as they are afraid that they might cut the skin, when in fact they are safer to use than scissors as the blades are always parallel to the skin.

Razors

Razors can be used when cutting the hair to remove bulk or to thin out the ends. They are especially good for creating textured looks. You have the choice when using a razor for cutting hair of an open razor, a safety razor, or a shaper as shown below.

A safety razor and a shaper

It is essential that you hold and use a razor correctly, not only for your own and the client's safety, but to prevent damage to the hair.

The safety guard must be facing you as you work

You must keep the hair wet at all times when cutting with a razor as this will allow the razor to slice into the hair and cut precisely. You should also ensure that your blade is extremely sharp. The advantage of modern razors is that you can change the blades frequently, especially if you are using them to shave excess hair from below the outline. For instance, in the nape area of a short cut, if you shave the hair away, you must replace the blade following your salon policy for disposal of sharps. This is to prevent the risk of cross-infection. Care must be taken as it is very easy to slice the skin when using a razor, especially when you are working around the eye or ear area.

An important point that you must make to your client is that there is a risk of ingrowing hairs after close razor or even clipper work. This can happen if the hair curls as it is growing and starts to grow back into the skin. It would be evident by a small lump in the skin that can become infected. They are, however, usually easy to remove by piercing the skin with a sterile surgical needle, allowing the hair to be freed. Ingrowing hairs are more likely to happen to a client with curly or African Caribbean hair. A client with dark skin will need to be advised about the changes that can happen to the skin with repeated use of close clipper or razor work. The area of skin that has been clippered or razored may start to thicken or darken, causing discoloration of the skin that will be very noticeable below the hairline: this is known as 'shadowing'.

Cutting techniques and effects

Now that you are aware of cutting tools and their uses, we can begin to look at the various cutting techniques in more detail.

Club cutting

This technique removes the hair length only. It gives the hair ends a very blunt look and is the most commonly used technique. Clubbing or blunt cutting allows you to cut very straight and precise lines, for example, in the cutting of a one-length bob.

When club cutting, it is the angle at which you hold the hair that determines the finished effect. You have to hold the hair firmly between the fingers with even tension and ensure each section is thoroughly combed to produce even cutting. You can club cut on wet or dry hair but it is more precise on wet. When you clipper cut the hair, you are also club cutting.

Thinning

This method of cutting is used to remove bulk from the hair but not length. It is more commonly carried out with thinning scissors; however, there are scissor-thinning techniques that you can use. For instance, chipping into the hair at the root area will remove bulk and the shorter hairs will help to provide style support to the longer lengths.

Keys to good practice

- Thinning scissors should be used only on dry hair to prevent too much hair from being removed. They should not be used on partings or around hairlines as short hairs can be seen protruding once the hair has been styled.
- Thinning scissors are not suitable for use on fine or thinning hair, but they are good for very thick or coarse hair. You can use the thinning scissors at any point along the hair length depending on the amount of hair you wish to remove and the effect you want to create.
- If you have cut hair very short and there are 'steps' in the haircut that you cannot remove, a good tip is to use thinning scissors to go over the hair ends to remove them.

Razoring

This technique has become very popular again as very textured and feathered looks are currently fashionable. Razors should only ever be used on wet hair as the hair ends can be easily damaged by using a razor on dry hair. It will also be uncomfortable for the client as it drags along the hair shaft, giving the feeling of hair being ripped out of the head. You must also make sure that your razor's edge is always sharp, again to prevent damage or discomfort. Razor cutting can be done anywhere in a haircut and removes bulk and/or length, depending on where you use the technique.

With razor cutting, the hair is held between the fingers and can be cut either on top or below the section, with the razor held at a slight angle to the hair shaft. The amount of pressure you apply will determine the amount of hair removed, so take care – it is much safer to remove a little at a time than to take off too much. Razor cutting is especially good for creating very textured looks or for blending short layers into very long layers.

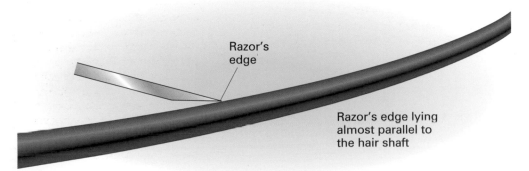

Razor's edge

Razor's edge lying almost parallel to the hair shaft

Free hand

This technique can be done on wet or dry hair and is carried out by cutting the hair without holding it between the fingers. The hair is just combed into place and the ends cut to allow it to fall in its natural lie. It is especially good when cutting the hair around unusual growth patterns. For example, if a client has a cowlick at the front hairline and you were to cut the fringe between the fingers, when you let go it would jump up and look uneven in length. Similarly, if you were cutting around nape whorls, it would look much better for the client if you cut it to its natural lie.

Texturising/point cutting

This can also be called chipping or point thinning. It can be carried out on wet or dry hair and is used to remove either length or bulk. The ends of the scissors are used to cut into the hair anywhere along the hair shaft from mid-lengths to ends, depending on the effect you are trying to create. It will give a look a much more choppy uneven finish, with softer broken edges. It can be incorporated into many different styles; for instance, a client with a very straight-edged look can require a softer fringe that has been point cut.

Tapering/slicing

This technique is used when you want to remove bulk or join together short layers with long layers. It can be done on wet hair if using a razor and dry if using scissors. The scissors are allowed to slide into the hair, as you slightly open and close the blades, in a backcombing type of movement. With the razor method, you scoop into the hair sections and apply pressure according to the amount of hair you want to remove. This method requires a great deal of accuracy and skill so as not to cut off too much hair.

Scissor-over-comb

Although more commonly used in men's hairdressing, it is inevitable that you will have to cut a short tapered neckline on a woman's haircut. It can be carried out on wet or dry hair. Care must be taken not to cut 'steps' into the hair. For this technique, you place the comb into the hair at the root area and pull out the comb away from the scalp up to the desired length. You cut the hair that protrudes through the teeth of the comb while maintaining a flowing movement; the scissors must open and close to cut at the same pace up the haircut or else lines will develop. Again, this type of cutting requires accuracy and a great deal of practice. Clipper-over-comb is done in exactly the same way, except the clipper blades are run over the hair protruding through the teeth of the comb.

Beveling

The beveling technique is used when you want to introduce graduation into your cutting line. The hair is held between the fingers but the fingers are turned over to allow the hair to wrap slightly around. This small amount of drag will provide slight graduation. It can be done on wet or dry hair but, as with most haircuts, it will be more precise if carried out on wet hair.

Free hand

Texturising/point cutting

Check it out

You can practise the movement of scissor-over-comb in the work-station mirror. Make sure that the comb follows the movement of the opening and closing scissor action and that you hold your comb in a way so that you can flip it over to comb down each section that you have just cut.

Creating a classic look: a step-by-step guide

Before the haircut.

A horizontal section is taken in the nape.

The base line is then point cut to the desired length.

The hair is held out from the scalp and angled slightly to give a slight graduation.

The section is point cut. Continue this until the back of the head is complete.

Take a section at the side of the head, parallel to the hairline. Angle the fingers up towards the face, using a guideline from the back, point cut the section.

When both sides are complete and blended with the back, the fringe is then point cut.

Texturise the fringe to give a 'softer' appearance.

Check the hair cut is even in length.

Cross-check the cut and assess the finished result.

Personalise the hair cut by texturising where necessary.

The finished result.

Creating a current look: a step-by-step guide

Before the haircut.

The first section is taken straight across the back, in the nape area.

The hair is then club cut to the desired length.

Subsequent sections are then introduced. The hair length is brought down and cut to this length – ensure that your sections are fine enough to see your guideline.

After the back sections have been cut to length, the side sections are cut following the back's guideline.

In order to introduce the razored layers, the hair is sectioned from halfway up the back of the head.

The hair is then razored from mid-lengths to ends, taking sections up the back of the head.

The side sections are also razored, taking horizontal sections up to the centre parting.

The front hairline sections are then taper cut to give a more textured look.

The length should be checked to ensure an even cut all over the head.

When the hair has dried you should point thin the ends to create a soft, flicky effect.

The finished look.

Creating an emerging look: a step-by-step guide

Before the haircut.

The top layers are sectioned out of the way. The undercut result is created by taking sections parallel to the hairline and cutting them short.

Subsequent sections are introduced ensuring that you can see the guideline before cutting.

Continue with the same pattern, sectioning around the head and behind the ear.

The back of the head has been cut so that a sloping section is visible from one side of the head to the other.

The top layers are then point cut at a much longer length to produce the undercut effect.

Continue around the head by bringing the top layers down and point cutting them.

As the hair length increases on one side, section layers are introduced, again point cutting to give a choppy effect.

Vertical sections are taken working through the longer length from back to front.

The underneath fringe is sectioned out of the hair and cut freehand to the desired length.

The longer fringe sections are then point cut to blend into the side layers.

The finished look can be accentuated by the addition of colours and creative styling.

Cutting angles, baselines and guidelines

Now that you have looked at all the cutting techniques, you need to familiarise yourself with the effects you will be creating by cutting angles. They fall into two main types: layering and graduation. You will no doubt be familiar with the terminology, but do you fully understand the difference between the two? Firstly, you will layer most haircuts, except for one-length cuts. The most common layering technique is the uniform layer – this is where the hair is cut at a 90-degree angle to the scalp and is cut to the same length all over the head, as shown in the illustration below.

Hair cut in a uniform layer

Graduation is when the hair is cut to varying lengths throughout the haircut. For example, the layers on top may be quite short but through the back they are substantially longer; this is known as increased graduation. To achieve increased graduation you need to over direct the layers through the back and sides, pulling them all over to the shorter length guidelines at the top. The cutting angle will fall anywhere between 90 to 180 degrees depending on the amount of graduation. Alternatively, when the layers through the top are much longer than the underneath layers, this is known as reverse graduation. For this type of graduation, the cutting angle will fall anywhere between 45 to 90 degrees, again, depending on the amount of graduation. Examples of these are shown in the illustrations below.

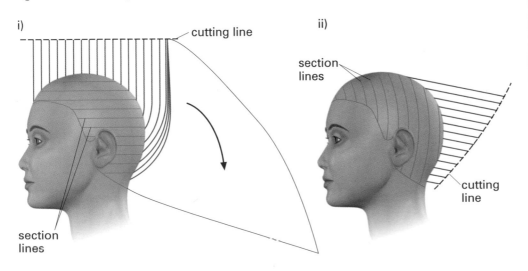

i)
cutting line
section lines

ii)
section lines
cutting line

Increased and reversed graduation

> ## Remember
>
>
> It is extremely important that throughout the cut you are aware of the cutting angles you are using, as they will affect the finished shape and balance of the hair. Not only is this important, but you must be accurate in the way that you section the haircut. It is not always necessary to start at the back, but be sure to section off the hair and follow neat and even sections throughout the cut. Good sectioning will allow you to follow your guideline and ensure that no areas are missed. This also looks professional to the client. It is also important to take clean sections to ensure you achieve the desired effect.

The initial guideline or baseline you cut will be important in determining the overall length, shape and balance of the cut. Sometimes you will cut the outer line of the hair first, as in a one-length cut, or you may cut the inner length of the hair first, as in a uniform layer cut. Either way, you will always have to cut both the outer and the inner lengths. Guide or baselines can be cut in a variety of shapes, each of which is detailed below.

- **Symmetric:** the haircut is evenly balanced over both sides, as in a hairstyle with a centre parting of equal lengths on both sides of the head.
- **Asymmetric:** the hair is unevenly balanced over both sides, for instance, if the hair has a side parting and more hair is distributed to one side of the head.
- **Straight:** the hair is cut to a straight baseline as in one-length looks.
- **Concave:** the baseline will be cut curving inwards or downward; think of a concave bob where the hair curves downwards towards the sides.
- **Convex:** the baseline is cut longer from the sides into the middle section, which gives a curve of longer in the back to shorter towards the front.

Look at each of the illustrations below to help you visualise them all.

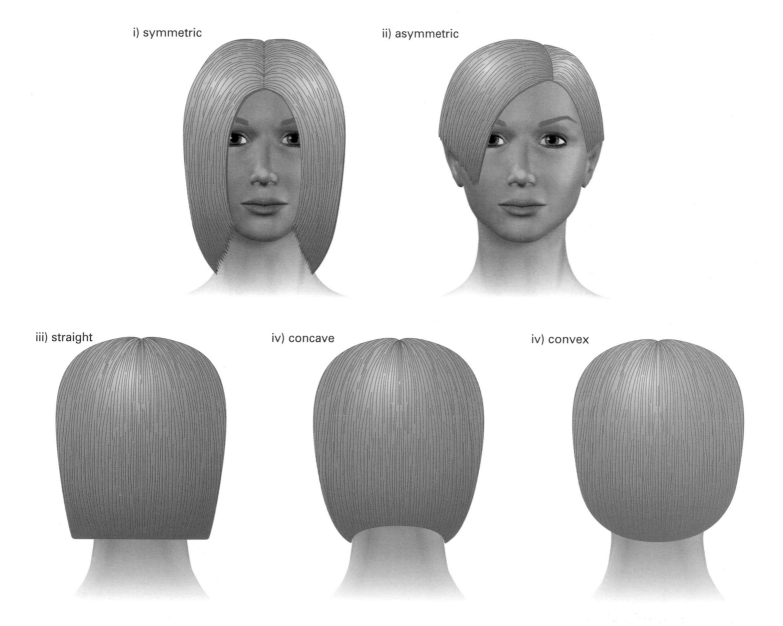

i) symmetric ii) asymmetric iii) straight iv) concave iv) convex

Cross-checking

While you are carrying out the cut, you must maintain the consultation throughout. You will find that as the cut builds up, you may have different ideas about where it is going and you need to check this out with the client before making those changes yourself. It is also vital to cross-check the cut and check the balance throughout to ensure you have not made any mistakes. When cross-checking, look at it the opposite way to how it was first cut. For instance, if you took vertical sections then take horizontal ones. Remove any hair only if you find it out of line. The point of cross-checking is to look for mistakes, not to re-cut the hair and take it another centimetre shorter. The client will not thank you for this and it is a waste of your time. Also, look at the length of the hair all over the head and make sure that you have not missed any areas.

Correct positioning of self and client

The positioning of yourself and your client during the cut is something that you must be aware of at all times. If the client is sitting awkwardly or slouching with his or her legs crossed, then this could affect your finished cut. If the client is slouching to one side then you could end up with the hair longer on that side. It is much easier to cut hair if you position the head correctly. For instance, in the difficult-to-reach areas, such as the nape of the neck, you must ensure the head is placed down as far as is comfortable for the client. Not only is the client's position an influencing factor, but also your own body stance is very important. If you are stooped over clients all day and not keeping your back straight, you will soon feel discomfort in your back. It is essential to prevent long-term injury or damage by ensuring that your own posture is good. Think about balancing the weight over your body when you stand and not leaning to one side for long periods. It is far too easy to put unnecessary strain on muscles and ligaments by over-reaching or stretching. However, this can be avoided by taking the time to adopt good posture while working. Eventually it will become habit to stand in the correct position and you will do it without realising.

Do not strain your back by leaning over your client

Keep your back straight and balance your weight correctly

In the salon

Marco was increasingly troubled with back pain that was causing him to take time off work. After several trips to see the doctor it became apparent that it was his posture that was causing the problem. When he thought about the way he stood whilst working, he realised that, because the salon chairs where large and bulky with a thick back, he was over-stretching to reach clients when working on them. Marco began to learn Tai'chi to enable him to correct his posture and also took the time to position his client so that he could keep his back straight whilst working. Within a few

months his back pain had gone and he was feeling much better. This prevented any long-term injury that could have affected him for the rest of his life.

- What lesson can be learned from this example?
- Take the time to look at your own posture while you are working. Are you positioning yourself and the client correctly?
- Ask someone you work with to look at the way you stand whilst working and check if it looks as if you are over-stretching or standing incorrectly.

Timings

Timing is very important while you are training. You should be checking the length of time it takes you to carry out services in the salon. As a guide, a cut and finish should take no longer than 45 minutes on short hair, and a re-style or long hair cut and finish should take about one hour. However, this may vary depending on the type of salon that you work in.

Check it out

Think about the timings allowed in the salon for all the cutting services that you offer. Do senior members of staff have a different time allowed to them from the junior staff?

Solving cutting problems

There are various types of problems that you may come across during the cut and you need to feel you can deal with these as they arise. Usually, they are because your consultation was not accurate. For instance, you begin to cut and then find that there is a conflicting hair growth pattern that is preventing you from getting the look you require. You will have to deal with problems such as these whenever they occur, but remember to keep the client informed, use your professional judgement, and be tactful in explaining the situation. If you have a confident manner then your client will feel confident in your ability, whereas if you are floundering and unsure, they will realise this and may begin to panic. This type of situation will get you nowhere; it will look totally unprofessional and could harm your reputation. Even if you are not fully confident, do not panic but just keep talking to the client while you plan your course of action.

Below is a table showing common cutting problems with possible remedies.

Cutting problem	Possible remedy
Sides are not even on finished cut	Cross-check, use the mirror and remove the longer length to even up
Cannot get close enough into the nape to cut to required length	Adjust the way you hold the hair for cutting or use a different cutting technique
Hair will not lie correctly around hairline	Adjust the finished style to incorporate the hairline's natural lie
Cut the client's or own skin	Stop immediately and clean the wound so it is free from hair (ensure you are wearing gloves to prevent cross-infection) and apply pressure to stop bleeding. Use a plaster if continuing
During the cut you notice head lice	Advise client to treat the hair as soon as possible

One problem that can easily be avoided is getting cut hair on the client's clothing. When you use a cutting gown, make sure it fits over all the client's clothing and that it is correctly fastened. You can use either a towel or cutting collar around the shoulders. The benefit of a cutting collar is that it fits well over the shoulders and does not get in the way when cutting around the shoulder or neck area as a towel might. It is also a good idea and looks professional if, at regular intervals throughout the cut, you remove any hair that has fallen onto the skin or shoulders. This will also help to prevent any hair going down the neck area and causing discomfort to the client.

> **Remember**
>
> A good tip if the cut hair is wet and sticking to the skin, is to use a little talcum powder on your neck brush to help to remove it.

Keys to good practice

- Remain aware of critical influencing factors such as growth patterns at all times.
- If cutting wet hair, keep it wet throughout, especially if using a razor.
- Always take neat, even sections.
- Ensure that your tension is good and even throughout the cut.
- Make sure you can see your guideline before you cut.
- Never cut shorter than your guideline.
- Check regularly throughout the cut that it is level.
- Always cross-check your cut.
- Do not cut off too much hair when cross-checking, only the hair you have missed.
- Maintain the consultation throughout with the client to check what you are doing is to their requirements.
- If things go wrong, do not let the client see that you are panicking.
- Remember, if you cut the hair too short, there is nothing you can do about it!

If you cut hair using these rules, you will not go far wrong. Make them your cutting commandments and you will have many happy clients!

Cutting techniques and effects: a quick reference guide

Technique	Effect	Cut on wet, dry or either	Best suited to straight or curly hair
Club cutting	Gives a blunt, straight edge to the hair ends	Either, but more precise on wet hair	Either, but will help to reduce curl
Clippering	Gives a blunt, straight edge to the hair ends	Dry	Can be used on either, but open the blades slightly to aid cutting on curly hair
Thinning	Removes bulk but not length	Dry	Either, but will encourage curl
Razoring	Removes bulk and length, good for texturising	Wet	Either, but will encourage curl
Free hand	Removes length and bulk	Either	Either
Point cutting/ texturising	Produces softer, broken edges	Either	Either
Slicing/tapering	Removes bulk, gives texture	Wet with razor and dry with scissors	Either
Scissor-over-comb	Club cutting on short hair	Either	Either
Beveling	Creates graduation at the ends of the hair	Either	Either

After the service

Once you have finished the client's hair, just sending them out of the salon is not enough. You need to discuss with them how to maintain the look and book them another appointment for the next service that you recommend. Include in your discussion any after-care advice or recommendations that you feel are relevant.

What you will learn

- Disposal of waste, including sharps
- Using styling products to finish
- Confirmation of the finished look
- Removing the client's protective clothing correctly
- Recommendations
- Intervals between cuts

Disposal of waste, including sharps

On immediately finishing the cut and checking with the client that it is what they require, it is most important that you remove any loose hair cuttings from the client's gown and skin so as to prevent any discomfort. If you brushed off the hair cuttings as you went along then this will be a small task. You can use the hairdryer to blast away any hair from the chair or skin that you cannot brush off. The more hair you remove from the client and surrounding area, the more professional it will look and there will be less chance of them becoming itchy.

At this point, you must also sweep up all the hair from the floor and dispose of it following your salon policy. Hair cuttings left on the floor can cause a slippery surface and this then becomes a hazard in the salon, both to you and the client when they stand up. Salons will dispose of hair cuttings in different ways, but generally it is more hygienic to ensure that they are placed in a covered bin and put in the outside bin in a tied-up bag to prevent it spilling out. At the end of the cutting service, you may need to dispose of sharps and again this must be done in line with salon policy. However, it is a strict health and safety rule that used sharps are disposed of in a sharps bin. This has to be a sealed container clearly labelled with its purpose.

Check it out

Visit your council offices and look up the local bylaws for the disposal of used sharps and waste to see if there are written codes of practice. You will usually find that they have them and you should be observing and following these.

Using styling products to finish

When you are styling the client's hair, you must select the correct styling products to complete the desired effect. It is also a great opportunity for recommending the products you use to sell to the client. Remember that it will be harder for them to style and maintain the look without the professional products that you are using in the salon. Let the client look at and feel the products and put a little in their hand for them to smell and feel. This will let them know that you have every confidence in the products that you are using and that you are proud to show off their quality. It is impossible to achieve a good finish using styling products of poor quality.

Let clients try different finishing products – it could encourage them to buy!

Know your styling products well – if you have thorough product knowledge, it will show your professionalism and will allow you to recommend with confidence. This is especially important if you work in a salon that pays you commission on your sales. This can be a good boost to your income. There are often other perks thrown in for the best salesperson such as free products.

Look at the table below. It lists several of the styling products available for use and the effects they will help you to achieve.

Styling product	Effect
Gel/gel spray	Firm to ultra hold
Mousse	Volume, natural to extra firm hold
Wax	Texture, defines curl
Hairspray	Natural to ultra firm hold
Dressing/styling crème	Adds shine, reduces static, defines curl
Gloss spray	Adds shine, reduces static
Blow-dry lotion	Volume, natural to firm hold
Straightening crème	Helps hair to stay straight, defies humidity

Any styling product that you use will need to be applied following the manufacturer's instructions. Take time out to read these on first use, as it will ensure that you get the maximum effect and best results from whatever you are using. If it says use a pea-sized amount then you should just use that much; however, you will need to judge if the hair is thick and abundant and requires more of the product, or if it is fine and requires less of the product.

Any products that you use in the salon must be stored, handled, used and disposed of following COSHH regulations (refer to Unit G1 for more detailed information). Following COSHH regulations will show professionalism, ensure that safety is of the utmost importance to you and sets a good example to other staff.

Keeping up to date

There are many different manufacturers and types of product available to aid styling. Usually you find products that you can rely on and trust and you will tend to stick to this particular manufacturer. However, new products are being developed all the time and you need to keep up to date on the latest developments by taking regular trips to the wholesalers or receiving visits from the company representative.

Check it out

When you have a spare few minutes in the salon, look at the products for sale and read the manufacturer's information to see if you have forgotten any of the benefits that they offer. Do this regularly, as it is easy to forget how good a product is when you use it day in and day out. It will help you sell to your client if you are fully conversant with what the products can do for their hair.

Remember

All of the styling products that you are using are likely to be flammable. You must take care that you do not use them near a naked flame, for example, near a cigarette lighter.

Remember

A good tip is to ask the wholesalers or company representative to let you try the products for free before you buy them for the salon. You need to judge for yourself if the styling products will deliver what they say they offer and who better to try them than you!

Confirmation of the finished look

When you have finished the blow-dry, you will need to check the balance of the finished style and confirm with the client that he or she likes the end result. Always look in the mirror and check the overall balance from every angle around the head, as this is what everyone will see of your client's look. Show the client the back, making sure that he or she can actually see through the back mirror. A good rule of thumb is if you can see the back or sides through the mirrors then your client will also.

Sometimes the cut will need a little adjusting after drying. Explain this to the client and keep him or her informed at all times of where and how much you are cutting off. You may find that the feathering is finer on one side; this is sometimes visible only on dry hair. You may find that a small piece of hair, when wet, was stuck behind the ear and you missed it. Do not be afraid to tell the client that you have spotted something that needs correcting. He or she will thank you in the long run and be happier with the style once he or she has left if it is corrected now instead of on the next cut.

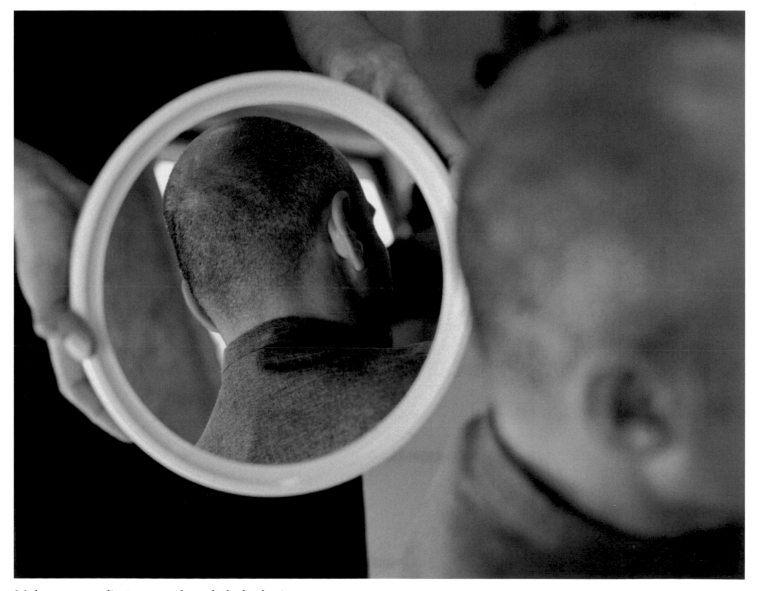

Make sure your client can see through the back mirror

Removing the client's protective clothing correctly

Once you have applied the styling products and are about to start blow-drying, you (or your client) may want to remove the gown, especially if it is a hot day in the salon. It is, however, important not to remove the gown before applying styling products so as to prevent any spillage onto the client's own clothes. If you do need to remove the gown at this stage, explain to the client that cut hair may still blow off the head during blow-drying and onto the clothing, causing discomfort later. They may reconsider if they have to go to work or go shopping and are unable to change soon.

When removing the gown, always take care to take it off properly. Unfasten it correctly and ensure that any cut hair is thrown from the gown onto the floor and not over the client's clothing. If you do find there is some on their clothes, offer them a clothes brush to remove it – never let them leave the salon with hair on their clothes. This looks messy and does not give a good impression of the salon. Remember that a client is looking for an all-round excellent service; they may think that although you have given them a fabulous haircut that your customer service skills leave a lot to be desired. It is likely that it will stick in their mind and is what they tell their friends about your salon.

Recommendations

Finishing off the style can be a very relaxing experience for clients and they often tell you that the blow-dry is the best part of the service. If it is a regular client that trusts you then he or she may just want to close his or her eyes and relax. Alternatively, he or she may want you to explain how you are drying it so he or she can re-create the look at home. As you are blow-drying, you can discuss with your client the drying techniques you are using and why and how the products are helping you to achieve the final look. Ensure you have a selection of brushes available for retail sale. A client may find it easier to style at home using the tools that you use and it is another good selling opportunity. Never shy away from giving clients advice on styling – it is a reflection of your salon's good name if their hair always looks good. They are, after all, a walking advertisement for you out on the streets.

Intervals between cuts

Remember to advise the client on when he or she will need to return to the salon for his or her next appointment. This may be for a service other than cutting, but generally, clients have their haircut maintained between every four to six weeks, unless they are growing their hair in which case they may want to leave a longer gap. Usually, no longer than ten weeks between cuts is advised. If it is left any longer, the ends of the hair become more susceptible to splitting and the style will begin to look messy, causing the client to have difficulty with it at home. Always ask the client to book his or her next appointment before he or she leaves; do not miss the opportunity while you still have the client in the salon. This will make sure they return to you and do not have the chance to go elsewhere in the meantime. It will also make them think that you care about keeping their hair in good condition and, if you work in a busy salon, they may need to book early to avoid the disappointment of you not being able to fit them in.

> ## Check it out
>
> Using a selection of pictures or photographs of your own work, describe how you achieved the overall look and incorporated different cutting techniques. In your descriptions, indicate the cutting angles and list the tools and equipment you used. State which products you used to create the looks.

Knowledge check

1. State your salon's requirements for client preparation when cutting.

2. State your salon's expected service times for cutting services.

3. Why is it important to avoid cross-infection and infestation?

4. Why must you maintain your consultation throughout the cutting service?

5. Why is it important to position your cutting tools for ease of use?

6. Why must you cross-check your cut on completion?

7. Why must you apply the correct degree of tension during the cut?

8. Why must you give the client after-care advice?

Create a variety of looks using barbering techniques

Unit H21

Introduction

Cutting hair, whether it is men's or women's, requires a high level of skill to be successful. This unit focuses on using and combining an extensive range of cutting techniques to create traditional, current and emerging looks for men. You will use the cutting techniques you have previously learnt but will adapt them to create a diverse range of men's styles. The principles of cutting are the same for men and women; the differences lie in the outline and neckline shapes.

What you will learn
• Preparing the client • Creating the look • After the service

You the stylist

You need to be skilled in creating three different looks: traditional, current and emerging. The step-by-step photographs in this unit demonstrate how to create a current look.

Traditional

This type of look uses traditional barber-styling techniques to create a classic men's style, for example, the short back and sides.

Current

This type of look is the current fashion, though styles can change quickly. Spiked and textured styles are the latest fashion for men.

Emerging

This type of look is very modern and eye-catching. These are the styles that are seen on the fashion catwalk and are usually beyond what is expected commercially.

Preparing the client

In this section you will learn about the fundamental principles of preparing a client for the cutting service.

What you will learn

- Thorough consultation
- Checking for contra-indications and influencing factors
- Personal hygiene
- Personal protective equipment
- Preparing your work area.

You must always observe and follow the salon's code of practice including any relevant health and safety laws, for example, the correct gowning procedure and the safe disposal of used sharps. With thorough preparation, not only will you present a professional image but also ensure the best use of the time available.

Keys to good practice

In order to present a professional image, you should always shampoo a man's hair prior to cutting. This will prevent any damage to your cutting tools by removing dirt or debris from the hair. Your client may have come straight from work and his hair may be dirty. It will also show your professionalism by preparing the hair correctly for the cutting service.

Thorough consultation

The consultation you carry out with your client will determine your client's requirements. It also creates an opportunity for you to use your imagination and recommend what you think will be suitable. There are certain factors that you must consider when creating a style for a client (Unit G9 covers this in much greater detail). However, when consulting with a male client, there are other factors that must be considered such as:

- the presence of male pattern baldness
- the presence of added hair.

Both these factors, if present, need to be addressed in your consultation.

Male pattern baldness

If a client has male pattern baldness then your styling of the hair will need to be adapted to take account of this. There are several different types of male pattern baldness.

Some men prefer the hair to be cut very short or even shaved off completely to help disguise any thinning areas. However, some men prefer to leave the hair longer and comb across the thinning area. As the stylist, it is your responsibility to determine the client's requirements and advise on whichever is the most suitable option.

If the client has added hair, for example, a toupee, then when you cut the hair you must take account of this and blend the two together, keeping it as natural looking as possible. However, the specialist who supplies the hairpiece usually carries out this type of cutting.

A crew cut can help disguise thinning areas

Your client may wear a full wig and may require you to cut the hair very short to prevent any hair from showing beneath; this must also be taken into consideration.

The age of your client is something that you should consider. For example, children often need short, easy-to-manage styles that require little or no styling. You must also check to see if your client is wearing spectacles or a hearing aid. Both can present problems as they interfere with the lie of the hair after the cut and you will need to take this into account.

Keys to good practice

- Take the time to have a thorough discussion with your client and find out their exact requirements.
- Use a stylebook to help to clarify the look you and your client have in mind. This will ensure there are no misunderstandings between you regarding the final outcome.

Checking for contra-indications and influencing factors

There are several contra-indications and influencing factors that you must consider. Each one has different effects on the haircut that you are creating.

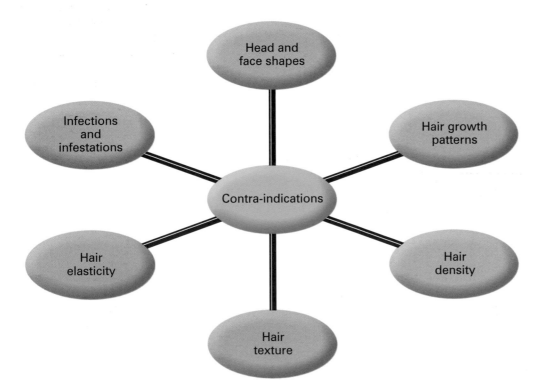

Each of these contra-indications and influencing factors has been addressed in greater detail in Unit G9.

As the majority of men have their hair cut short, the growth pattern in the nape area will determine the type of neckline you can achieve. The client will have great difficulty maintaining the style if the growth pattern conflicts. For example, if a strong nape whorl is present then it would create a problem for the client when the hair begins to grow, especially if cut into a round neckline.

Nape whorls

Check it out

List the methods of sterilisation used in your salon. Next, look at Unit G1 to remind yourself of the all the methods available and decide if you are using the correct methods for your salon's requirements.

Remember

If you follow strict rules of health and hygiene in the salon, the chances of passing on an infection or infestations will be greatly reduced.

Looking for infections and infestations is very important (see Unit G9). If you suspect the presence of these, you must inform the client of your suspicions immediately. You should then sterilise any tools and equipment that you have used to prevent the risk of cross-infection. Infections and infestations are illustrated on pages 51–2 in unit G9.

Personal hygiene

It is imperative to present a professional image at all times. This can be achieved only by maintaining high standards within the salon. You need to consider your own standards of hygiene as well as those of the salon. Washing regularly and using a good deodorant will ensure you always smell fresh. As you are working in close proximity to your client, your body odour and breath will be unmistakable. It is therefore essential to have fresh breath at all times, especially after lunch or a cigarette break. Strong odours such as onions or nicotine can be offensive to a client. Check that your hands and nails are also clean, as dirty fingernails will not convey a high standard of hygiene.

Personal protective equipment

Protecting yourself and the client should always be a high priority. When cutting a male client's hair, it is essential to ensure that you adequately protect their clothes from loose hair cuttings. The only protective equipment needed will be for the client's benefit, for example, the gown, cutting collar, or neck strip. You must be sure before you begin the cut that the gown covers all the clothing and no areas are left exposed that may become covered in hair. Secure the gown properly to prevent it slipping off. Always use some other type of protection over the gown, following your salon's requirements. For example, using a towel, cutting collar, or neck strip around the shoulders will provide added protection and help to prevent any loose hair from falling down the neck of the gown.

Your client should be gowned correctly

Keys to good practice

You must continue checking throughout the haircut that the personal protective equipment used still effectively covers your client. This will continue to protect the client's clothing from hair cuttings.

Preparing your work area

It is essential that you be fully prepared for the service that you are carrying out. The salon junior will play a vital role in ensuring that your work area is ready for you. Their training is of great importance and should be initially taught by watching you prepare the work area.

There are several aspects of preparation that must be checked prior to commencement.

- Make sure you have everything you will need with you.
- Check all tools and equipment are fit for purpose.
- Visually check any electrical equipment prior to use.
- Sterilise any necessary tools and equipment.
- Check the surrounding work areas are clean, tidy and free of excess hair.

Being fully prepared for your client will save you time in the long run. It also presents a professional image to the client if you are ready for the service. Having to excuse yourself to find something you forgot not only slows you down but can also irritate the client.

Check it out

What are the salon's rules regarding correct storage and handling of cutting tools and equipment?

In the salon

A client called into a salon and asked for a quick trim during a break from work. Simon decided he would carry out the cut and offered the client a seat at his workstation. The client stressed that, as it was his break from work, he would have to be quick and time was of the essence. Simon then went into the staff room and finished off his sandwich quickly because it was also his lunch break. When he came back, the client again stressed his limited time and asked him to be as quick as possible. Simon went to get a gown from reception but answered the phone whilst there, which delayed him even longer. When he had put the gown on the client, he realised that he had left his tool wrap and equipment on the workstation at the other side of the salon where he had been working last. He again excused himself and went to retrieve them. By this time, the client's patience had expired and he got up, removed his gown and left the salon in a rather disgruntled mood.

- Should Simon have offered to carry out the client's cut during his lunch break?
- Was Simon fully prepared for his client?
- What could a situation like this do for the salon's reputation?

Creating the look

In this section you will be looking at how to carry out men's hairdressing across a variety of looks, including the traditional, current and avant-garde looks.

What you will learn
• Cutting tools and their uses • Cutting techniques and effects • Neckline shapes • Cutting angles, guidelines and outlines • Correct positioning of self and client • Timings • Solving cutting problems

The act of cutting hair, whether it is men's or women's, demands a high level of skill. When cutting men's hair, you must be able to meet the demands of your client, whatever style he requires. To be successful, you need to have a sound knowledge of all the cutting tools available. You must also be able to achieve a variety of looks by adapting cutting techniques.

Cutting tools and their uses

There are many cutting tools available for use. You need to be familiar with each one and the effects you can achieve using them. Below is a table showing cutting tools and their uses.

Cutting tools	Uses	
Scissors	Used for a variety of techniques, e.g. club cutting, slicing, texturising or thinning	
Thinning scissors	Used to remove bulk but not length; only on dry hair	
Razors	Used to remove bulk or length, especially good for texturising; only on wet hair	
Clippers	Used for club cutting, especially good for creating very short styles	

Scissors

The scissors you use must be extremely sharp to function correctly. A good-quality pair need not be the most expensive, but always choose a pair that feels comfortable to use. When cutting men's hair, the majority of haircuts that you carry out are on short styles, which will require a lot of scissor-over-comb work. The length of the blade on your scissors is therefore very important. You will find it much easier to carry out good scissor-over-comb work using a pair of scissors with longer-length blades. As a guide, a minimum of six inches should be used. If you use scissors with a short-length blade then it may cause 'steps' within the haircut. Although these 'steps' are often removable, it will prolong the time that you spend on carrying out the haircut.

Thinning scissors

As well as straight-edged scissors, there are thinning scissors with serrated edges; these can also be called aesculaps or texturising scissors. This type of scissor is used to remove bulk but not length from the hair and should be used only on hair that is dry. They can be bought in a variety of styles, with either one or both of the blades having a serrated edge. The degree of serration may also vary and this will allow you to produce a variety of different effects. For example, thinning scissors with only one blade serrated will remove less bulk from the hair. However, if both blades are serrated then more bulk can be removed and, if the degree of serration is increased, a very textured look can be achieved.

> ### Keys to good practice
>
> - Thinning scissors can be used to remove 'steps' within the haircut if used on the ends of the hair.
> - Never use thinning scissors around the hairline, crown or near a parting. It may leave exposed, short spiky hairs that protrude off the head. Thinning scissors are especially good for use on thick hair but do not produce particularly good results on fine hair.

> ### Remember
>
> Any scissors that you use must be handled with care and well maintained in order to prolong their working life and to ensure they give you the best possible results with each cut. Blunt scissors can cause damage to the hair ends by splitting them. Each time you use your scissors, wipe them when you have finished the cut. Using light oil on the hinge regularly will prevent them from rusting or seizing up. You must sterilise them to prevent the passing on of infection or infestation. Due to the fact you are using them so close to the hair and skin, it is inevitable that they pick up bacteria from one client that could easily be passed onto another.

Razors

Razors are used in hairdressing to remove bulk and length and should be used only on wet hair. They are especially good at thinning the hair ends, producing particularly good textured looks. There are a variety of razors available for use and you will have to decide which one is right for you. The table below shows the types of razors available, with a description of each.

Type of razor	Description
Open razor	This type of razor has a fixed blade and needs to be stropped and honed to sharpen (see Unit H19); must be sterilised between clients
Safety razor	This type of razor has removable blades, making it more hygienic
Shaper	This type of razor is used only in hair cutting and is favoured in cutting women's hair

It is essential that you hold and use a razor correctly, not only for your own and your client's safety, but also to prevent damage to the hair.

The blade of the razor must be extremely sharp; this will prevent any damage to the hair ends or discomfort to the client. The hair must be kept thoroughly wet whilst cutting to allow the razor to slice into the hair more easily and again to prevent discomfort to the client.

In the salon

Asia was carrying out a short razor cut on a man's hair one day in the salon. He was a regular client and they were also friends socially. They were chatting and laughing about a recent night out they had both been on. Asia was telling her client a story about one of their mutual friends and she was being quite animated in her description. Unfortunately, whilst demonstrating the actions, she flung out her arms and dropped the razor from her hand. As it fell to the floor, it cut her leg quite deeply. She had to receive medical treatment for the wound and was unable to carry on at work that day.

- Was Asia taking the care necessary with her use of the razor?
- How could she have avoided this accident occurring?

You should always inform the client of the risk of ingrowing hairs after close razor or even clipper work. This can happen if the hair curls as it is growing and starts to grow back into the skin. It would be evident by a small lump in the skin that can become infected. They are, however, usually easy to remove by piercing the skin with a sterile surgical needle, allowing the hair to be freed. Ingrowing hairs are more likely to happen to a client with curly or African Caribbean hair. A client with dark skin will need to be advised about the changes that can happen to the skin with repeated use of razor work or even close clipper work. The area of skin that has been clippered or razored may start to thicken or darken causing discoloration of the skin that will be very noticeable below the hairline: this is known as 'shadowing'.

Clippers

Clippers are used a great deal in the cutting of men's hair, as they can produce very short styles. Clippers have two blades with serrated edges and during use one of the blades moves over the other to cut the hair.

Using clippers to produce a very short style

Check it out

Look at this photo of the correct method of holding a razor. You must practise holding the razor this way to ensure safety of use.

Check it out

Try using your razor to shave off a few hairs on your arm or leg whilst the hair is dry. Take care not to cut yourself! It feels like the hair is being ripped out and is most uncomfortable. This is what your client is feeling on their head if you razor cut dry hair.

Remember

Great care must be taken when using a razor; the risk of cutting the skin when using sharp implements must never be forgotten. This must also be remembered when cutting short hair around the eye or ear area. You will need to concentrate and not allow yourself to be distracted from your work.

Remember

Depending on the type of razor you use, you will either have to dispose of the blade or sterilise the razor after each use. You must follow the salon's rules regarding the disposal of used sharps. This will prevent the risk of harm or injury and also cross-infection.

Due to the style of the blades, it is essential that specialist services carry out the sharpening of the clipper blades (usually the manufacturer). The clipper blades must be cleaned after each use and are usually supplied on purchase with a cleaning kit, containing a small hard bristle brush and lubricating oil. The brush should be used to remove any loose hair cuttings and occasional use of the oil will ensure smooth running of the equipment.

Remember

As clippers are electrical, they must be used in line with the Electricity at Work Regulations.

Keys to good practice

If you are using clippers on thick or curly hair, you must open the blades using the lever on the side. This will allow the clippers to glide through the hair and will prevent pulling or dragging, which causes discomfort.

Cutting combs

There are two different types of cutting comb used in men's hairdressing. The traditional cutting comb is probably the most commonly used.

However, the barber styling comb is also used for cutting and is particularly useful for fine graduation, for example, tapering in the neckline or sides of the head. This is due to the fine teeth, which allow close-up work in confined areas, such as around the ears.

Clipper with attachments

Traditional cutting comb

Barber styling comb

Cutting techniques and effects

There are several cutting techniques used in the cutting of men's hair that you will need to become familiar with. The cutting techniques used in men's and women's hairdressing are exactly the same. It is the overall style produced that differs.

Club cutting

This technique removes the hair length only and gives the hair ends a very blunt look. Clubbing or blunt cutting allows you to cut very straight and precise lines. When club cutting, it is the angle at which you hold the hair that determines the finished effect. For example, if you wish to produce graduation, you will need to over direct the hair and hold at an angle above 45 degrees to achieve this. You have to hold the hair firmly between the fingers with even tension and ensure each section is thoroughly combed; this will produce an even cut. You can club cut on wet or dry hair, but it is more precise on wet. When you clipper cut the hair, you are also club cutting.

Scissor- and clipper-over-comb

Scissor-over-comb is most commonly used in men's hairdressing. It allows you to cut the hair very short and is especially good for blending short areas of graduation. To carry out this technique, you place the comb into the hair at the root area and pull out the comb away from the scalp up to the desired length. It is important to keep a flowing movement as you cut the hair that protrudes through the teeth of the comb. The scissors must open and close to cut at the same pace up the haircut or else lines will develop, known as 'steps'. Again, this type of cutting requires accuracy and a great deal of practice. Clipper-over-comb is done in exactly the same way, except the clipper blades are run over the hair protruding through the teeth of the comb. (Look at the step-by-step photographs on pages 187–8 to see an example of scissor- and clipper-over-comb.) Clipper-over-comb is better used on thick hair or when there is a lot of bulk to be removed. This technique is quicker and saves time.

> ### Check it out
>
> You can practise the movement of scissor-over-comb in the workstation mirror. Make sure that the comb follows the movement of the opening and closing scissor action and that you hold your comb in a way so that you can flip it over to comb down each section that you have just cut.

Tapering

This technique is used when you want to remove bulk or join together short and long layers. It can be done on wet hair if using a razor and dry if using scissors. The scissors slide into the hair and, as you slightly open and close the blades, care must be taken not to close the blade together or the hair will be cut straight across. With the razor method, you scoop into the hair sections and apply pressure according to the amount of hair you want to remove. This method requires a great deal of accuracy and skill so as not to cut off too much hair. Tapering will produce a textured look on short hair or blend short to long layers as in feathering.

Thinning

This method of cutting is used to remove bulk from the hair but not length. It is more commonly carried out with thinning scissors; however, there are scissor-thinning techniques that you can use. For instance, chipping into the hair at the root area will remove bulk and the shorter hairs will help to provide style support to the longer lengths.

Remember

If you have cut hair very short and there are 'steps' in the haircut that you cannot remove, a good tip is to use thinning scissors to go over the hair ends to remove them.

When barber stylists are seen using thinning scissors on longer length hair, instead of sectioning the hair off, they use the end of the blades to lift the hair up before placing the comb into the section. You must be sure that the blades are fully closed to prevent them cutting the hair if using this method. Look at the step-by-step photographs on page 188 to see an example of thinning.

Razoring

Razor cutting can be done anywhere in a haircut and removes bulk or length, depending on where you use the technique. With razor cutting, the hair is held between the fingers and can be cut either on top or below the section, with the razor held at a slight angle to the hair shaft. The amount of pressure you apply will determine the amount of hair removed, so take care – it is much safer to remove a little at a time than to take off too much. Razor cutting is especially good for creating very textured looks or for blending short layers into very long layers.

Check it out

Visit your council offices and look up the local bylaws for the use of fixed blade razors. This should give you information on safe practice.

Free hand

Cutting the hair without holding it between the fingers or comb is known as free-hand cutting. Free hand can be carried out on wet or dry hair. The hair is combed into place and cut without any tension being applied. It is particularly useful when cutting around an unusual growth pattern, for example, around a nape whorl. You must allow the hair to lie as it will without applying any pressure, and then cut. This will allow the hair to fall into its natural lie and will not look uneven when finished.

Texturising

Texturising is used to remove both length and bulk and can be carried out on wet or dry hair. The ends of the scissors are used to cut into the hair anywhere along the hair shaft, from mid-lengths to ends, depending on the effect you are trying to create. You can use it to produce a much more choppy, uneven finish or just to give softer broken edges. It can be incorporated into many different styles; for instance, when cutting a straight-edged one-length look, you can texture the ends to soften the edges.

Creating a current look: a step-be-step guide

Before the haircut.

The hair is cut using clipper-over-comb, working up the back of the head.

The sides are also cut using clipper-over-comb to reduce length.

Starting at the crown the hair is club cut to the desired length, working towards the front hairline.

Taking vertical sections and working around the head from the back to the front hairline, blend the hair into the side sections.

Once the club cutting is complete, the ends are point cut to create texture.

Any 'steps' between the shorter and the longer length are blended using scissor-over-comb.

The outline cut is done using taper clippers and the arching technique over the ears.

The nape line is then tapered using clipper-over-comb to produce fine graduation.

Any neck hair below the outline is removed using the taper clippers.

Once the hair has been dried off, bulk is removed using thinning scissors.

The finished look, styled using gel and wax.

Creating traditional looks

When creating traditional looks you will use traditional cutting techniques: scissor- and clipper-over-comb and club cutting. A commonly requested traditional look is a short back and sides. This style requires the barber stylist to cut the back and the sides to a much shorter length than the top sections. On the shorter lengths (the back and side sections) you will use scissor- or clipper-over-comb and for the longer lengths (the top sections) use the club cut technique. If the hair is thick then consider using the thinning scissors through the top to reduce bulk.

A short back and sides look

Creating avant-garde looks

When creating avant-garde looks you will need to use a variety of cutting techniques depending on the look you want to create. To create extreme looks it will be necessary to adapt your cutting techniques to allow for imagination in your work, for example, using a razor to produce extremes of short to longer lengths within a cut. All of the cutting techniques within the range can be used in a variety of ways to produce creativity and flair in your work, such as using clippers freehand to cut patterns into the hair, but this takes a lot of skill and practice to ensure accuracy.

Neckline shapes

When cutting men's hair, there are a variety of neckline shapes that can be created. They can be used together and separately to create many different effects. For example, a client may require a square neckline that has also been tapered. It is usually the client's choice that determines the neckline shape, as most men have a personal preference. However, other influencing factors must be considered, for example, hair growth patterns. The most common have been listed in the table below.

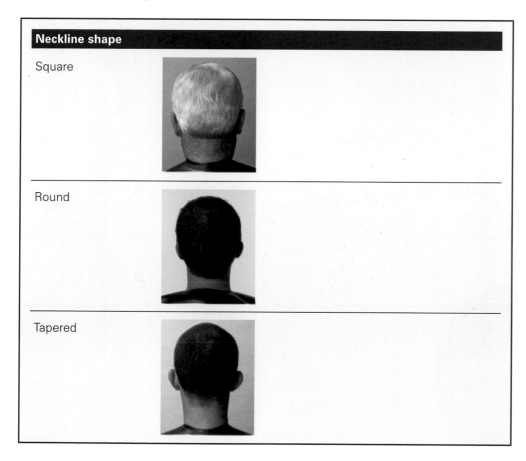

Neckline shape
Square
Round
Tapered

Keys to good practice

When cutting the neckline shape, always cut the sides of the neckline first and then across the neckline to join the two sides. This will allow you to judge the correct height at which to cut the neckline length.

Cutting angles, guidelines and outlines

It is extremely important that throughout the cut you are aware of the cutting angles you are using, as they will affect the finished shape and balance of the hair. It is also important that you are accurate in the way that you section the haircut. It is not always necessary to start at the back, but be sure to section off the hair and follow neat and even sections throughout the cut. Good sectioning will allow you to follow your guideline and ensure that no areas are missed; this looks professional to the client and results in the haircut being even at the end.

Below are some examples of the cutting angles used.

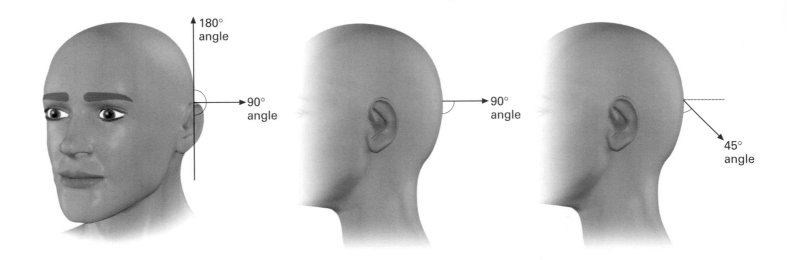

Different cutting angles

Most men's haircuts can be divided into three sections, as shown in the illustration below.

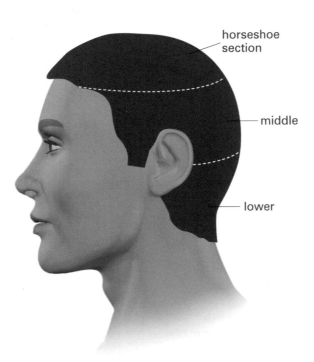

Men's haircuts can be divided into three sections

The lower section, into the nape of the head, is usually cut first, followed by the middle section, and then finally the horseshoe section from the temple, round the crown, and back to the temple on the other side. Each of these sections is blended into the other during cutting. Outlining a short or medium-length man's cut is essential to create a professional finish. Cutting around and over the ears is known as the arching technique and this is demonstrated in the step-by-step photographs on page 186. Any hair below the outline must be removed by using either the clippers or a razor to shave the hair away. If using the clippers then the small taper clippers are ideal as they cut closer to the skin.

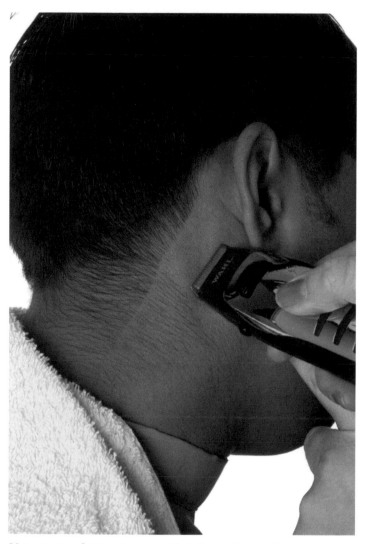

Using taper clippers to remove hair below the outline.

Remember

When using a razor blade on a client, the blade must be disposed of or sterilised after each use in line with your salon's policies. This will reduce the risk of cross-infection.

Check it out

What is your salon's policy for the safe disposal of used sharps? Does it adequately cover the lawful requirements of safe disposal?

Correct positioning of self and client

The correct position of your client is extremely important whilst carrying out the haircut. You must ensure that you position your client and their head in the correct way. This will prevent you from being restricted whilst cutting in difficult-to-reach areas such as the nape. You must make certain that your client is seated upright and not slouching. As you work your way around the haircut, be sure to position the client's head in a way that will assist you, without causing them any discomfort. If your client is not positioned correctly, it will not only restrict your cutting but could produce an uneven finished result.

Your own stance while working must also be considered at all times. The way that you stand to work will affect your posture and can lead to muscle fatigue if incorrect. Think about balancing the weight over your body when you stand and not leaning to one side for long periods. It is far too easy to put unnecessary strain on muscles and ligaments by over-reaching or stretching. However, this can be avoided by taking the time to adopt a good posture whilst working. Eventually it will become habit to stand in the correct position and you will soon do it without realising.

Look back at the 'In the salon' feature on Marco on page 169 of Unit H27. This is a good example of how poor posture can affect you over a period of time; you must take your posture seriously.

Timings

The time that you spend on a haircut will differ from client to client. However, the salon you work in will usually have expected service times and it is important that you are aware of these and work within them.

Check it out

Find out the expected service times in your salon for cutting services. Do both senior and junior staff work to the same expected service times?

Solving cutting problems

If any problems arise during the cutting service, it is essential that you are aware of the methods used to solve them. Usually problems arise because your consultation was not accurate. For instance, you begin the cut and then find that there is a conflicting hair growth pattern that is preventing you from getting the look you require. You will have to deal with problems such as these whenever they occur, but keep the client informed, use your professional judgement, and be tactful in explaining the situation. You must remain confident in your approach, stay calm, and never panic. This will serve only to alarm your client and they in turn will lose confidence in your ability. Below is a table of cutting problems and possible remedies that you may come across during the cutting process.

Cutting problem	Possible remedy
Sides are not even on finished cut	Cross-check; use the mirror and remove the longer length to even up
Cannot get close enough into the nape to cut to required length	Adjust the way you hold the hair for cutting or use a different cutting technique
Hair will not lie correctly around hairline	Adjust the finished style to incorporate the hairline's natural lie
Cut the client's or own skin	Stop immediately and clean the wound so that it is free from hair and apply pressure to stop bleeding; use a plaster if continuing

Another common problem is loose hair cuttings being allowed to fall onto the client's clothing. This can easily be avoided by securely fastening the gown and checking it throughout the cut to ensure it is still in place. Removing the cut hair during the cutting process also helps to prevent a build-up around the neckline.

Thorough preparation and staying focused on the service you are carrying out will help to prevent any problems arising.

Remember

A good tip if the cut hair is wet and sticking to the skin, is to use a little talcum powder on your neck brush to help to remove it.

Keys to good practice

- Be aware of critical influencing factors, such as growth patterns, at all times.
- If cutting wet hair, keep it wet throughout, especially if using a razor.
- Always take neat, even sections.
- Ensure that your tension is good and even throughout the cut.
- Make sure you can see your guideline before you cut a section.
- Never cut shorter than your guideline.
- Check regularly throughout the cut that it is level.
- Always cross-check your cut.
- Do not cut off too much hair when cross-checking, only the hair you have missed.
- Maintain the consultation throughout with the client to check what you are doing is to his requirements.
- If things go wrong, do not let the client see you are panicking.
- Remember, if you cut the hair too short, there is nothing you can do about it!

Cutting techniques and effects: a quick reference guide

Technique	Effect	Cut on wet, dry or either	Best suited to straight or curly hair
Club cutting	Gives a blunt, straight edge to the hair ends	Either, but more precise on wet hair	Either, but will help to reduce curl
Clippering	Gives a blunt, straight edge to the hair ends	Dry	Can be used on either, but open the blades slightly to aid cutting on curly hair
Thinning	Removes bulk but not length	Dry	Either, but will encourage curl
Razoring	Removes bulk and length; good for texturising	Wet	Either, but will encourage curl
Free hand	Removes length and bulk	Either	Either
Texturising	Produces softer, broken edges	Either	Either
Tapering	Removes bulk, gives texture	Wet with razor and dry with scissors	Either
Scissor-over-comb	Club cutting on short hair	Either	Either

After the service

This section is about completing the service in a manner that ensures the client leaves the salon fully satisfied. This may involve making recommendations for styling products for home use or making further appointments.

What you will learn

- Using styling products to finish
- Confirmation of the finished look
- Correct removal of the protective clothing
- Recommendations and intervals between cuts
- Disposal of waste, including sharps

Using styling products to finish

It is likely that the salon has a particular product range that you use and are familiar with. However, you must keep abreast of new developments within the styling range in order to ensure that your knowledge is up to date. There are several ways of doing this; for example, reading trade magazines, checking at the wholesale suppliers when you visit, or talking to technical representatives when they call into the salon with information on offers and developments.

There are several product companies that are dedicated to selling only men's styling products, but if your salon is unisex, you may wish to stock a range that caters for both men and women. Men are less likely to ask about how to maintain the style at home and it is your responsibility as the stylist to recommend the correct product for them to use. There are many styling products available and they each serve a different purpose; however, they can usually be categorised into whether they provide hold and/or shine for the hair. A client may have a preference as to the look they require or they may be looking for advice from you. Discuss your client's requirements and determine what the finished look requires the product to do – you will then be able to recommend something suitable.

The table below lists several men's styling products available for use and the effects they will help you to achieve.

A finishing product can help your client to maintain his hairstyle at home

Styling product	Effect achieved
Wax	Gives texture and will define curl
Dressing/styling crème	Will add shine to the hair; reduces static and will define curl
Hairspray	Will hold the hair in place; natural to ultra firm hold
Gel/gel spray	Will provide extreme hold, ranging from firm to ultra

---

Remember

Any products that you use in the salon must be stored, handled, used and disposed of following COSHH regulations (see Unit G1 for more detailed information). Following COSHH regulations shows professionalism, ensures that safety is of the utmost importance to you, and sets a good example to other staff.

Confirmation of the finished look

Confirming your client's satisfaction with his finished look is no less important than the rest of the service. Take the time to show the client the back and sides of the cut, using the back mirror. Check to be sure the client can see through the back mirror and adjust the angle of the mirror if necessary. Usually, if you can see through the mirrors then your client will also.

If the cut needs adjusting to the client's specific requirements, do not take this as a dislike of your finished work. You must look at it from the client's point of view – he wants the finished look to meet his expectations. Minor adjustments should be made but never a re-cut of the whole head. This should be left to another appointment. Do not be afraid to correct any mistakes, for example, a few longer hairs left above the ear. The client will thank you in the long run if he leaves the salon with a perfect cut.

Correct removal of the protective clothing

When removing the gown, always take care to take it off properly. Unfasten it correctly and ensure that any cut hair is thrown from the gown onto the floor and not over the client's clothing. If you do find there is some on his clothes, offer him a clothes brush to remove it but never let him leave the salon with hair on his clothes. This looks unprofessional and does not give a good impression of the salon. Remember that a client is looking for an all-round excellent service; he may think that although you have given him a fabulous haircut, your customer service skills leave a lot to be desired.

Recommendations and intervals between cuts

Never be afraid to give the client advice on styling, as it is a reflection on your salon's good name if his hair always looks good. He is, after all, a walking advertisement for you out on the streets. As you are finishing off, you can discuss with your client the styling techniques you are using and why and how the products are helping you to achieve the final look. Ensure you have a selection of brushes available for retail sale. A client may find it easier to style his hair at home using the tools that you use and it is another good selling opportunity.

Advise the client on when he will need to return to the salon for his next appointment. This may be for a service other than cutting, but generally, clients have their haircut maintained between every three to six weeks, unless they are growing their hair at which point they may want to leave a longer gap. Usually, no more than ten weeks is advised. If it is left any longer, the ends of the hair become more susceptible to splitting.

Disposal of waste, including sharps

There are different types of waste that must be disposed of safely in the salon. However, after a cutting service, it is only likely to be hair cuttings, used sharps, and empty product containers. Hair cuttings left on the floor can cause a slippery surface and this then becomes a hazard in the salon, both to you and the client when they stand up. Salons dispose of hair cuttings in different ways, but it is more hygienic to ensure that they are placed in a covered bin and put in the outside bin in a tied-up bag to prevent it spilling out.

A *sharps bin*

Used sharps must be disposed of with extreme care due to the risk of injury or cross-infection. A sharps bin must be used and this should be a sealed container with a clear label stating its purpose. You must follow the salon policy for the safe disposal of empty product containers; usually they are placed in a covered bin and put outside for refuse collection. However, in today's environmentally friendly society, recycling is becoming increasingly popular and your salon may be adopting a policy for this.

Remember

Aerosol containers, even when they feel empty, can still contain flammable materials. There is also a risk of them exploding if punctured or overheated so care must be taken with regards to their safe disposal.

Check it out

Using a selection of pictures or photographs of your own work, describe how you achieved the overall look and incorporated different cutting techniques. In your descriptions, indicate the cutting angles and list the tools and equipment you used. State which products you used to create the looks.

Knowledge check

1. Where would you find information on the use limitations of fixed blade razors?

2. What safety considerations must be taken into account when cutting men's hair?

3. What visual aids may be used during consultation to help ascertain the client's requirements?

4. What effects might close clipper or razor work have on dark skin?

5. Why is it important to cut to the client's natural hairline?

6. Why do you need to establish, and follow, a guideline during cutting?

7. What are the expected service times for cutting men's hair within your salon?

8. What are the recommended time intervals between men's haircuts?

Perm hair using a variety of techniques

Unit H29

Introduction

This unit is concerned with providing fashion-related perming services to clients. You will need an understanding of how to create movement in the hair using a variety of advanced winding techniques. The ability to personalise and adapt winding techniques to create current and emerging looks is essential. Consideration must be given to the condition of the client's hair, especially when working with sensitised hair, and this should be reflected in the perming techniques and products used.

Over the last decade, the popularity of perming hair has drastically reduced. However, both product manufacturers and the hairdressing industry have realised the enormous earning potential of perming becoming fashionable again. Every effort is now being made to educate the public in the benefits of permanently adding movement to the hair. Modern perm lotions are much gentler on the hair and most contain conditioning properties, allowing a more natural-looking curl or wave to be introduced.

Create beautiful natural-looking curls with perming techniques

What you will learn
• Preparing the client
• Creating the look
• After the service

You the stylist

You have a responsibility as a hairdresser to be aware of the latest developments in perming techniques and products and sell the benefits of these to your clients.

Preparing the client

In this section you will learn about requirements for preparing both yourself and the client for the perming process including:

What you will learn
• Thorough consultation
• Contra-indications and influencing factors
• Tests and testing
• Safe working practices
• Preparation of products, tools and equipment

Thorough consultation

The initial consultation with the client prior to any perming service should be carried out with rigour and accuracy. No detail should be left out; this will not only serve to fully inform you of the look the client requires, but allow you to thoroughly assess the client's hair. Establishing both the type of curl or wave required and the client's expectations of the new look will enable you to determine the correct winding technique and products to use on the hair.

You should be aware of your salon's expected service times and always work within them. It could help to let the client know how long the service might take, especially if it is a complicated wind or the hair is long, and you feel it may take longer than a regular perm. This will prevent any upset for the client if they are expecting to be finished by a certain time.

Keys to good practice

The use of visual aids, such as style magazines, will help to clarify what look the client requires and also assist you to demonstrate the look you feel is achievable with the client's hair.

It is during the consultation that you should be deciding which tests need to be carried out on the hair in order to determine its condition and previous history. A record of the conversation and the outcomes of any tests should be recorded on a consultation sheet along with the client's record card. This would prove extremely useful if you were faced with legal action following a perming disaster. You cannot always trust a client to be completely truthful about what has previously been used on her hair. You must stress to the client the importance of having a good knowledge of the hair and how this affects the products you are using.

In the salon

Mrs Hussein, one of Natalie's regular clients had made an appointment for a perm. Although Natalie had previously cut and styled Mrs Hussein's hair, she had never permed it. Mrs Hussein arrived for her appointment and Natalie was thorough in her consultation. She discussed with Mrs Hussein what her requirements were and asked her if she had used anything on her hair that Natalie should know about. Mrs Hussein was sure that she had not used anything on her hair and convinced Natalie that her hair was virgin. Natalie proceeded with the perming process without carrying out an incompatibility test, as she did not feel there was anything to be suspicious about.

When Natalie began to rinse the hair after the perm had developed, Mrs Hussein's hair just broke off with the perm rods still wound until all the hair had completely broken off her head. Natalie was horrified and very upset. She explained to Mrs Hussein what had happened and brought over the manager. Mrs Hussein was very distressed that she had no hair left on her head and was in complete shock. The manager immediately went out to buy her a wig and told Natalie to keep hold of the hair, as it would have to be tested.

Mrs Hussein was adamant that she had put nothing on her hair prior to the appointment, but the manager explained that there must have been something used on the hair that was incompatible.

When Mrs Hussein left the salon she went straight to a solicitor to seek legal advice, leaving the salon facing legal action. On completion of tests on the hair samples by the product manufacturer, it appeared that Mrs Hussein had henna in her hair and this had proved to be incompatible with the perm solution. Although this had not been disclosed to Natalie, she was, however, at fault for not carrying out an incompatibility test. This negligence caused the salon to have to pay the client compensation.

- How could this situation have been avoided?
- Is it more professional to trust what a client is telling you or to carry out tests regardless of what they say?
- Do you think the consultation sheet and record card would have been used here to help prove the stylist had asked the right questions during consultation?
- Even though the client had been somewhat at fault, what effect has this incident had on the salon's reputation?

Contra-indications and influencing factors

Both contra-indications and influencing factors play a vital role in determining the perming process and outcome. Although contra-indications and influencing factors can be very similar, they are not exactly the same. A contra-indication would prevent you from continuing with the service, whereas influencing factors may not necessarily prevent you, but would need to be considered in all the decisions you make while the perming service is taking place.

Contra-indications

Contra-indications should never be overlooked. If this happens, you could be presented with problems that you did not foresee. Below is table of contra-indications and how to detect their presence.

Contra-indication	How to detect their presence
Skin sensitivities	Thorough discussion with the client; look at the previous record card; ask about any known allergies or reactions
Previous history of allergic reaction to perming products	Ask the client during consultation; look at the previous record card or consultation sheet information
Known allergies	Ask the client during consultation
Skin disorders	Thoroughly check the skin and scalp prior to commencing the perming service
Incompatible products	Carry out an incompatibility test on the hair
Specific medical advice or instructions	Ask the client during consultation about any medical advice or prescribed drug use and, if you are unsure, ask them to seek further guidance from their GP

Influencing factors

These are just as important as any contra-indications and will have an effect on the outcome of the perming process. By giving careful consideration to these, you can ensure perfect perming results.

Temperature

The temperature in the salon will affect the speed of the development of the perm. If the room is cold then it will slow it down; alternatively, if the salon is hot this will speed up development. If you are using heat to accelerate the development time, you must consider the hair's condition. If the hair is porous or sensitised then the use of heat is likely to cause over-processing and irreparable damage to the hair's internal structure. Always follow the manufacturer's instructions as some perms require heat to develop.

Direction, degree and extent of movement required

The direction, degree and extent of movement required must be carefully considered. It will determine the choice of winding technique, the size and type of rod used, and the type of perm solution. In fact, it is crucial to determine your client's exact requirements in order to achieve a successful result.

Hair condition

The hair's condition will need to be given great consideration to prevent any damage to the hair. The condition will affect the choice of perm rod, solution and development times. If the porosity of the hair is misjudged, this can lead to over-processing and either breakage or a frizzy result. Alternatively, if you do not assess the hair's resistance tendency correctly, you may find a weak curl result and the hair left with a dull appearance.

Hair texture

The hair's texture should be determined to assist you with the choice of rod size and perm solution. If the hair is fine, it may accept perm solution more readily and a weaker solution will need to be used. However, if the hair is coarse, it can prove to be more resistant, which would necessitate the use of a stronger perm solution. Determining the texture correctly will prevent an unsatisfactory curl result.

Hair density

The hair's abundance will have to be taken into account when perming. If the hair is particularly thick and dense, it will affect the time taken to wind the hair and the amount of product used. It can also restrict the choice of winding technique for both finer and denser hair. With both of these extremes, consider the time and product used. This should be reflected in the price charged to the client.

Hair length

The length of the client's hair will not only affect the time spent and the amount of product used, but also the suitability of the winding technique and application of perm solution. If you are dealing with long hair and carrying out a spiral wind then you may have to wind with solution to ensure that perm solution reaches to the ends of the hair.

Keys to good practice

- Consider the time taken to wind and the effect the perm solution will have on the hair over a long period of time. This could be overcome by using a weak solution on the hair ends whilst winding.
- You may want to set the price for perming services according to hair length in order to maximise your profitability.

Growth patterns

Any growth patterns over the head should be taken into consideration to prevent problems arising during winding. You must ensure that the growth pattern does not conflict with how you wish the hair to be wound. Conflicting growth patterns can prevent a suitable result from being achieved by preventing the hair from lying correctly.

Haircut

Perming the hair should enhance and personalise a haircut. You should always balance the hairstyle with your perm choice. On completion, the perm should accentuate the features of the haircut, working with the style and showing off the haircut's best features. The amount of movement added to the hair should improve the look of the haircut, not work against it. This should be considered in the direction, degree and extent of movement you add to the hair.

Tests and testing

The tests carried out on the hair both prior to and during the perming service are essential in order to preserve the hair's condition and to reach a satisfactory result. The results of tests that are carried out may influence the decisions you make, especially if they reveal contra-indications. You will need to think carefully about the results and what your course of action will be in order to achieve success. Never underestimate the usefulness of testing the hair, as the potential consequences of failing to test can be catastrophic.

There are several tests that must be carried out and these are:

- elasticity
- porosity
- incompatibility
- development test curl
- skin test for African Caribbean clients or clients with sensitive skin.

Each of these tests has been thoroughly covered in Unit G9.

Safe working practices

While completing perming services in the salon, adhering to safe working practices is crucial in order to prevent the risk of harm or injury to yourself or your client. You have responsibilities under certain legislation to maintain safe working practices. For example, the products you use are covered by COSHH Regulations and any electrical equipment must be used in line with the Electricity at Work Regulations (see Unit G1).

Your own health is important and working while unwell is not recommended due to the risk of cross-infection. Keep yourself fresh and clean at all times – this will increase your stamina to work for long periods in the salon and will impress clients. Maintaining good posture while working will prevent the risk of long-term injury. As you will be standing for long periods of time whilst working in the salon, you will soon become fatigued and stressed if you adopt an unhealthy posture.

Always use the correct personal protective equipment whilst carrying out perming services. The gown, plastic cape, cotton wool and towel used on a client all serve to protect during the perming process. As the stylist, you should use an apron and gloves to protect yourself from the harmful effects of prolonged use of perm solution on the skin.

Preparation of products, tools and equipment

Organising the preparation of everything required before the service begins will demonstrate your professionalism and save time. You must ensure that the products are available for you to use (via a regular stock check), and that the tools and equipment used are clean, safe for use and at hand. Correct sterilisation of the tools you are using will serve to prevent the spread of bacteria (see Unit G1 to recap on sterilisation methods used in the salon).

Your salon assistant, if trained correctly, should support you in preparation. Initially, observing you prepare for perming will educate the assistant in what is required. Once he or she are aware of how this is done, it will save you time if your assistant prepares for you. It is crucial that you maintain clear and detailed communication with your assistant to prevent the misunderstanding of instructions. You may find it useful to ask the assistant to relay back any instructions given to allow you to clarify his or her understanding.

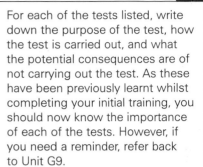

Check it out

For each of the tests listed, write down the purpose of the test, how the test is carried out, and what the potential consequences are of not carrying out the test. As these have been previously learnt whilst completing your initial training, you should now know the importance of each of the tests. However, if you need a reminder, refer back to Unit G9.

Remember

You must accurately record the outcomes of any tests that you carry out. Not only could this prove to be useful if a problem occurs, but it will also serve to assist you with further hairdressing services that you provide for the client. Consideration should be given to your responsibility under the Data Protection Act – any information you store on a client must remain confidential.

Check it out

Are you adopting and using the correct personal protective equipment when carrying out perming services in the salon?

Remember

Leaving the client unattended while you find the items needed for the service will waste valuable time and will make you look unprepared. This can be avoided by being thoroughly prepared.

Creating the look

This section contains information on how to carry out the perming process and the chemical effects on the hair structure. The benefits of creating movement in the hair should be impressed upon your clients, especially given the fact that perming has been less popular in recent years.

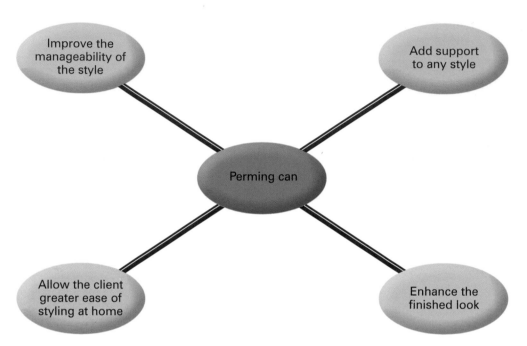

By stressing these important points, you may sway your client's decision on whether to proceed with a perming service.

What you will learn
• Perming science • Products, equipment and their use • Sectioning and winding techniques • Solving perming problems

Perming science

In this section you will learn about the chemical processes and the effects of perm lotions and neutralisers on the molecular structure of hair. It is essential that you fully understand what is happening to the hair structure during the perming process in order to ensure accuracy and success when carrying out perms. If you are not fully aware of the effects of the chemicals you are using, serious problems may arise that could result in you facing legal action.

Structure of the hair

Although you will have learnt about the processes of perming during your initial training, it is easy to forget about the structure of the hair and how it is affected during perming. The illustration opposite shows the structure of polypeptide chains inside the cortex and the disulphide linkages that are affected during the perming process.

Remember
It is essential to read the manufacturer's instructions and ensure you fully understand them before proceeding with any perming services.

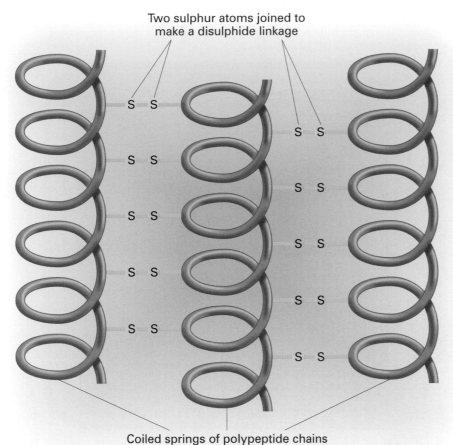

Two sulphur atoms joined to
make a disulphide linkage

Coiled springs of polypeptide chains

The breakage of the linkages allows the hair
to be moulded to the shape of the perm rod.

The structure of polypeptide chains inside the cortex

The disulphide linkages within the cortex are very strong and can be broken only by
chemical intervention. As you can see from the illustration above, they link together
the polypeptide chains within the hair's structure. A disulphide bond is also known as
a molecule of cystine, which is a bond of two amino acids joined together, that is, two
atoms of sulphur joining to form a disulphide bond.

During the reduction process when the disulphide bonds are broken by the addition
of hydrogen, the one molecule of cystine becomes two molecules of cysteine, as
indicated in the illustration below.

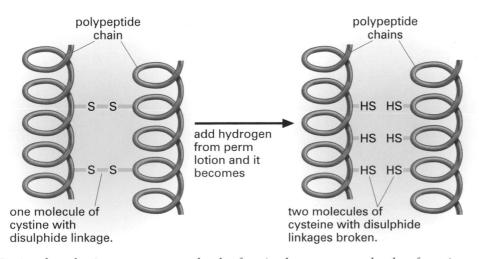

polypeptide
chain

polypeptide
chains

add hydrogen
from perm
lotion and it
becomes

one molecule of
cystine with
disulphide linkage.

two molecules of
cysteine with disulphide
linkages broken.

During the reduction process, one molecule of cystine becomes two molecules of cysteine

There are three stages to the perming process.

1   **Softening** – when perm lotion is applied to wound hair, it will initially swell the cuticle scales allowing the chemicals to easily enter into the hair's cortex.

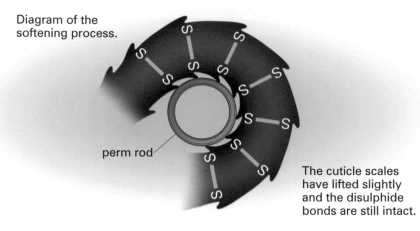

Diagram of the softening process.

perm rod

The cuticle scales have lifted slightly and the disulphide bonds are still intact.

2   **Reduction** – the reducing agent in perm solution adds hydrogen to the hair, which breaks the disulphide linkages allowing the hair to mould into the new shape created by winding around a perm rod.

Diagram of the reduction process.

By the addition of hydrogen. 25–30% of the disulphide linkages are broken during the reduction process

3   **Oxidation** – the neutralising process adds oxygen to the hair that attracts the hydrogen, leaving the sulphur bonds to re-form into disulphide linkages. The new shape has now become fixed.

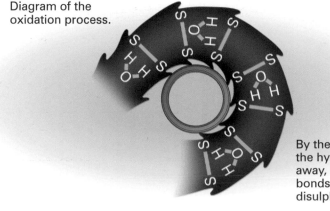

Diagram of the oxidation process.

By the addition of oxygen the hydrogen is attracted away, allowing the sulphur bonds to reform into disulphide linkages.

When carrying out the perming process, accurate timing and thorough rinsing of products is crucial. If care is not taken on both these points it may result in a weak curl, for example, not enough sulphur bonds re-forming during the neutralising process or chemical damage to the hair if left on too long.

The importance of the hair's condition

Once you understand the way in which perm solution works within the hair's structure, it is easy to see why there are perm solutions of varying types and strengths. For example, a client with coarse, virgin hair is likely to require a stronger, alkaline solution to allow the chemicals to enter into the tightly packed cuticle scales. Alternatively, a client with sensitised hair will need a weaker, acid-type lotion to prevent further damage occurring.

If you consider the hair's condition carefully before you begin then you can tailor your solution choice to the hair's needs. That is why pre-perm tests are crucial. If chemical processes or heat have previously weakened the hair, this will be detected by testing. You must give consideration to the condition of the cuticle layer and the structure within the cortex. If damage is apparent then great caution must be taken, as the hair will accept the perm solution more readily, which can lead to irreparable damage or even breakage of the hair.

The effects of temperature

The perming process can be affected in two ways by temperature. Firstly, if the room is too cold then this will slow down the process or even prevent the perm solution from working. Secondly, heat will speed up the process, which can serve to save time. However, you need to take care not to over-process the hair causing damage.

Differing types and strengths of lotion

There are many different types of lotions available for use and you will probably have found your preferences. Try not to become narrow-minded and think that the only perm solution you use should be the one you already know. New products are being developed all the time and you should regularly update your knowledge by attending training events or asking technical representatives for advice.

Due to the vast choice we have available to us, you need to be aware of the chemical composition of perm lotions and how they affect your choice for use on different hair types.

> ### Remember
>
> Only 25–30 per cent of the disulphide linkages should be broken during the perming process. If the solution is left on too long and more than 30 per cent are broken, this will result in irreparable damage to the hair's internal structure.

> ### Remember
>
> If the hair is already sensitised, the addition of heat is not advised, as the perming process will be quite speedy due to the weakened state of the hair.

Type of perm lotion	Chemical composition	Additional information
Alkaline	Aqueous alkaline solution of reducing agents; ammonium thioglycolate	Stronger and more likely to give a firmer curl; useful on resistant hair
Acid	Thioglycolic acid activator and alkaline base lotion, ammonia or sodium hydroxide	Particularly useful on previously chemically treated or sensitised hair due to its acidic nature
Exothermic	Aqueous alkaline solution of reducing agents; ammonium thioglycolate	Needs additional heat to activate the buffer ingredient

Pre- and post-perm conditioners

The use of a conditioner before a perm may sound like a contradiction in terms because we always think of conditioners as creating a barrier to the perm solution by coating the cuticle scales. This is, in effect, true and if a surface conditioner were to be used prior to a perming service then it would create a barrier to the solution entering the cortex. However, if the hair has been previously chemically treated or is sensitised, the use of a restructurant conditioner will help to prevent any further damage. The restructurant works by balancing out the porosity in the hair and allowing the perm solution to work evenly on the hair structure, thus preventing any further chemical damage by over-processing.

Following all perming services, irrespective of the type, it is essential to restore the hair to its natural pH balance. This can be done by the use of a pH balancing conditioner, which also serves to prevent creeping oxidation. These are known as anti-oxidant conditioners. When used, they not only help to stop the oxidation process, but they add moisture to the hair and restore it to its natural acidic pH balance.

Products, equipment and their use

This section is divided into two parts: products and equipment. There are many products and types of equipment available for use when perming and it would be impossible to have a working knowledge of every one. You will, however, be familiar with the ones you have chosen to work with in your salon. You should not let this familiarity become a barrier to you trying new products or equipment – you could be missing out on something extremely beneficial to you.

Products

When carrying out perming services in the salon, you must ensure that you are familiar with how to use all the products correctly. This will demonstrate your professionalism and reduce the risk of wastage. Using products economically will ensure cost effectiveness since throwing away waste products is throwing away money! Care should be taken when measuring out products and overuse should also be avoided. You have a responsibility to ensure that all staff, including junior staff, are trained in the correct use of the products.

The products you choose to use when carrying out perming services are likely to be the ones you have a good knowledge of, particularly if your salon uses only one product manufacturer. Do not let this familiarity cloud your judgement on other products available; you may try one that is not only more economical to use, but gives better results. In the table on page 207, you will see listed all the products you need to use when perming hair with a description of their uses. (A cross-section of product manufacturers has been represented.)

Many manufacturers produce products suitable for permed stlyes

Product	Uses
Barrier cream	Used to protect the client's skin from the harmful effects of perming chemicals
Pre-perm treatments	Used to even out the porosity of hair prior to a perm being carried out
Perm lotion	Used to break the disulphide linkages in order to mould the hair into a new shape
Neutraliser	Used to re-form the disulphide linkages in order to fix the hair into a new shape
Post-perm treatments	Used to prevent creeping oxidation and to restore moisture and pH balance after the perming process

Keys to good practice

Never be afraid to show the client that you are reading the manufacturer's instructions, especially if you are not familiar with the product. Explain that you want to be sure you are using the product to its best advantage on their hair. This will help to boost their confidence in your ability and show your professionalism.

Types of perm lotions

When choosing the type of lotion to use, you need to consider the hair's condition, previous chemical treatments, and the results of any tests you have carried out. This will help to determine which lotion will give you the best results.

Check it out

Look at the following case studies and decide which type of lotion you feel will give you the best results or whether you think the hair will be suitable for perming. Consider also the use of pre-perm treatments.

Case study 1

The client has below-shoulder-length hair in good condition; however, the last six centimetres still have the remnants of a previous perm. She would like a spiral perm that has a firm curl.

Case study 2

The client has above-shoulder-length, layered hair, with bleached highlights that were last touched up only two weeks ago. She would like a perm to add body and volume but not curl.

Case study 3

The client has a shoulder-length bob but has a full-head permanent tint to cover over white hair. She would like a perm to add body to her lank hair.

Case study 4

The client has below-shoulder-length, layered hair and has recently had a full head of bleached and high-lift tinted highlights. She uses straightening irons daily, which has caused heat damage, and would like a perm to add movement and wave that she can straighten easily if required.

Types of neutraliser

You have read about the various types of perm lotions, but you will also find several types of neutralisers available for use. Some require you to dilute them with water on a 1:1 ratio and you must read the instructions carefully to ensure correct use. The neutraliser you use may be a foam-before-use type that is applied using a sponge and bowl, or the type that is applied straight from the bottle that it is supplied in.

Pre- and post-perm conditioners

Although these have been previously covered on page 207, it is important to consider the different types available for use. Pre-perm conditioners, also known as restructurants, are available in small bottles for individual use or larger bottles for bulk usage. Whichever you feel is more suitable for you will determine which one you buy. You need to consider that a large bottle will allow you the benefit of no wastage on shorter or finer hair while an individual bottle can be sold to a client for use at home.

Restructurants can also be used to aid the hair's manageability following chemical or heat damage, or for use before and after colouring services, making it a versatile product. Post-perm treatments are essential to return the hair to its natural acidic pH balance and will also close the cuticle scales that have been lifted during the perming process, thereby restoring moisture to the hair. They are known as anti-oxidant conditioners and can also be used after colouring services, as this again is an oxidation process. A post-perm treatment will serve to prevent creeping oxidation; this is when the oxidation process continues working in the hair's structure and can cause chemical damage. They are usually bought in bulk for use at the back-wash area and are an essential part of the perming process.

Equipment

There are many different types of rod available for use when perming. You may be familiar with a wide range that is already used within your salon or you may be looking to expand your knowledge and experience.

The table below shows a range of the types of rod available and their uses. Look at the photographs in this unit to see how they are used in the hair to create different effects.

Type of rod	Uses of rod
Traditional	This type of rod is the most commonly used and can be used in a variety of ways to produce many different effects
Spiral	This type of rod is used to create spiral curls on medium to longer-length hair
Wella Formers	Used to create soft waves on medium-length hair
L'Oreal Techni-wavers	Used to give volume or soft waves on shorter-length hair
Bendies	Used to create various effects, including spirals, curls and waves, on most hair lengths
Pin-curl clips	Used to create volume and lift on shorter hair; must be plastic as metal clips may react with chemicals used during perming process

Sectioning and winding techniques

The way in which you section and wind the hair will have been decided following a thorough and detailed consultation with your client. This section contains photographs of various winds, all of which you will have to carry out to complete the range.

Piggyback

This wind is carried out by taking fine sections with a section of hair between two rods left out and wound on top of the two rods underneath. This will allow the rod to sit on top of the two underneath, as shown in the photograph below. They are usually wound from the nape up to the front. This wind is useful when you want to put plenty of volume and curl into the hair, particularly if the hair is abundant. You can alternate the size of rod used to create curls of varying tightness over the head.

Spiral

This wind can be carried out using a variety of tools, for example, spiral rods, traditional rods, bendies or chopsticks. It is usually wound from the nape up to the front. It is used to create spiral-type curls, can be carried out on medium to shoulder-length hair and is best suited to a style with some layering.

Weaving

This type of wind is carried out by winding the hair in any direction but weaving to leave out some as you go along. It can be used on hair of any length and is useful to achieve different textures throughout the hair. Care must be taken when applying perm lotion and neutraliser to prevent it from touching the weaved-out sections, as this hair should remain un-permed. Using conditioner on the hair and wrapping it in packets or clingfilm will serve to protect the weaved-out sections.

Stack

A stack wind is carried out by winding from the nape up. The effect you want to achieve is curl on the ends and straighter mid-lengths and roots. Therefore, as you wind up the head, the rods are wound leaving more of the root and mid-length out, allowing it to stack out in this way. It is particularly useful if the client requires curl on the ends of the hair only.

Root

This type of wind is used to give volume and style support at the root area. It is most commonly used on shorter styles, although if a client has very long hair and has a perm that is considerably grown out, you may just need to perm the root area to avoid over-perming the mid-lengths and ends. The ends of the hair can be blocked out by the use of conditioner and wrapping in clingfilm or packets, or alternatively, the hair can be wound leaving the ends out but protected. Great care must be taken to prevent any chemicals from touching the ends.

Hopscotch

This wind is carried out on any length of hair, except very short, and produces an extremely textured look with curl or wave going in various directions. The hair is wound, leaving out a fine section between each rod. The hair that is then left out is wound over the top of these rods in a conflicting direction, as demonstrated in the photograph. It is usually wound from the nape up to the front.

Double wind

This type of wind is carried out by starting to wind the hair as normal and then introducing another rod along the section to give the effect of a tighter curl on the end and a looser curl at the root area. It is used on longer-length hair to create varying curl along the length of the hair. It is useful if a client requires a loose wave at the root area and tighter curl towards the ends of the hair. It is usually wound from the nape up to the front.

Keys to good practice

Although most perm winds can be started anywhere on the head, if you are winding longer-length hair, it is much easier to wind starting at the nape and working up the head, as this will allow you to section hair out of the way while you are working and build up the wind as you go.

Consideration must be given to your application, development and neutralising of differing winds. You will need to judge the requirements of the product you are using and the outcomes of your consultation and tests to determine how to apply the lotion. It may be necessary to wind with solution; however, if the wind is complicated or the hair is sensitised, then application of the lotion after winding may be required. Whilst developing the perm, you may be required to carry out a development test curl and this must be done without disturbing the rest of the wind. Care should be taken not only to test hair in several places over the head, but also to prevent the pattern of the wind from being disrupted.

Once development is complete and the neutralising process is being carried out, you will again have to consider the wind used. It may be necessary to rinse the lotion at the front washbasin if the position of the rods prevents access at the nape or to prevent lotion from being rinsed over untreated hair. Care should be taken to ensure that all rods are both rinsed well and completely covered with neutraliser to prevent chemical damage or straight pieces. This will be more relevant with winds such as piggyback, hopscotch or double, where an extensive number of rods are used.

Remember

It is crucial to take great care when working on sensitised hair to protect the hair from further damage. It is imperative to use a winding technique suitable for the hair's condition and consider the hair's needs during application, development and neutralising. For example, using a solution or particular wind that requires you to wind the hair with solution, would not be an option on sensitised hair. The importance of taking special care cannot be stressed enough.

Solving perming problems

As perming is a detailed process, there are several problems that may arise. Even an experienced stylist can make mistakes and, if you are aware of how to deal with problems if and when they occur, you will never feel overwhelmed by them. Most importantly, any faults should be identified and dealt with as soon as possible. The table below identifies several faults and the possible causes and remedies of each.

Fault	Possible cause	Remedy
Fish hooks	Hair ends not wrapped around the rod correctly	Cut them off
Straight pieces	Perm lotion or neutraliser not applied evenly; an uneven wind	If hair condition allows, re-perm the straight pieces
Uneven curl result	Perm lotion or neutraliser not applied evenly; uneven winding technique; uneven tension on the wind	If the hair condition allows, re-perm the affected areas
Skin/scalp irritation	Chemicals used are too strong or have been left in contact with the skin	Rinse affected area immediately with cool water and seek medical advice if serious
Frizz	Lotion used too strong; over-processed or excessive tension used on winding	Re-style to remove some of frizz; apply restructurant or course of penetrating conditioning treatments
Hair too curly	Lotion too strong; over-processed; rods used were too small	If hair condition allows, reduce curl by relaxing
Hair not curly enough	Lotion too weak; under-processed; rods used were too large; poor neutralising	If hair condition allows, re-perm
Discoloration of hair	Metal tools allowed contact with the hair; presence of metallic dyes in hair	Colour over the affected areas with suitable colouring products
Pull burn	Tension on wind allows perm solution to enter follicle	Rinse immediately with cool water and seek medical advice if serious
Perm drops out	Poor neutralising; excessive tension used when drying hair	If hair condition allows, re-perm
Breakage	Over-processed; lotion too strong; too much tension applied on wind; bands placed incorrectly on rod	Use a restructurant or course of penetrating conditioning treatments
Band marks	Rubber bands placed incorrectly on rod	Use a restructurant or course of penetrating conditioning treatments

Although many difficulties may arise during perming, thorough consultation and preparation will help to prevent them. Most are easily remedied and worrying about what might happen should not put you off. You must, however, consider the role of your assistant and you should feel confident that you have fully prepared him or her to deal with his or her role in the process, making him or her aware of the consequences of not carrying out your instructions correctly.

Check it out

Look at the four case studies below and decide for yourself how each problem could have been avoided and what remedial action could be taken.

Case study 1

A client has had a perm a couple of days previously and has returned to the salon to complain, as she feels there is little curl left in her hair.

Case study 2

On completion of a perm, while blow-drying, you are having difficulty curling the hair. The hair is frizzing and feels dry and brittle.

Case study 3

After neutralisng a perm, you notice that the front section on the side of the head appears to have little or no curl in it.

Case study 4

While a perm is processing, a client complains that the lotion feels as if it is burning her scalp. On inspection you notice the scalp looks very red.

After the service

After the service you will need to dispose of any waste materials or products safely and complete an accurate record of the service carried out. You must also give your client advice on how to maintain and care for the perm at home.

What you will learn

- Disposal of waste
- After-care advice
- Completion of the record card

Disposal of waste

On completion of the service, you must dispose of waste following your salon's policies and legislative requirements. Waste chemicals should be washed down the sink and not put into the general waste bin; this will prevent the risk of contact by an unsuspecting person. Any other waste, such as end papers or cotton wool, must be placed in a covered bin along with empty containers.

After-care advice

You have a duty to your client to ensure that she understands how to look after her new look. How she maintains her hair on leaving the salon will advertise your work. Initially, the hair will be fragile after perming and care must be taken when styling not to apply too much tension. This might not only cause the hair to stretch and possibly break, but you also run the risk of pulling out the perm, leaving the hair straight again.

You should be advising the client to use a suitable shampoo and conditioner for curly/permed hair and also recommending the correct styling products to use to create the finished look. Successful management of the permed look will depend on using the correct styling products and how the hair is styled into place. There are products available specifically for permed and curly hair such as mousses, defining jelly and serum.

Completion of the record card

Completing the record card after the service is an essential requirement. It will keep a record of what has previously been used on a client's hair, providing you with a history, which is important when making further decisions on chemical processes. The diagram below indicates the minimum amount of information that should be stored on the card.

You should advise your client to use products specifically for permed hair

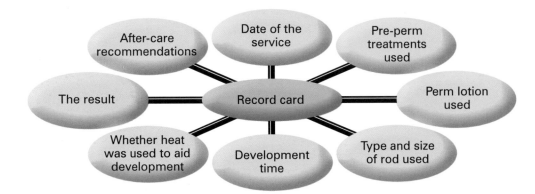

This information needs to be accurate, legible and up to date. Under the Data Protection Act, you are responsible for maintaining the information and ensuring its confidentiality. If any problems arise from the perming service, the information contained on the card will prove to be useful, especially if the client takes legal action against you. Accurate information could help to prove your competence.

Knowledge check

1. Why is it important to record client responses to questioning during a consultation?

2. What important influencing factors must be taken into consideration before the perming service?

3. List the five tests carried out before the perming service, and briefly state their purpose.

4. List the personal protective equipment used during the perming service for both the client and the stylist.

5. Which strong bonds are broken during the reduction process?

6. What factors might cause the hair to over-process during perming?

7. Why would you use a pre-perm treatment?

8. What is the effect on the hair of using an anti-oxidant conditioner?

Colour hair using a variety of techniques

Unit H30

Introduction

This unit is concerned with combining, adapting and personalising colouring techniques. You will need to be able to produce a variety of fashion effects in a way that complements the style you are creating. You will also be required to restore depth and tone of colour and neutralise unwanted colour tones. Colouring the hair will allow you to use your artistic flair and represent the looks you are creating in an innovative way. In terms of chemical treatments, colouring the hair has become substantially more popular than perming over the last decade and, with this in mind, product manufacturers have developed many more interesting and expansive colour ranges and treatments. This gives you, the stylist, a broader spectrum of choice when colouring a client's hair, allowing you more versatility in the work you produce.

You should consider all the reasons why a client may come to the salon for a colour. This will help you to realise the importance of colouring in the salon.

Colour allows you to create more innovative looks

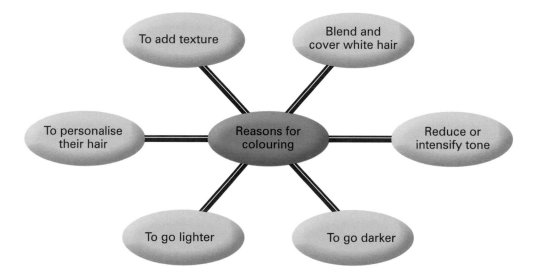

What you will learn

- Preparing the client
- Preparing for the colouring service
- Colouring techniques
- Solving colouring problems
- After the service

You the stylist

While carrying out your initial training, you will have learnt the importance of the shade chart and the international colouring system. In building on this foundation of knowledge, you must now move forward and develop your colouring skills further to allow you vision and diversity in your colouring work. The more confidence you build in your ability, the more inspirational your work will become.

Preparing the client

Preparation is the key to success when colouring. Thorough preparation will prevent problems arising such as running out of a colouring product or incompatibility of the product you are using with the client's hair. Ensuring you are fully prepared and ready for the service will not only present a professional image, but also allow you to work within the expected service times for your salon.

Check it out

What are your salon's expected service times for colouring work?

What you will learn

- Thorough consultation
- Contra-indications and influencing factors
- Tests and testing
- Safe working practices
- Preparation of products, tools and equipment

Thorough consultation

Before providing colouring services to your clients, the consultation you carry out is essential to extract the correct information, allowing you to proceed with the correct colour choice and techniques. Remember, the use of visual aids, such as shade charts, are very useful in helping the client choose a colour. You will have to rely on your excellent communication skills, as clients are not always aware of the consequences of misinforming the stylist regarding any previous colour treatments they have had. To ensure your success, you should complete a consultation sheet with your client. This will not only prevent you from forgetting to ask an important question, but will serve as a written record of the discussion you have had. This could prove to be extremely useful if you are faced with legal action as a result of a colouring service.

Shade charts can help your client to choose a colour

Keys to good practice

If a client wants a particular colour treatment and you suspect there is something on the hair that may cause a problem, you cannot always trust a client to tell you the truth, even if you have explained the consequences. Therefore, any written record of the consultation will prove useful if the client challenges you later.

During the consultation you will need to assess how the client's hair needs to be prepared for the service. If you are unsure, always check the manufacturer's instructions, as it may be a requirement that the colour is applied to clean, freshly shampooed hair. The way the hair is prepared for the service will play a vital role in the colour result and, if you prepare the hair incorrectly, the results may not be as you or the client expected. This would cause both yourself and your client to feel unhappy and dissatisfied and you may lose the client, along with your confidence in your ability to colour hair.

Contra-indications and influencing factors

Although these two can be very similar, they are not exactly the same. A contra-indication would prevent you from continuing with the service, whereas influencing factors may not necessarily prevent you but must be considered in all the decisions you make while the colouring service is taking place. Influencing factors can sometimes prove to be contra-indications. For example, if a client is suffering from an adverse skin condition and it proves to be infectious, this would present you with a contra-indication that would prevent you from continuing.

Contra-indications

It is important that you question your client to ascertain whether they have any contra-indications to the colouring service, as sometimes they may not be apparent by observation alone. A few minutes spent questioning your client may save hours of time and possibly money should there be problems (which could have been avoided) during or after the service.

Contra-indications should always be carefully considered. Never overlook their presence, as this could present you with problems that you did not foresee. The table below shows contra-indications and methods that may be used to assess the problem.

Contra-indication	How to assess the problem
Skin sensitivities	Carry out a skin test prior to the colouring service
Previous history of allergic reaction to permanent colouring services	Ask the client during consultation and look at previous record card or consultation sheet information
Known allergies	Ask the client during consultation and record any known allergies
Skin disorders	Thoroughly check the skin and scalp prior to commencing the colouring service
Incompatible products	Ask the client about any colour products they may have used in between visits. Carry out an incompatibility test on the hair
Medical advice or instructions	Ask the client during the consultation about any medical problems they may have that could prove problematic. If necessary, ask for notification from their GP

In the salon

Margaret came into the salon for a colour service. She did not want a permanent colour, as the condition of her hair was quite poor due to several bleached highlight services. Her hair was very fine and below the shoulder in length, and her skin was quite pink in colour. She thought an overall colour might be more suitable until the condition of her hair had improved and a quasi-colour was recommended. The stylist did not carry out a skin test, as she did not think it was necessary because she was not using a permanent colour.

The stylist applied the colour and, during the development, Margaret complained that her scalp felt quite sensitive and itchy. The stylist removed the colour immediately with cool water and noted the hairline and scalp were very red and looked quite 'angry'. However, she assured Margaret it would subside and not to worry. Margaret had in fact had an allergic reaction to the colourant.

- How could this have been avoided?

Influencing factors

Influencing factors should never be overlooked. Giving full consideration to these will help to produce perfect colouring results.

Temperature

As you have previously learned in your hairdressing training, the temperature of the salon will influence the processing time. A cold salon may slow down the processing time while warm temperatures will speed up the process. Use of heat to develop colours quickly is useful; however, the porosity and condition of the hair needs to be considered, as hair in poor condition will accept colour more readily. You should take extra care when developing bleach using an additional heat source, as the bleach may develop more quickly than you expected, resulting in over-processed hair.

Keys to good practice
Always check the manufacturer's instructions to establish whether the colouring products should be developed using additional heat.

Body temperature plays an important role when carrying out a full head colour, as the colour on the roots of the hair will process more quickly than the colour on the end. This is because its development is speeded up by the addition of body heat. Therefore, when carrying out a full-head lightening or full-head red application, you should apply the colour to the mid-lengths and ends first, and the roots last. This will prevent the colour being too light at the roots (in the instance of a lightening application) and will prevent root glare when using 'reds'.

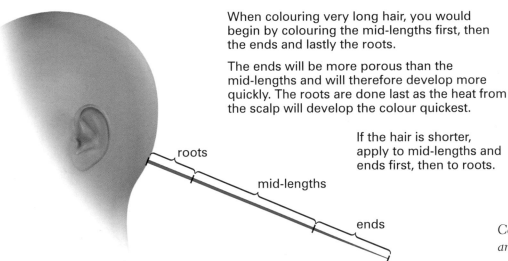

When colouring very long hair, you would begin by colouring the mid-lengths first, then the ends and lastly the roots.

The ends will be more porous than the mid-lengths and will therefore develop more quickly. The roots are done last as the heat from the scalp will develop the colour quickest.

If the hair is shorter, apply to mid-lengths and ends first, then to roots.

roots

mid-lengths

ends

Colour being added to the lengths and ends of the hair

Existing colour of hair

The depth of hair colour needs to be considered, as permanent tint will only lift 3 to 5 shades. Therefore, if you have chosen a colour that needs to be lifted 6 or 7 shades, this cannot be achieved by permanent colouring and bleaching will have to be advised. You should always consider the capabilities of the products you are choosing from, for example, a quasi-permanent colour is not designed to lighten the hair, but is intended to add tone to the existing hair colour. Determining the hair's existing colour is important to ensure you choose the correct colour to apply and the correct hydrogen peroxide strength.

If the hair has previously been coloured, this must also be taken into consideration, as it will both affect and determine the choice of colouring products that you may use. Test cuttings are very useful in these instances.

Hair condition

It is essential that you determine the condition of the client's hair, as it will affect your colour choice and development times, and possibly your method of application. You must also consider whether the hair's condition is actually good enough to accept the service, as in some cases the addition of more chemicals will cause the condition to deteriorate. In this instance, you may need to use a pre-colouring treatment. These treatments even out the porosity of the hair and help to rebuild the internal fibres.

As previously stated, hair in poor condition accepts colour more readily; however, if the hair is in good condition, there is a greater chance of resistance. If you feel the hair may be resistant to the colour application then you should consider pre-softening the hair to open the cuticle scales, allowing the colour molecules into the cortex. The hair's condition will also influence the advice you give regarding care of the hair. For example, the use of a good-quality shampoo and conditioner for colour-treated hair will help the colour to retain its vibrancy and tone.

In the salon

John was very busy in the salon and had fallen behind due to several late clients. Suzanne arrived at the salon to have bleached highlights. As John was very busy, he did not carry out a thorough consultation. Suzanne's hair was 'mousy' brown and he felt bleached highlights would be fine. He applied the foils quickly and left the colour to develop whilst he finished his previous client.

He went back to Suzanne to check on the colour development and discovered her blonde highlights were in fact pale pink. He then asked Suzanne if she had coloured her hair recently, to which she replied, 'No.' After lots of searching questions, Suzanne finally admitted that she had in fact coloured her hair black and did not like it so she bleached it blonde. After a few weeks, she decided she did not want to be blonde any more, so she coloured it brown. Fortunately, John was able to correct the colour for Suzanne, who eventually left the salon quite a few hours later.

- What went wrong?
- How could this situation have been avoided?

Length of hair

You need to consider the length of the client's hair before colouring as it may affect the price and the time allocated for the colour treatment. For example, long hair will require more product and more of your time, whereas shorter hair will be quicker to complete and use less product; this should be reflected in the price. Another factor is the technique you use to apply the colour. If a client has very long hair and requires bleached highlights, you will need to bear in mind that bleach develops at varying times. Consideration would have to be given as to where on the head you started and which technique you used. Alternatively, if a client had very short hair, trying to wrap colour in foil packets could prove difficult and you may consider a polishing technique. Polishing is applying colour by placing it on a piece of foil and lightly brushing it over the hair, which deposits colour anywhere you choose.

Polishing service taking place on short hair

Haircut

Colouring the hair should enhance and personalise a haircut. You should always balance the hairstyle with your colour choice. On completion, the colour should accentuate the features of the haircut and be working with the style. In addition, it should accentuate the client's best features, for example, the colour of their eyes.

Hair density

If a client has particularly thick, dense hair then you will have to consider the cost of using more of the products and the time it may take. Again, the technique may be affected; if you need to apply the colour quickly, will you be able to on thick hair? Alternatively, if the hair is sparse and fine then great care needs to be taken to prevent staining of the skin and scalp, which would be clearly visible through fine hair.

> **Keys to good practice**
>
> When selecting colour, the hair density should be considered. Colour on thick, dense hair may appear darker than the same colour used on fine, sparse hair, as there is a greater concentration of colour present.

Percentage of white hair

The percentage of white hair will influence the type of colour and hydrogen peroxide choice. As the hair has no colour pigment, you are always darkening it; therefore, 20 volume, or 6 per cent hydrogen peroxide, should always be used when colouring the hair permanently. You will also need to be able to determine the percentage of white and decide the ratio of base shade to tonal shade. This is especially important when using strong fashion tones, as failure to add base with the fashion tone may lead to a more vibrant result, especially on the white hair. The table below shows the basic rules for mixing colour for use on white hair; however, always check with the product manufacturer's recommendations.

Percentage of white	Ratio of base shade to tonal
25–50%	25% base to 75% tonal
50–75%	50% base to 50% tonal
75–100%	75% base to 25% tonal

> **Keys to good practice**
>
> • Remember that white hair can often be more resistant and the use of pre-softening can prove to be beneficial, especially on an area of concentrated white hair, such as around the front hairline.
> • Some manufacturers have a permanent colour range specifically for resistant hair to ensure good coverage; this may affect your choice of product.

Tests and testing

The results from the tests that you carry out on the hair will play an important role in any colouring decisions you make. If the outcome of any test proves to be undesirable, this will have a restrictive effect on the services you can offer. For example, redness and itching of the skin following a skin test would prevent you from using permanent colouring products on a client. The results of any tests carried out, either prior to or during the colour service, should be noted on the client's record card. If you have any doubts regarding the suitability of the client's hair, carry out pre-service testing.

The tests required before colouring include:

- skin test
- test cutting
- incompatibility test
- porosity test
- elasticity test.

See Unit G9 for more information on these tests.

When carrying out a skin test, it is essential that you follow the manufacturer's instructions. If you fail to follow the instructions and your client has a reaction to the colour, you may find yourself liable in a court of law. Some clients may be upset if they react to a skin test, as this will undisputedly mean they may not have their hair coloured. However, if your salon carries more than one product range, it may be possible to try a different manufacturer. In all other cases, you must advise your client against the chosen colouring service and suggest an alternative, for example, a semi-permanent colour (remember to check the manufacturer's instructions, as some semi-permanent colours require skin testing prior to application).

An allergic skin reaction to permanent colour

You should forewarn your client about the possibility of a positive reaction to a skin test and advise them accordingly. This may be to wash the area with warm soapy water and then apply a soothing lotion, such as calamine lotion. If this has no effect, they may need to seek medical advice. It is essential that you note on the client record card any positive reactions to tests, as the information must be communicated to any stylist who may intend to colour the client's hair in the future and also to comply with the requirements of the Data Protection Act 1998 (refer to Unit G9 for more information).

Safe working practices

During colouring services in the salon there are several health and safety considerations that you must be aware of. Your own personal health and hygiene are important. If you are feeling unwell or rundown then it will be difficult for you to keep up the pace in the salon and you run the risk of passing an infection on to others. You should keep yourself clean and fresh at all times to avoid causing offence to your clients or colleagues.

Your posture while working in the salon is another important consideration. You will soon become fatigued and stressed if you adopt an unhealthy posture whilst working. Bear this in mind and it will prevent any long-term stress or injury to your body. You should avoid standing in the same position for too long and move about as much as you can. If you are finding it difficult to access certain parts of the head during colour application, you must ask the client to assist you by moving their head. This will prevent you from working in an awkward position and help to maintain good posture.

The personal protective equipment that you need to use while colouring is essential to prevent the risk of harm or accidents to both yourself and the client. Permanent colourants are known to cause dermatitis and it is essential that you protect your hands when working. Personal protective equipment will protect both the skin and clothes from staining. In addition, barrier cream should be available to protect the client's skin when applying colour, especially if the client has a history of sensitivity around the front hairline or if you are using a dark colour.

Many clients are sensitive around the front hairline, but not on the scalp itself. This may be due to the fact that the hairline is cleaned along with the face several times a day, whereas the scalp should have a protective layer of dirt and grease to protect it from the colouring products. Care must be taken to avoid getting barrier cream onto the hair itself, as it will cause a barrier and the colour will not penetrate.

In addition to the above safe working practices, you have responsibilities under the COSHH Regulations and the Electricity at Work Regulations (see Unit G1). In relation to the requirements of COSHH, there are specific safety considerations relating to the use of powder bleach. Powder bleach should be mixed in a well-ventilated area as inhalation of the powder may cause coughing, choking, and/or breathlessness. This could prove to be hazardous, especially in the case of someone suffering from asthma. Personal protective equipment should be worn at all times, as powder bleach is a known irritant and may cause skin sensitisation. A protective facemask may be worn when mixing the bleach to prevent inhalation of the powder. Some manufacturers now make 'dust free' powder bleaches to help alleviate the problem.

Preparation of products, tools and equipment

The salon assistant will play a vital role in the preparation of products, tools and equipment used for colouring services. It is essential that you have trained him or her fully in how to prepare for all colouring services and this is best done, initially, by observing your working practices. As your assistant will have less technical knowledge than you, you must ensure any instructions given to your assistant are clear and accurate, as this will prevent any misunderstandings and potential problems.

> ### Keys to good practice
>
> - When giving instructions to your assistant, ask him or her to repeat back to you what you have instructed him or her to do to clarify his or her understanding.
> - When preparing and using colouring products in the salon, it is essential that you follow the manufacturer's instructions, as this will ensure optimum results. Failure to follow the specified instructions could lead to an unwanted or undesirable outcome.

Mixing colours

When mixing colours, you must ensure you measure the correct quantities of colour and hydrogen peroxide; nothing should be left to chance. Most product manufacturers indicate quantities of colour down the side of the tint tubes; others provide applicators that also act as a measure, which may be used for both the colourant and oxidant. When measuring liquids such as hydrogen peroxide, this should always be carried out with the measuring cylinder on a stable flat surface that is at eye level, as this will give an accurate reading. When using cream hydrogen peroxide, make sure all the hydrogen peroxide is poured into the mixing bowl. As the

Check it out

Write a list of all the PPE that you use in the salon whilst colouring. Write down next to each one what its purpose is and what it serves to protect. Use the photo below as a prompt.

Check it out

Are you aware of your responsibilities under the current COSHH Regulations and Electricity at Work Regulations? If you are not sure, refer back Unit G1.

cream hydrogen peroxide is of a thicker consistency, it is very easy to leave 10 ml of peroxide in the measure, meaning your working mixture has not been prepared to the manufacturer's specifications.

Keys to good practice

When applying a full-head colour or bleached highlights on long hair, you will need to mix a second (or possibly third) batch of product to ensure the colourant you are using is fresh and working at full strength. Mix only the amount you need, as any leftover products will be washed down the drain along with your employer's money!

If you are not fully prepared when you begin the service and have to keep leaving the client unattended to find what you need, this will present an unprofessional image and will waste your valuable time. You will need to be sure that the necessary products are available for you to use and that the tools and equipment used are clean and sterilised, as this will ensure you minimise the risk of cross-infection. (More detailed information regarding the sterilisation of tools and equipment may be found in Unit G1.) All tools and equipment should be checked prior to use to ensure they are fit for purpose, which will minimise the risk of harm to yourself and others. They should be at hand to enable you to give a professional and efficient service and to avoid any unnecessary stretching or twisting of the body.

Check it out

Make a list of the products, materials, tools and equipment used in your salon for all the colouring services that you offer. State the purpose of each item on the list. This will ensure you are fully aware of everything available for use in your salon.

Preparing for the colouring service

There are benefits for both the salon and the client when colouring hair. For the client, the benefits might be:

- to complement or accentuate a haircut
- to give individual or personalised results
- to create fashion effects
- to have an up-to-date service.

For the salon, the benefits might be:

- to create client loyalty
- profitability
- to enhance the salon's professional image
- to create variety in your working day
- to give job satisfaction
- to allow for inspiration in your work.

All of these benefits will help to motivate you in your colouring work and encourage you to be a successful colourist.

Check it out

Choose four different styles and decide how the hair should be coloured to accentuate the features of the hair cut. Which colours would you use and why?

What you will learn

- The effects of light and artificial lighting on the appearance of colour
- Natural colour pigment
- Principles of colour selection
- The effects on the hair structure of different colouring and lightening products
- Colouring techniques

The effects of light and artificial lighting on the appearance of colour

In an ideal world, all colouring would take place in natural daylight, in the middle of the day, as this gives a truer indication of a colour result. However, as the day progresses towards dusk, the colour of the natural light alters to a warmer colour, altering the appearance of the hair colour.

In the salon, the lighting must be given special consideration to ensure the colours seen are as true as possible with no shadow. This is especially important when colour matching. Incandescent light, from an ordinary light bulb, can be quite yellow and this would be undesirable within the salon, especially when colouring white or blonde hair. However, the higher the wattage, the whiter the light becomes. Fluorescent tubes are made in a variety of colours. Those marked as 'warm white' or 'warm white daylight' are most suitable for colouring work, as they give off a strong white light with some slightly warm tones.

The intensity of the lighting in the salon must be strong enough to judge colour without any glare. Many salons now use spotlights as a means of lighting the salon. Again, these are available in a variety of colours, including 'warm daylight'. However, spotlights can cast shadows and leave dark areas in the salon. This may be overcome by the use of specific types of reflectors.

The salon décor plays its own part in how you perceive colour. Afterimages and competing colours can influence and interfere with your colour vision. White is not considered ideal for walls, as it can be very bright and harsh. Softer colours such as beige, cream or pale peach, are ideal for use in the colouring area.

Correct lighting in a salon gives a truer indication of colour

Natural colour pigment

The hair's natural colour pigments are found in the cortex and are seen as such because the cuticles are colourless. The hair contains both melanin (black and brown pigment) and pheomelanin (red and yellow pigment) in varying degrees. Therefore, you could expect someone with dark hair to have more melanin than pheomelanin and someone with naturally fair hair to have predominantly pheomelanin.

However, when looking at the client's natural hair colour, remember that there may not be a uniform colour, but individual hairs that may be quite different; for example, a client with dark hair may have some individual hairs that are quite red. Hairs that have no melanin or pheomelanin are colourless but are seen by the naked eye as being white. This is usually due to age but may be attributed to illness or hereditary influences.

How natural pigmentation affects the colouring process

The hair's natural pigmentation must be considered to ensure the chosen colour is achievable. You must check the client's natural depth and tone. Darker hair may not lift as easily or as much as you would like and you will need to consider the products you are to use. If a client with naturally red/copper-coloured hair wants all vestige of warmth removed, you must consider your colour choice very carefully (reds are not always easy to tone down).

Principles of colour selection

Before applying any colouring products on a client's hair, there are a number of points that must be considered to ensure the best results for your client.

- The client's natural depth and tone
- The target shade (is it achievable given the client's natural depth and tone?)
- The type of colouring service required (slices, woven highlights, etc.)
- The percentage of white hair
- Strength of hydrogen peroxide needed
- The condition of the hair (elasticity)
- The porosity of the hair
- The hair texture
- The hair density
- Previous chemical history
- The results of any tests carried out
- The length of the client's hair
- Will the chosen colour complement the client's skin tones? (Warm skin tones suit warm colours, whereas pink skin tones suit cooler colours.)
- Any contra-indications?
- Client image and lifestyle
- The haircut
- The temperature in the salon.

When you have answers to all of the above, you should have sufficient information to choose your colourant, oxidant and colouring technique.

The effects on the hair structure of different colouring and lightening products

Semi-permanent colours

A *range of colour charts*

A true semi-permanent colour comes ready to use and is not mixed with any type of oxidant; always check the manufacturer's instructions first. Semi-permanent colourants work by depositing small colour molecules into the cuticle and outer part of the cortex. The colour will last between six to eight washes, unless the hair is porous, in which case it may last longer.

small molecules are deposited into the cuticle and outer edge of the cortex

The effects of semi-permanent colour on the hair structure

Semi-permanent colours are not designed to lighten the natural hair colour, but to add tone and depth. Because they have a conditioning base, they add shine to the hair. They are not meant to cover large amounts of white hair, but many will cover up to 30 per cent. Remember, if the hair is unevenly porous, the result may be patchy and the colour molecules will remain in the hair for more than six to eight washes.

Quasi-permanent colours

Quasi-permanent colours are mixed with a low-volume oxidant, usually on a 1:2 ratio. They work in a similar way to permanent colour (see below), in as much as the colour molecules are oxidised. However, as the oxidant is very mild, the colour molecules do not become as large (as permanent colour molecules) and are able to be washed out of the hair over a period of time. The colour is designed to fade gradually over a period of twelve weeks, without giving a re-growth.

Permanent colour

Permanent colours have a wide range of uses in the salon and are available in a variety of colours, from subtle, natural colours, through to striking and bold colours that add individuality and flair to your work.

Permanent colours can lighten or darken the hair and they can also be used to add tone. They may be used to achieve a number of different effects and are designed to cover white hair. Permanent colours may be mixed with 10, 20, 30 or 40 volume hydrogen peroxide, depending on the desired results. Remember to read the manufacturer's instructions to check which hydrogen peroxide strength will give the optimum results, given the base shade you are working on.

Permanent colours may also be referred to as para dyes or oxidation tints. They work by depositing small (usually colourless) molecules into the hair cortex along with the hydrogen peroxide. The hydrogen peroxide (which is an oxidising agent) begins to break down, releasing nascent oxygen, which joins together with the small molecules, to form larger, coloured molecules. As the molecules become larger, they are unable to pass back through the cuticle as they become trapped between the polypeptide chains within the cortex.

A permanent and quasi colour board

Using a colour shade chart during a consultation

small colourless molecules mixed with oxidant penetrate the cuticle, into the cortex

small molecules swell and become larger due to the nascent oxygen

The effect of permanent colour on the hair structure

Remember

If the hair is too porous and the cuticles are damaged or have been destroyed, even the larger molecules may be washed out of the hair, resulting in colour fade.

Bleach

Bleaching may occur through exposure to the sun and salt water, or artificially by using bleaching products in the salon. Bleach is usually used when other colouring products, for example, high-lift tints, cannot achieve the required amount of lift. It is also used when lightening hair that has already been coloured with tint and for pre-lightening.

Bleaching is the process of changing the natural colour pigments, melanin and pheomelanin, by a process of oxidation into colourless oxymelanin and oxypheomelanin.

1 **Hair prior to bleach application**

2 **Hair after bleaching**

natural colour pigment

colourless, oxymelanin

The effect of bleaching on the hair structure

Melanin (black and brown pigments) are oxidised more easily than pheomelanin (red and yellow), therefore the oxidisation process takes place in three stages.

1   The black and brown pigments are oxidised.
2   The red pigment is oxidised.
3   The yellow pigment is oxidised.

By watching the colour changes that occur during the bleaching process, the sequence of oxidation may be easily seen.

Hydrogen peroxide

Hydrogen peroxide is the oxidising agent used in permanent, quasi-permanent, lightening and bleaching services. It comes in different strengths and each strength has a specific purpose.

Check it out

Using 3 test cuttings of hair, apply a mixture of bleach powder and 9% H_2O_2. Leave the first cutting to develop for 10 minutes, the next for 20 minutes and the last for 30 minutes. Can you identify the different colour pigments being lightened within the hair?

Hydrogen peroxide strength	Purpose
10 vol (3%)	Used for refreshing faded ends; giving maximum depth of colour (tinting darker than the natural colour)
20 vol (6%)	Used for permanent colouring when adding depth and/or tone; will give up to 1 shade of lift on a base 6 or above
30 vol (9%)	Used for permanent colouring; will give up to 3 shades of lift on a base 6 or lighter
40 vol (12%)	Used for permanent colouring when using high-lift tints; will give up to 5 shades of lift on a base 6

The above table is a guide to choosing the correct volume strength; however, you should always check the manufacturer's instructions.

Keys to good practice

When measuring hydrogen peroxide, if you accidentally pour out too much, you must pour it down the sink. Putting it back into its original container may cause the hydrogen peroxide to start to deteriorate.

Hydrogen peroxide is made up from two parts of hydrogen and two parts of oxygen and is recognised as H_2O_2. It is classed as an unstable substance as it decomposes easily to form water and oxygen ($H_2O + O$). Stabilisers are added during its manufacture to avoid the loss of oxygen during storage. However, during colouring, bleaching and neutralising, the decomposition of the hydrogen peroxide is necessary as the newly formed oxygen (nascent oxygen) does all the work.

When mixing colouring products with hydrogen peroxide, you must follow the manufacturer's instructions regarding the mixing ratios. Some colourants are mixed on a 1:1 ratio, for example, 30 ml of oxidant to 30 ml of colourant, whereas others, such as high-lift tints and quasi-permanent colours, may be mixed on a 2:1 ratio, for example, 60 ml of oxidant to 30 ml of colourant.

There are occasions when the salon may not have the correct strength of oxidant in stock. Diluting the hydrogen peroxide with water may readily solve this problem. For example, if you only have 40 vol (or 12%) but need 30 vol (9%):

$\frac{30}{40} = \frac{3}{4}$

You would need to use three parts H_2O_2 to one part water to achieve 30 vol.

To dilute 40 vol (12%) to 20 vol (6%):

$\frac{20}{40} = \frac{2}{4} = \frac{1}{2}$ You would need to use one part H_2O_2 to one part water.

Check it out

If you have only 30 vol (9%) H_2O_2 in the salon but need 20 vol (6%), what ratio of H_2O_2 to water would you need to use to dilute the 30 vol?

Block colour and slicing techniques: a step-by-step guide

Before the colouring service.

The top hair is sectioned and the underneath section is dampened using a water spray.

Quasi-permanent colour is applied to underneath, section by section.

Wraps are placed over the section to prevent the colour from touching the top layer during development.

Back-to-back slices are then put into the top section, using 3 different colours.

The colour is developed according to the manufacturer's instructions.

The underneath, darker colour is removed first to prevent the colours from running.

The back-to-back slices are rinsed individually, before shampooing, to prevent the colours from bleeding.

The finished look.

Weaving and slicing techniques: a step-by-step guide

Before the service.

The hair is sectioned. The 1st section was taken from just above the ears, into a 'v' shape in the lower occipital region.

A diagonal sub-section was taken, then woven. A red colour was then applied to the hair on the foil.

Sub-sections were continually taken and woven, as step 3, until the 1st section was complete.

A 2nd section was taken from above the temples to just below the crown. The sub-sections were taken in the opposite diagonal direction to those taken in steps 3 & 4 and a copper colour applied.

The second section completed.

A gold colour was then applied from the crown to front hairline in slices.

The full head complete.

The finished result.

The table below shows some of the materials used for colouring.

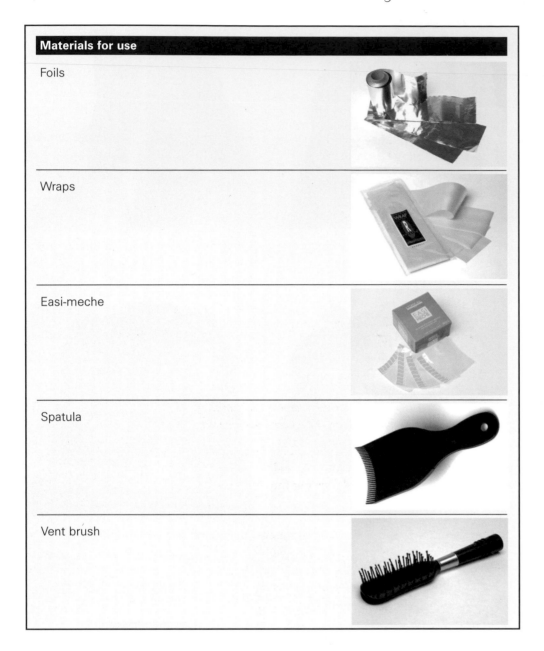

Materials for use	
Foils	
Wraps	
Easi-meche	
Spatula	
Vent brush	

Monitoring development and removing colour

Careful monitoring of the colour development must be carried out, especially when using bleaching products, as they do not have a set development time and may easily over-process if not checked frequently enough. If a client has very long hair and requires bleached highlights, you will need to bear in mind that bleach develops at varying times. Consideration would have to be given as to where on the head you started and which technique you used.

You must also consider that the bleach may be fully developed at your starting point before you have completed the whole application and would need to be removed with extreme care so as not to disturb the areas that are still developing. When using bleach and permanent colours, care must be taken so the permanent colour does not 'bleed' into the bleached hair. This may be achieved by removing the permanent colour first, taking care not to disturb the bleached areas.

*Take extra care when removing
bleach and permanent colours*

When the colour has fully developed, it must be entirely removed from the hair and scalp. Failure to do so will cause scalp irritation. Always remove colour following the manufacturer's instructions.

In the salon

Philippe, the stylist, had completed a full head of foil highlights using alternate slices of bleach and a vibrant red permanent colour. When the colours had developed, he asked Jenny the junior to remove the colour and shampoo the client's hair. Jenny was used to removing foils, but she had only ever removed permanent colour. Philippe was now busy with his next client and left Jenny to it. She removed all the foils and then began to rinse the colour from the hair. During the shampooing process she noticed the hair looked quite pink in places and called Philippe over to look at the client's hair. The red colour had bled into the bleach, leaving pink slices where the bleach should have been.

- What went wrong?
- How could this have been avoided?

---

pH values of colouring products

The pH value indicates the level of acidity or alkalinity within a product. The pH value of colouring products is an important factor to consider, as acidic products are kinder to the hair since they help to close the cuticles, whereas alkaline products will open the cuticles.

pH values and their effect on cuticles

The more alkaline the product, the more damage it will cause to the hair; therefore, you should consider the products you are using and the potential damage they may cause.

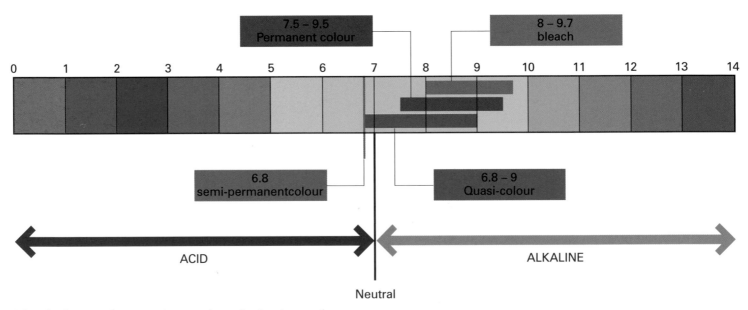

pH scale showing the approximate values of colouring products

As most colouring products are alkaline (they open the cuticles), it is essential that an anti-oxidant conditioner be used after the colour has been shampooed off the hair. An anti-oxidant conditioner will:

- return the hair back to its normal pH of 4.5–5.5 (slightly acid)
- add moisture to the hair
- stop any further oxidation taking place (continuing oxidation will cause unnecessary damage to the hair)
- close the cuticles.

Remember

Remember to keep the salon clean and tidy throughout the service, as this will maintain your professional image and help to prevent cross-infection. All remaining colouring products and used materials must be disposed of correctly.

Solving colouring problems

There may be times when colouring or bleaching problems occur in the salon and it is essential that you know why the problems have occurred and how they may be rectified. If you do not have a good understanding of why the problems have occurred, it may prove very difficult to remedy the situation to produce a satisfactory result.

What you will learn
• Restoring depth and tone • Neutralising colour tone • Colouring resistant hair • Using bleach to pre-lighten the hair • Pre-pigmentation

There are several problems that you may encounter while colouring that are easily solved, such as restoring depth and tone or neutralising colour tone. However, if you feel the level of colour correction is above your ability then you may need to refer the client to another stylist in the salon for specialist correction work. When dealing with a colour problem, you need to accurately identify the hair's condition and what has previously been used on the hair. You will need to use questioning and/or observation in addition to testing the hair to establish the exact nature of the problem and determine the best course of action.

Once you have determined the problem and assessed your client's needs, you can present to him or her the options available to resolve the predicament. Ensure you present all the options and thoroughly discuss the outcomes and consequences of each to enable yourself and your client to agree a course of action.

Restoring depth and tone

Depth and tone may be lost for several reasons; for example, a client may have been on holiday and exposed his or her hair to the sun. Another reason might be that the client has very porous hair that cannot hold on to colour. If the cuticles are badly damaged or non-existent, the hair may not be able to 'hold' the colour molecules in the cortex, resulting in colour fade. This may also occur if permanent colour is not left on the hair for the full development time, as the molecules do not have sufficient time to join together to form the larger molecules and may be 'washed away'.

If the client has lost depth and tone out of their hair colour, you have several options available to help with this problem. If the hair is sensitised, in order to prevent any further chemical damage, the use of temporary or semi-permanent colours may be necessary. These will stain the cuticle layer and will not affect the elasticity of the hair. Remember that if the hair is extremely porous, they may last longer than a few shampoos.

The most commonly used solution is to refresh the tired hair with the usual colour. Several product manufacturers now produce their own colour refreshers; however, other companies still use the most common method of diluting their permanent hair colours. There may be instances where the loss of depth and tone is so great that pre-pigmentation is necessary prior to the usual colouring service.

Check it out

List the tests you might carry out on a client's hair prior to colour correction work. State the purpose of the test and what the expected outcomes might be (see Unit G9).

Keys to good practice

Always follow the product manufacturer's instructions. If you are unsure, telephone the technical helpline.

Neutralising colour tone

From time to time you may come across a client who has developed unwanted tones in his or her hair. This can be due to a number of influencing factors, for example, smoking can leave a yellow tinge in the hair and swimming in water containing chlorine can place a green cast on the hair. In your initial colour training, you will have learnt about the colour star and the fact that opposite colours neutralise each other; however, you must remember to consider the intensity of the colours.

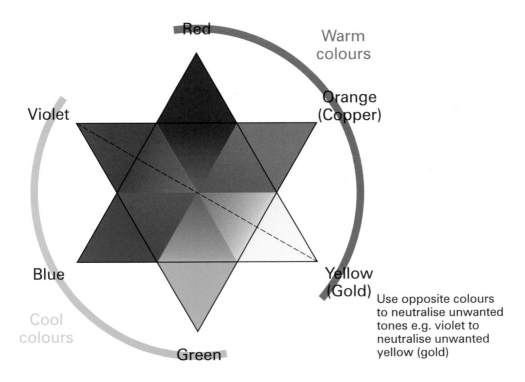

Use opposite colours to neutralise unwanted tones e.g. violet to neutralise unwanted yellow (gold)

You will need to be aware of this when using a colour to neutralise unwanted tone. There are shampoos available to neutralise colour tone, the most common being a purple shampoo that neutralises yellow. If you do not already retail these, consider stocking them for sale, as it would provide a good selling opportunity. Due to the high levels of pollution in our towns and cities, most clients with blonde colours in their hair will benefit from infrequent use of 'brightening' shampoos.

Keys to good practice

Take care not to use a darker or more vibrant colour tone than is necessary or the outcome could be undesirable. Assess the depth of the client's hair colour and use a slightly lighter depth, but make sure that the intensity of the tone is the same; for example, if you wanted to remove nicotine staining on white hair, you would use a silver colour rather than a colour with intense violet tones.

Colouring resistant hair

The resistance of a client's hair is due to the cuticle scales being flat and smooth; this is usually found in hair in good condition. Some hair, such as Oriental hair, falls into this category, as it has more layers of cuticle scales than either European or African Caribbean hair and does not allow the colour to penetrate into the cortex and develop. You can overcome this by pre-softening the hair, which lifts the cuticle scales, allowing colour molecules to enter the cortex.

Hair with tightly-packed cuticles   *Hair with raised cuticles*

Pre-softening the hair is a relatively quick and simple process. It involves applying neat 10 vol or 3% hydrogen peroxide to the resistant areas, drying the H_2O_2 into the hair, and then proceeding with the colouring service. You may find it easier to use cream hydrogen peroxide as it has a thicker consistency and is therefore easier to work with.

You will need to carefully assess the hair's porosity to determine its resistant tendencies. Consider also that naturally white hair is often more resistant and this can be overcome not only by pre-softening, but also by the use of permanent colour with extra depth added. Most product manufacturers now produce colours with intense depth for improved coverage on resistant white hair.

Using bleach to pre-lighten the hair

If you cannot achieve the required amount of lift using permanent colour or a high-lift tint, it may be necessary to pre-lighten the base using bleach. However, many hairdressers make the mistake of bleaching the hair to almost white before applying the target colour. This will cause unnecessary damage to the hair. The hair should be lightened only to the corresponding depth and used as an undercoat. The target shade should then be applied on top of the undercoat.

A client with a natural depth of 4 (medium brown), who wants highlights of 7/43, would need to be pre-lightened only to an orange/yellow base as this corresponds to the depth of 7. However if pre-lightening hair that is to be coloured blue, it is essential to bleach the hair to almost white first. If there is any yellow left in the hair it will give a green result when it is mixed with the blue colour!

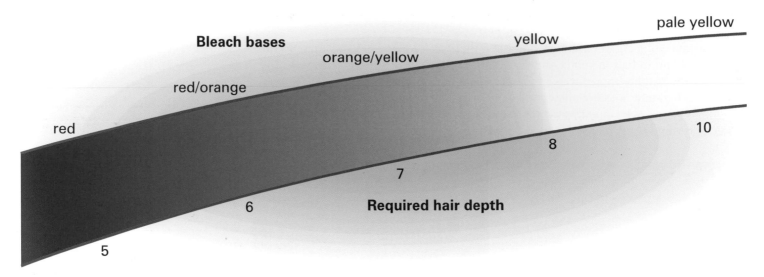

Bleach bases and their corresponding depths

Pre-pigmentation

Pre-pigmentation is the term used to describe restoring lost pigment to pale hair that needs to be made darker and/or warmer. An example of this is a client with bleached hair who wishes to go back to his or her natural colour. As bleaching removes the warm tones (red and yellow) from the hair, these tones must be replaced prior to applying the target shade or the finished result will have a green cast.

Pre-pigmenting may be done using temporary, semi-permanent, quasi-permanent or permanent colour; however, the porosity of the hair must be taken into consideration when choosing the correct product. The pre-colour may be either red, copper or gold, depending on the depth of the target shade; for example, a light colour would usually require a gold pre-colour, whereas darker hair would require a red pre-colour. Look at the illustration above of bleach bases and corresponding depths for an indication of the correct colour to use. Always remember to follow the manufacturer's instructions.

Keys to good practice	

When taking clients back to their natural colour, always use one shade lighter than the target shade, as you can add colour to the hair at any time, but it is more difficult to remove colour from previously treated hair.

Check it out	

Which pre-service tests should be carried out prior to taking a client back to his or her natural colour?

Pre-pigmentation may be carried out in a number of ways and this should be checked using the manufacturer's instructions. Below is a simple and effective method of pre-pigmenting the hair.

1 Prepare yourself and the client.
2 Make all the necessary preparations as per any colour application.
3 Prepare the hair (by shampooing) if required.
4 Apply the correct pre-colour evenly to the hair, avoiding the re-growth area.
5 Allow the colour to develop fully.
6 Wipe off any excess colour using cotton wool.
7 Mix permanent colour (one shade lighter than target shade) following the manufacturer's instructions and apply directly over the pre-coloured hair and develop as normal.
8 Remove the colour and apply an anti-oxidant conditioner. (Refer to H28.)

Colouring problems do occur from time to time and it is essential that you have a good understanding of the common faults that may arise.

Colouring problems and remedies

Problem	Cause	Remedy
Over-processing	Usually caused by incorrect timing during the development of the colour/bleach, e.g. the product has been left on the hair for too long	Remove colour immediately; use a restructuring conditioner to help to rebuild some of the internal fibres; cut off as much of the over-processed hair as possible; give the client effective and accurate after-care advice
Under-processing	Usually caused by incorrect timing, e.g. the colouring product has not been left on long enough	Check the condition of the hair and re-apply the product if the condition allows
Skin staining	This may be due to several reasons: poor application; seepage of products; excessively dry skin that has not been protected (especially when using dark or red colours)	Use a skin stain remover
Deterioration of hair condition	This may be due to several reasons: the product used was too strong; the colour has been over-developed; the condition of the hair prior to colour application was very poor	Remove colour immediately; use a restructuring conditioner to help to rebuild some of the internal fibres; give the client effective and accurate after-care advice
Uneven results	This may be due to several reasons: the application was uneven; the sections taken were too large; when mixing two or more colours together, the colours weren't mixed sufficiently, giving an uneven result	Spot colour the darker or uncoloured areas
Product seepage	This may be caused by: using too much product, which then seeps out of the foil/ packet; incorrect mixing, e.g. the product is too runny	Spot colour the areas of seepage
Scalp sensitivity	This may be caused by: an allergy to the products used, high strength of the hydrogen peroxide used on the scalp, or the over-use of chemicals on the scalp e.g. permanent colour used directly after a bleaching service.	Rinse immediately with cool water and no further chemical processing should be carried out. Some product manufacturers have scalp sensitivity products that may be used for this purpose, but ensure there is no evidence of broken skin.

After the service

When any colour service is complete, it is imperative to give the client the correct advice. This will serve to ensure long-lasting results and client satisfaction. It is also a good selling opportunity; following any colour treatment, the correct hair care advice will give your client the optimum, long-lasting result.

Once the colour treatment is complete, you must discuss with your client how to care for the hair and the colour. During the initial and ongoing consultation, you will have determined your client's lifestyle and given advice about how often to shampoo and condition. You should make sure the client understands the importance of looking after his or her hair in order to maintain the colour.

Discuss the features and benefits of the shampoo and conditioning products that have been specifically designed for use after colour treatments. Ensure the client understands not only how these products help to maintain their hair in good condition, but how and when to use them.

You should recommend that your client uses products for colour-treated hair

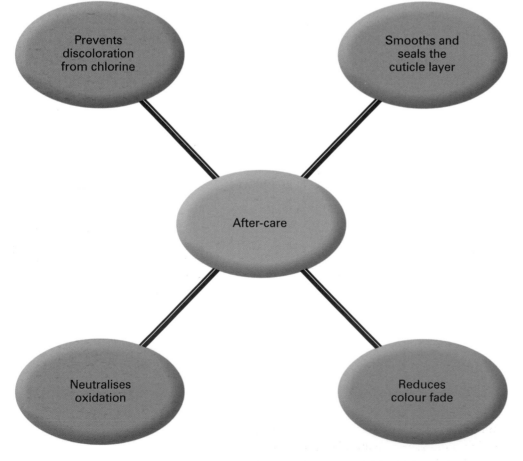

Prevents discoloration from chlorine

Smooths and seals the cuticle layer

After-care

Neutralises oxidation

Reduces colour fade

Check it out

What products does your salon retail that will help the client to maintain the colour intensity between visits?

Intervals between colour appointments

The client's hair growth and the type of colour treatment will determine the length of time between the colour appointments. Most clients hate to see their re-growth visible and are usually counting the days until their next colour appointment. However, this is not always the case and if a client has a large re-growth when they return to the salon then there are implications for this. For instance, the hair ends will have changed colour over time and an accurate colour match may be more difficult. Implications such as these should be explained when giving advice on the client's return visit.

Temporary colours usually last only one shampoo and the client will need this treatment each time he or she have his or her hair blow-dried or set. Semi-permanent colours will last between six and eight shampoos; therefore, consideration will need to be given to how often a client shampoos his or her hair in determining the next colour appointment. A quasi-permanent colour can last on the hair between sixteen and twenty-two shampoos, giving the client the option of a colour treatment every few months. These colours are designed to fade and they should not leave a visible re-growth. If your client is having a quasi-colour every four weeks, you should ask yourself whether your product choice is correct. Permanent colours and bleach both grow out of the hair and the next colour treatment will be determined by the client's hair growth. However, most clients will require a re-touch every four to six weeks.

Encourage your clients to make their next appointment before leaving the salon, as this will help to reinforce the professionalism of the salon and ensure a return visit.

Completion of the record card

Completion of a record card can prove to be useful if there are any repercussions following a colour treatment. It is your responsibility to ensure the card is completed both accurately and legibly. Not only is it vital to be able to read and understand the information on it for the next appointment, but it could also be needed as proof of your professionalism. The information contained on the client record card must be clear to other stylists who may colour the client's hair in the future and should include:

- the client's name, address, and contact number
- the client's natural depth and tone
- the percentage of white hair and whether the white hair is scattered across the head or confined to one area
- the date of the client's skin test
- the results of any pre-service tests that have been carried out
- the colour/s used
- the volume or percentage strength used with each colour
- how or where the colours were used (for example, alternate slices of colour)
- the length of time the colour/s was developed
- the final result
- any retail sales made.

> **Check it out**
>
> List the eight principles of the Data Protection Act and summarise your responsibilities under this piece of legislation.

Consider also your responsibilities under the Data Protection Act. Remember that you have to store and use this information in line with the requirements of the Act.

Disposal of waste

At the end of the colour service, any waste products and materials must be disposed of carefully and in a safe manner. You have legal and moral responsibilities under the Environmental Protection Act 1990 to dispose of waste in a safe manner that will not cause harm to others or the environment.

Knowledge check

1. In what way does colouring hair benefit the salon?

2. State what you would do to ensure your client did not have any of the following contra-indications to a colouring service: skin sensitivities; previous history of allergic reaction to permanent colouring services; known allergies; skin disorders; incompatible products or medical advice or instructions?

3. State the effects temperature has on the colouring process.

4. What advice would you give to a client whilst carrying out a skin test?

5. Why is it important to accurately monitor colour development in the salon?

6. Draw and label the colour star and state its uses.

7. Why is it important that your client record cards are accurate and up to date?

Provide colour correction services   Unit H28

Introduction

Colour correction is carried out for a number of reasons:

- To lighten the hair
- To darken the hair
- To change the tone of the hair

Hair colour problems can occur no matter how experienced you are as a stylist. The majority of colour problems are the result of human error which stresses the importance of following the correct procedures. Colour problems can be varied and there are no hard and fast solutions to correcting these problems, as the desired outcome and influencing factors will differ from client to client. This unit is about the advanced skills you will need to develop in order to determine and correct complex colouring problems.

What you will learn	
• Preparing the client • Preparing for the colour correction service • Correcting the colour problem • After the service	

You the stylist

This unit aims to give you possible solutions to colouring problems but you must make your own decisions regarding the most suitable course of action to take in a range of different circumstances. You must always ensure that your clients are aware of the length of time required to perform this kind of service and the cost.

Preparing the client

What you will learn	
• Thorough consultation to determine the problem • Plan and agree a course of action to correct colour • Contra-indications and influencing factors • Pre-service tests and examination • Maintain effective and safe methods of working	

Thorough consultation to determine the problem

One of the most important factors to consider is a thorough and effective consultation in order to determine the problem. This will ensure that you have all the necessary facts to enable you to select the most appropriate products and techniques to perform the service to a satisfactory standard. You will need to draw on your communication skills to ensure you elicit the correct information from your client. If you fail to gain all the necessary information you may not achieve a satisfactory result. You must establish:

- The nature of the colouring problem
- The extent of the problem
- The condition of the client's hair and scalp
- The extent of artificial and natural colour on the one head
- The results the client would like to see (using visual aids may help at this point)
- The most suitable products and techniques to achieve the desired result
- If the client's desired result is achievable. If not you will need to discuss and negotiate with your client until you reach a satisfactory outcome.

This information may be obtained by asking the client a series of probing questions to find out the exact nature and the extent of the problem. You must also establish whether your client has any known contra-indications. Some contra-indications are easily identified by observation; however, others may not be so apparent. Therefore it is essential that you question your client beforehand and any responses must be logged on the client's record card. This is not only good practice but may also be required at a later date should the client decide to start legal proceedings against the salon. You should at this point establish the client's requirements regarding the expected outcome.

You should make reference to the client's existing record card, as this should hold the client's complete colouring history (providing the client is an existing client). This information may affect the colour correction service you are able to offer and the products you may use, e.g. the client's natural base shade and products previously used on the hair.

Keys to good practice

The information contained on a record card should be accurate and up to date to comply with the Data Protection Act 1998. This includes the responses from your clients when questioned about contra-indications, etc. See Unit G9 for more information on the Data Protection Act 1998.

The extent of the problem may be identified by observation. In addition you should question your client to gain their perspective on the problem, using both factual and feeling questions. As an experienced hairdresser, you should be able to recognize a number of different colouring problems.

In this unit, the problems you must effectively correct are:

- Removing artificial colour on a full head
- Removing bands of colour
- Re-colouring bleached hair using pre-pigmentation and permanent colour over at least 60% of the head
- Re-colouring hair that has had artificial colour removed by reduction on a full head
- Correcting highlights and lowlights

Plan and agree a course of action to correct colour

Once you have all the necessary information, you must decide on the most suitable course of action to take. This should include the products and techniques you intend to use to achieve the optimum result for your client. There may be more than one possible course of action, in which case these should be presented to your client using non-technical language that he or she can readily understand. Explain to your client the reasons behind your recommendations, in other words, the results of your analysis. Be honest with your client and explain the likelihood of achieving the colour result he or she wants. There may be times when you know it is highly unlikely that you will be able to achieve the required colour and it is better that the client is aware of this from the onset than for it to be a shock at the end of the service. This also gives you both the opportunity to explore other possibilities with a more acceptable outcome. You must also discuss maintaining the colour result; this should include plenty of home-care advice on product usage and general maintenance.

You must explain to your client the implications that the colour correction service may have on future hairdressing services, e.g. following colour removal by reduction and subsequent re-colouring of the hair, a permanent wave would be unadvisable as the hair may not be able to withstand further chemical treatments.

Keys to good practice

When the client is in possession of all the facts regarding the colour correction service (e.g. the products you intend to use, the cost and duration of the service and the expected outcome), and you have his or her consent to continue, this should be recorded on the client's record card. In the event of an unexpected problem occurring, you have documented evidence to prove you have followed the correct procedures.

Contra-indications and influencing factors

Contra-indications

A contra-indication is something that would prevent you from continuing with the service. Therefore you must question your client and record the responses.

Contra-indications should always be carefully considered. Below is table of contra-indications and the reasons how and why they can affect the delivery of colour correction services.

Contra-indication	How and why they can affect the delivery of colour correction services
Skin sensitivities	Every client must have a skin test prior to a colouring service to test for an allergic reaction to the colourant. Any reaction to the colourant would result in the colouring service not being able to take place or possibly an alternative product would need to be used. You should ask your clients if they have ever had any sensitivity to hairdressing products and record their answers on the client record card.
Previous history of allergic reaction to permanent colouring services	Once a client has developed sensitivity to permanent colouring products, this is unlikely to ever change. If placed in this situation, you will need to use non-permanent colouring products, but you must carry out a skin test using the products you intend to use.
Known allergies	Some allergies may prevent services taking place. You should ask your clients: • If they have any known allergies • If they have ever been referred to see a dermatologist for patch testing and, if so, the number of known allergies they may have. A client with a history of allergies or sensitivity is more likely to react to hairdressing products.

Contra-indication	How and why they can affect the delivery of colour correction services
Skin disorders	Any skin disorders must be identified prior to application. An infectious skin disease would obviously mean that you could not carry out the colour correction service. With others, such as psoriasis, the service may continue as long as the skin is not broken. If in doubt, ask for confirmation from the client's GP.
Incompatible products	Any products used prior to the colour correction service that contain metallic salts will have an adverse reaction when mixed with hydrogen peroxide. Therefore, any products that contain or are mixed with hydrogen peroxide must not be used.
Medical advice instructions	Certain drugs/medication may affect the final outcome of the colour correction service. Therefore you should ask your client for confirmation from their GP that their medication will not affect the outcome before you colour the hair.

Influencing factors

An influencing factor may not necessarily prevent you from performing a colour correction service but must be considered in all the decisions you make both prior to and during the service. Some of the influencing factors are also contra-indications.

Temperature

The temperature of the salon will influence the processing time. A cold salon may slow down the processing time and warm temperatures will speed up the process. The use of heat to develop colours quickly is a good technique; however, the porosity and condition of the hair needs to be considered, especially during colour correction services, as careful monitoring of colour development may be necessary to prevent additional problems such as over-processing.

Using additional heat can speed up the colouring process

Existing colour of hair

The existing colour of the client's hair, both the natural colour and any artificial colour present, must be taken into consideration when carrying out a colour correction service. The outcome of the consultation will determine the most suitable products to use to enable you to achieve the required result. For example:

Client's natural base	6
Colour on mid-lengths and ends	4.45 (medium warm brown)
Target shade	7.1

Permanent colour would not be an option here, as a tint will not lighten another tint. The options open to you in this instance would be to remove the artificial colour by either reduction or oxidation.

You must be aware of the potential problems that may arise when colouring hair that has previously been coloured, e.g. deterioration of the hair condition, or on occasion, unexpected results, due to the presence of incompatible products. However, if all pre-service testing has been carried out, these problems can be kept to a minimum. Test cuttings are very useful in these instances.

Hair condition

It is essential that you determine the condition of the client's hair before the colour correction service, as it will affect your colour choice and development time, and possibly your method of application. You must also consider whether the hair's condition is actually good enough to accept the service, as in some cases the addition of more chemicals will cause the condition to deteriorate. In this instance you may need to use a pre-colouring treatment. These treatments even out the porosity of the hair and help to rebuild the internal fibres. Hair in poor condition accepts colour more readily but if the hair is overly porous, there is a good chance the hair won't hold the colour and it will fade very quickly. This is because when the cuticles are open or non-existent, there is nothing to trap the colour into the cortex.

If the hair is in good condition, it may be resistant to colour; this would necessitate pre-softening the hair to open the cuticle scales allowing the colour molecules into the cortex.

Test results

The results of any pre-service testing must be considered, as this will enable you to take the most appropriate course of action. You will need to think about the choice of products you can use or even the possibility that the colour correction service cannot be carried out due to poor hair condition, or the presence of incompatible products. All test results must be recorded on the client's record card.

Length of hair

The length of the hair will dictate the time you need to allocate for the service and the price you should charge for the service. The mid-lengths and ends of longer hair will be more porous, therefore this may affect your method and sequence of application.

Hair density

The hair density will also determine the amount of product you need to use. A client with an abundance of hair will require more product to be used than a client with sparse hair. The size of your sections must also be considered. When colouring the hair of a client with a great density of hair, the size of the sections should be finer to ensure a thorough application. It may also affect your application techniques.

Percentage of white hair

The percentage of white hair must be taken into consideration, especially the re-growth area, as although you may not need to colour correct the roots, they may be resistant to the subsequent colour being used. In this instance you may need to pre-soften the re-growth area.

Sequence of application

When applying colouring products, you may need to consider the sequence of application. Body temperature plays an important role when carrying out a full-head colour. The colour on the roots of the hair will process more quickly than the colour on the ends because its development is speeded up by the addition of body heat. Therefore, when carrying out a full-head lightening or full-head red application, you should apply the colour to the mid-lengths and ends first, and the roots last. This will prevent the colour being too light at the roots (in the instance of a lightening application) and will prevent root glare when using 'reds'.

However, when carrying out a colour correction service, such as removing colour by reduction, you may need to start your application at the darkest point.

Scalp sensitivity

Scalp sensitivity may affect your choice of product or application technique. A client with sensitivity to permanent colouring products will obviously limit your choices.

Pre-service tests and examinations

It is essential that you establish the condition of the client's hair, skin and scalp prior to performing a colour correction service. You should carry out a thorough examination of the hair, skin and scalp, checking for cuts and abrasions and any other known contra-indications to ensure suitability.

You are also required to carry out pre-service tests. The results from the tests that you carry out on the hair will be an important factor in any decision you make. If the outcome of any test proves to be undesirable, this may limit the services you can offer. For example, if when testing the elasticity of the client's hair, it stretches, but does not return to its original length, this indicates damage in the cortex. Extreme caution should be observed, as use of the incorrect product may cause the hair condition to deteriorate still further. The results of any tests carried out should be noted on the client's record card. Refer to Unit G9 for more information on pre-service tests.

Maintain effective and safe methods of working when correcting hair colour

Personal protective equipment

When carrying out any colour correction, it is essential that personal protective equipment is worn by both you and your client. You must ensure your client's clothing is protected throughout the whole of the service to prevent any colouring products from staining their clothes. Barrier cream may also be applied around the hairline to prevent skin staining, especially when using dark colours or if the client has very dry skin. You should be wearing gloves to protect your hands from the colouring products, and to prevent skin irritation (dermatitis). You should also wear an apron to protect your own clothes from staining.

You must wear the correct personal protective equipment, and ensure the client also has protective equipment on

> **Check it out**
>
> What are your salon's requirements for client preparation?

Working safely in the salon

When working with any colouring products, you must ensure compliance with COSHH regulations. Your responsibilities in relation to this piece of legislation are to:

- Maintain your protective equipment and report its loss or demise to your employer
- Comply with your salon's policies for safe handling, usage, storage and disposal of hazardous substances
- Report any hazards you cannot deal with yourself, to the designated person within your salon
- Follow the manufacturers' instructions relating to the colouring, lightening and bleaching products you are using.

There are specific safety considerations relating to the use of powder bleach under the COSHH regulations. Powder bleach should be mixed in a well-ventilated area as inhalation of the powder may cause coughing, choking and/or breathlessness. This could prove to be hazardous, especially in the case of someone suffering from asthma. Personal protective equipment should be worn at all times as powder bleach is a known irritant and may cause skin sensitisation. A protective facemask may be worn when mixing the bleach to prevent inhalation of the powder. Some manufacturers now make 'dust free' powder bleaches to help alleviate the problem.

All tools and equipment that you use during the service must be checked prior to use to make sure they are safe and fit for purpose. This includes items of electrical equipment used to aid the colouring process, e.g. clymazone, rollerball, etc. Using tools and equipment for their intended purpose will reduce the risk of damage to such equipment and minimise the risk of harm or injury to yourself and others.

Checklist for preparing your work area

What to do	Why/how?
All the necessary tools and equipment for the service should be prepared beforehand	Saves time and conveys professional image to the client
Any products needed for the service should be available and ready to use	Regular and effective stocktaking will ensure that all products are available
Work area must be clean and tidy	Prevents accidents occurring, reduces risk of cross-infection and promotes a professional image
Instruct junior staff to prepare the work area correctly	Saves time. Make sure that you clearly communicate what is required – a short list of instructions may be given to junior staff
Tools and equipment should be clean, sterilised and fit for the purpose	The appropriate method of sterilisation should be used and equipment should be checked for defects
Electrical equipment should be used in compliance with health and safety legislation	Ensure that junior staff are complying with the safe use of electrical equipment (see Unit G1). This is your responsibility.

Checklist for personal health and hygiene

What to do	Why/how?
Make sure your body and clothes smell clean and fresh	The client will feel more comfortable in your presence. Daily washing and the use of a good deodorant are essential.
Make sure your breath smells nice	Use a breath freshener. This will help to combat odours from strong-smelling foods or smoking
Do not work if you are feeling unwell	Infections can be spread in the salon. Keep yourself fit and healthy to ensure that you produce the best work possible.
Maintain a good posture while working. Think about whether your client is positioned correctly for your needs as well as their own comfort.	This will minimise the risk of injury and fatigue. Make sure you keep your back straight and balance your weight evenly. Having your tools and equipment close to hand will prevent you from overstretching.

Maintaining stock levels

Stocktaking should be carried out on a regular basis. This may be weekly, fortnightly or monthly, depending on the amount of stock you carry/use and the amount of storage space available in the salon. When carrying out colour correction services, you may not necessarily know precisely which products and/or materials you will be using. Therefore it is essential that you maintain adequate stock levels at all times.

Remember

Use all colouring products economically, e.g. prepare only the amount you actually need, as this will ensure you are working cost-effectively and minimising the wastage of the products.

Preparing for the colour correction service

Your client's hair should be prepared for the colour correction service. You must consider the products you will be using e.g. are they applied to dry hair or hair that has been shampooed and towel dried? All products must be prepared (mixed and measured) and used following the manufacturer's instructions to ensure the best results. You should be able to estimate the amount of product you will need to enable you to carry out the service. It is important that you use products economically (but use a sufficient amount to achieve the desired results) as this will have a positive effect on the salon's finances. The hair should then be sectioned off in a way that is suitable for the colour correction service. Your sectioning should be clean to enable you to work efficiently and precisely throughout the colour correction service.

Remember

If necessary, adjust the position of your client to enable you to gain access to all areas of the head. This will not only make your job easier, but also prevent you from working in awkward positions that have the potential to cause you injury.

What you will learn

- Colouring products
- Principles of colour correction
- Effects on the hair structure of different colouring products

Check it out

List the products, tools and equipment that may be used when colouring hair and state the reasons why you would use them. Refer to Unit H30 if you need a reminder.

Colouring products

You must be aware of the full range of colouring products available for use in the salon and their effects on the hair structure. Your choice of product will depend on:

- The intended result
- The condition of the hair, both elasticity and porosity
- The existing hair colour
- The products previously used on the hair.

Principles of colour correction

Before applying any colouring products on a client's hair, there are a number of points that you must consider to ensure the best results for your client.

1 The client's natural depth and tone
2 The target shade (is it achievable given the client's natural depth and tone?)
3 The type of colouring service required (slices, woven highlights, etc.)
4 The percentage of white hair
5 Strength of hydrogen peroxide needed
6 The condition of the hair (elasticity)
7 The porosity of the hair
8 The hair texture
9 The hair density
10 Previous chemical history
11 The results of any tests carried out
12 The length of the client's hair
13 Will the chosen colour complement the client's skin tones? (Warm skin tones suit warm colours, whereas pink skin tones suit cooler colours.)
14 Are there any contra-indications?
15 Client image and lifestyle
16 The haircut
17 The temperature in the salon.

When you have answers to all of the above, you should have sufficient information to choose your colourant, oxidant and colouring technique.

Reduction and oxidation

Oxidation is the term given to a chemical process that involves the addition of oxygen. In hairdressing, oxygen is used during permanent colouring processes, bleaching and when neutralising a perm. It is also used in some quasi-colours. The oxygen used in these processes comes from hydrogen peroxide.

Hydrogen peroxide is made up from two parts of hydrogen and two parts of oxygen and is recognized as H_2O_2. It is classed as an unstable substance as it decomposes easily to form water and oxygen ($H_2O + O$). The additional part of oxygen (nascent oxygen) is necessary when colouring the hair. The stronger the volume or percentage of hydrogen peroxide, the greater amount of nascent oxygen can be found.

Reduction is the opposite of oxidation. A process of reduction sees the addition of hydrogen and the removal of oxygen. Artificial colour may be removed from the hair by using a colour reducer that works by a process of reduction. As permanent colour works by a process of oxidation, it may be removed by using the opposite kind of chemical reaction.

Melanin

The hair's natural colour pigments are found in the cortex and are seen as such because the cuticles are colourless. The hair contains both melanin (black and brown pigment) and pheomelanin (red and yellow pigment) in varying degrees. Therefore, you could expect someone with dark hair to have more melanin than pheomelanin and someone with naturally fair hair to have predominantly pheomelanin.

Sometimes it is not easy to tell what your client's natural colour is

However, when looking at the client's natural hair colour, remember that there may not be a uniform colour, but individual hairs that may be quite different; for example, a client with dark hair may have some individual hairs that are quite red. Hairs that have no melanin or pheomelanin are colourless but are seen by the naked eye as being white. This is usually due to age but may be attributed to illness or hereditary influences.

Light and lighting

In an ideal world, all colouring would take place in natural daylight, in the middle of the day, as this gives a truer indication of a colour result. However, as the day progresses towards dusk, the colour of the natural light alters to a warmer colour, altering the appearance of the hair colour.

In the salon, the lighting must be given special consideration to ensure the colours seen are as true as possible with no shadow. This is especially important when colour matching. Incandescent light, from an ordinary light bulb, can be quite yellow and this would be undesirable within the salon, especially when colouring white or blonde hair. However, the higher the wattage, the whiter the light becomes. Fluorescent tubes are made in a variety of colours. Those marked as 'warm white' or 'warm white daylight' are most suitable for colouring work, as they give off a strong white light with some slightly warm tones.

The intensity of the lighting in the salon must be strong enough to judge colour without any glare. Many salons now use spotlights as a means of lighting the salon. Again, these are available in a variety of colours, including 'warm daylight'. However, spotlights can cast shadows and leave dark areas in the salon. This may be overcome by the use of specific types of reflectors.

How natural pigmentation affects the colouring process

The hair's natural pigmentation must be considered to ensure the chosen colour is achievable. You must check the client's natural depth and tone. Darker hair may not lift as easily or as much as you would like and you would need to consider the products you are to use. If a client with naturally red/copper coloured hair wants all vestige of warmth removed, you must consider your colour choice very carefully (as reds are not always easy to tone down).

Effects on the hair structure of different colouring products

Semi-permanent colours

A true semi-permanent colour comes ready to use and is not mixed with any type of oxidant; always check the manufacturer's instructions first. Semi-permanent colourants work by depositing small colour molecules into the cuticle and outer part of the cortex. The colour will last between six and eight washes, unless the hair is porous, in which case it may last longer.

Semi-permanent colours are not designed to lighten the natural hair colour, but to add tone and depth. Because they have a conditioning base, they add shine to the hair. They are not meant to cover large amounts of white hair, but many will cover up to 30 per cent. Remember, if the hair is unevenly porous, the result may be patchy and the colour molecules will remain in the hair for more than six to eight washes.

Quasi-permanent colours

Quasi-permanent colours are mixed with a low-volume oxidant, usually on a 1:2 ratio. They work in a similar way to permanent colour (see below), in as much as the colour molecules are oxidised. However, as the oxidant is very mild, the colour molecules do not become as large (as permanent colour molecules) and are able to be washed out of the hair over a period of time. The colour is designed to fade gradually over a period of twelve weeks, not giving a re-growth.

Permanent colour

Permanent colours have a wide range of uses in the salon and are available in a variety of colours, from subtle, natural colours, through to striking and bold colours that add individuality and flair to your work.

Permanent colours can lighten or darken the hair and they can also be used to add tone. They may be used to achieve a number of different effects and are designed to cover white hair. Permanent colours may be mixed with 10, 20, 30 or 40 volume hydrogen peroxide, depending on the desired results. Remember to read the manufacturer's instructions to check which hydrogen peroxide strength will give the optimum results, given the base shade you are working on.

Permanent colours may also be referred to as para dyes or oxidation tints. They work by depositing small (usually colourless) molecules into the hair cortex along with the hydrogen peroxide. The hydrogen peroxide (which is an oxidising agent) begins to break down, releasing nascent oxygen, which joins together with the small molecules, to form larger, coloured molecules. As the molecules become larger, they are unable to pass back through the cuticle as they become trapped between the polypeptide chains within the cortex.

Bold colours add flair to your work

Remember

If the hair is too porous and the cuticles are damaged or have been destroyed, even the larger molecules may be washed out of the hair, resulting in colour fade.

Hydrogen peroxide

Hydrogen peroxide is the oxidising agent used in permanent, quasi-permanent, lightening and bleaching services. It comes in different strengths and each strength has a specific purpose. The table below is a guide to choosing the correct volume strength; however, you should always check with the manufacturer's instructions.

Hydrogen peroxide strength	Purpose
10 vol (3%)	Used for refreshing faded ends; giving maximum depth of colour (tinting darker than the natural colour)
20 vol (6%)	Used for permanent colouring when adding depth and/or tone; will give up to 1 shade of lift on a base 6 or above
30 vol (9%)	Used for permanent colouring; will give up to 3 shades of lift on a base 6 or lighter
40 vol (12%)	Used for permanent colouring when using high-lift tints; will give up to 5 shades of lift on a base 6

Keys to good practice

When measuring hydrogen peroxide, if you accidentally pour out too much, you must pour it down the sink. Putting it back into its original container may cause the hydrogen peroxide to start to deteriorate.

Hydrogen peroxide is made up from two parts of hydrogen and two parts of oxygen and is recognised as H_2O_2. It is classed as an unstable substance as it decomposes easily to form water and oxygen ($H_2O + O$). Stabilisers are added during its manufacture to avoid the loss of oxygen during storage. However, during colouring, bleaching and neutralising, the decomposition of the hydrogen peroxide is necessary as the newly formed oxygen (nascent oxygen) does all the work.

When mixing colouring products with hydrogen peroxide, you must follow the manufacturer's instructions regarding the mixing ratios. Some colourants are mixed on a 1:1 ratio, for example, 30 ml of oxidant to 30 ml of colourant, whereas others, such as high-lift tints and quasi-permanent colours, may be mixed on a 2:1 ratio, for example, 60 ml of oxidant to 30 ml of colourant.

There are occasions when the salon may not have the correct strength of oxidant in stock. Diluting the hydrogen peroxide with water may readily solve this problem. For example, if you only have 40 vol (or 12%) but need 30 vol (9%):

$\frac{30}{40} = \frac{3}{4}$ You would need to use three parts H_2O_2 to one part water to achieve 30 vol.

To dilute 40 vol (12%) to 20 vol (6%):

$\frac{20}{40} = \frac{2}{4} = \frac{1}{2}$ You would need to use one part H_2O_2 to one part water.

pH

The pH value indicates the levels of acidity or alkalinity within a product. The pH value of colouring products is an important factor to consider; acidic products are kinder to the hair as they help to close the cuticles, whereas alkali products will open the cuticles. The more alkaline the product, the more damage it will cause to the hair, therefore you should consider the products you are using and the potential damage they may cause.

As most colouring products are alkali (they open the cuticles), it is essential that an anti-oxidant conditioner be used after the colour has been shampooed off the hair. An anti-oxidant conditioner will:

- return the hair back to its normal pH of 4.5–5.5 (slightly acid)
- add moisture to the hair
- stop any further oxidation taking place (continuing oxidation will cause unnecessary damage to the hair)
- close the cuticles.

Remember

Remember to keep the salon clean and tidy throughout the service, as this will maintain your professional image and help to prevent cross-infection. All remaining colouring products and used materials must be disposed of correctly.

Correcting the colour problem

Removing the colour

There will be times during colouring services when some of the hair has achieved the desired result and therefore the colour needs to be removed to prevent over-processing. This is particularly so when carrying out a full head of bleached foil/packet highlights. Great care must be taken when removing the foils that have reached the desired degree of lift, to ensure that the hair that is still processing is not disturbed. If care isn't taken, the colour may bleed (causing an unnecessary colour correction service to take place).

It is important when removing colouring and lightening products from the hair that the hair and scalp are thoroughly clean and devoid of any residual products. Failure to ensure the hair and scalp are clean can lead to scalp irritation and chemical damage.

If you have a junior member of staff working with you, it is essential that this and other relevant information be given clearly and accurately to him or her, as this will ensure a good final result. Failure to give clear and accurate information to less experienced members of staff will ultimately lead to mistakes and client dissatisfaction.

Using different products to remove artificial colour

Removing artificial colour

Artificial colour is usually removed from the hair because the colour is too dark. It is much easier to add depth to hair that is too light, but removing artificial colour requires knowledge and skill. As tint will not lighten hair that already has tint on it, the tint must be removed first. Artificial colour may be removed from the hair either by reduction or bleaching.

Removing colour by reduction

This involves removing artificial colour (tint) from the hair. As you already know, permanent colour works by depositing small colourless molecules into the cortex along with the hydrogen peroxide. The hydrogen peroxide (which is an oxidising agent) begins to break down, releasing nascent oxygen, which joins together with the small molecules, to form larger, coloured molecules. As the molecules become larger, they are unable to pass back through the cuticle as they become trapped between the polypeptide chains within the cortex.

The process of removing the permanent colour requires the colour reducer to penetrate the cortex and break down the large molecules into smaller molecules that can then be passed through the cuticles and rinsed away.

This service is usually carried out if the hair has a build-up of colouring products or it is too dark. The client's hair may be too dark due to applying an incorrect colour or because the client has decided to change the colour of the hair to a lighter shade.

Use reduction or bleaching to remove colour that is too dark

Before carrying out a colour reduction service, all tests should be performed and results assessed, especially porosity and elasticity tests, to ensure the hair is strong enough to endure the harsh treatment that will follow. This should be continued throughout the service, so that you are aware of any sudden deterioration in the hair's condition.

Keys to good practice

Test cuttings carried out prior to the application will give a good indication of the outcome of the service.

As a general rule, colour reducers may be mixed with either water or hydrogen peroxide, depending on the amount of lift required. You must assess the condition of the hair, as the more damaged the hair, the weaker the mixture would normally be.

To 'clean out' a build-up of colour, the colour reducer would usually be mixed with either water or 3% hydrogen peroxide. However, if you need to remove the colour to lighten the hair, 6% or 9% hydrogen peroxide may be used. When using colour reducers, the manufacturer's instructions must always be followed.

The application of the colour reducer should always be started where the colour is darkest and/or the hair most resistant. This is to allow more time for the colour reducer to work in these areas. Your application should be carried out as quickly as possible, but taking care to apply the colour reducer methodically to ensure all intended areas are covered. Care must be taken to avoid the re-growth area.

Keys to good practice

Use strips of cotton wool between the sections to ensure the re-growth area doesn't come into contact with the colour reducer.

It is highly unlikely that you will achieve an even base to work on. As the hair's porosity will have been uneven before application, the colour will be removed more quickly from the areas that are most porous, thus giving an uneven result.

While the colour reducer is developing, you should remain with your client and monitor the development as the colour may lighten unexpectedly. When development is complete, remove the colour reducer by rinsing the hair with cool water and shampoo the hair thoroughly. The hair should now be dried and the results assessed to ensure a satisfactory result. The colour is likely to be very warm and this may be quite alarming to your client. Therefore you may need to reassure your client that this is not the end of the service and not to worry. At this point the colour result may not be satisfactory and remedial action will be necessary before applying the target colour.

1. If the result is patchy, it may be necessary to re-apply the colour reducer to the darker areas to even out the colour.
2. If the result is excessively warm you may either:
   - Use a mild bleach mixture to remove the warm tones in the hair.
   - Choose a matt/ash tone to neutralize the warmth.

Re-colouring the hair

Removing colour by oxidation

All pre-service tests must be carried out prior to the application to ensure the hair is suitable for the service. Test cuttings taken before the service will give a clear indication of the final colour result and the condition of the hair afterwards.

Removing colour by oxidation is carried out in much the same way as removing colour by reduction, in that the darkest or most resistant areas are treated first. The main difference is the products that are used work by oxidation. These products are bleach preparations and they will not only lighten the artificial colour, but the natural hair colour as well. For this reason, the re-growth area should be avoided. An even base may not be achieved on the first application and it may be necessary to re-bleach any darker areas with a second application to ensure an even base.

If your client requests a warm target shade, you may bleach the hair to its corresponding depth, and then apply the target colour.

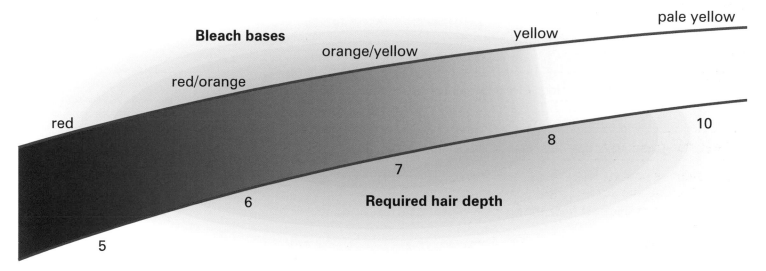

Bleach bases and their corresponding depths

However, if the client chooses an ashen or matt tone, the hair should be bleached lighter to remove excess warmth from the hair. In both instances, you may wish to add a little base to the target colour to ensure the colour adequately covers the hair and does not result in a translucent effect.

This method of removing artificial colour from the hair is most commonly used to 'break up' a full-head colour, e.g. highlights. Throughout the service you must check the elasticity of the hair at regular intervals to ensure the hair condition is not deteriorating. After the service, the client's hair will be extremely porous and the internal fibres may have experienced some distress; therefore it is essential you give the client extensive after-care advice on how to maintain the colour and condition.

Removing bands of colour

Bands of colour usually appear as a direct result of incorrect application or choice of colour when selecting or matching the existing hair colour. The banding may be either darker or lighter than the rest of the hair and needs to be corrected. When carrying out any colour correction service, pre-service testing and research into the

client's chemical history should be carried out. This includes even the most
experienced hairdressers. If the bands of colour were lighter than the rest of the hair,
spot colouring the hair using a tint to match would correct this; however, you must
consider whether it is necessary to add warm tones into the hair (this may be necessary
if the banded hair is lacking warmth, possibly as a result of a bleach application).

If the colour is too dark, it will need to be lightened sufficiently to match the existing
hair. This may be carried out in several ways, depending on the degree of lift
required. Many manufacturers recommend using their lightest tint, usually a 10/0
mixed with either 6, 9 or 12 % hydrogen peroxide and applied to the darker bands.
Development must be closely monitored and when the colour reaches the desired
shade, blot off any excess product and apply your target shade.

Darker banding may also be removed from the hair by mixing powder bleach with
water and a little shampoo to give a good consistency to work with. This is then
applied to the darker bands and must be monitored carefully until the desired
amount of lift has been reached. The key to correcting banding has to be precision in
your product application, e.g. no overlapping.

Re-colouring hair after the reduction process

Before re-colouring the hair, you must consider the condition of the hair. The hair
will be very porous and therefore you should choose the colouring products you use
very carefully. Immediately after the colour reduction service, the cuticles of the hair
will be open and receptive to colour. On occasion this may result in the final colour
result being darker than expected. Therefore it may be wise to opt for a slightly lighter
shade to ensure client satisfaction.

The condition of the client's hair will have suffered during the process and effective
after-care advice must be given.

Re-colouring bleached hair using pre-pigmentation and permanent colour

Pre-pigmentation is the term used to describe restoring lost pigment to pale hair that
needs to be made darker and/or warmer. An example of this is a client with bleached
hair who wishes to go back to her natural colour. As bleaching removes the warm
tones (red and yellow) from the hair, these tones must be replaced prior to applying
the target shade or the finished result will have a green cast.

Pre-pigmenting may be carried out using semi-permanent, quasi-permanent or
permanent colour; however the porosity of the hair must be taken into consideration
when choosing the correct product. The pre-colour may be either red, copper or gold,
depending on the depth of the target shade, e.g. a light colour would usually require a
gold pre-colour, whereas darker hair would require a red pre-colour. The diagram on
page 259 indicates the correct colour to use. Always follow the manufacturer's instructions.

Keys to good practice

When taking clients back to their natural colour, always use one shade
lighter than the target shade. You can add colour to the hair at any time but it
is more difficult to remove colour from processed hair.

Colour correction: a step-by-step guide

Before the service.

A copper semi-permanent colour was applied to the hair, avoiding the re-growth area.

Cotton wool was placed between each section to prevent the colour from touching the re-growth area.

The colour was left to develop.

Excess colour was wiped off to check development.

The hair after pre-pigmentation.

A dark golden blonde permanent colour was applied to the re-growth.

The permanent colour was applied to the mid-lengths and ends.

The finished result.

Correcting highlights and lowlights

In the salon

Cheryl was a very quiet, traditional client who attended the salon every three months for fine bleached highlights to brighten her hair, but she didn't want anything too noticeable. She cancelled her next appointment at the salon without giving a reason, but said she would phone again soon for a cut and blow dry. A few days later she telephoned the salon, asking for an immediate colour appointment. When she entered the salon, it appeared that she had a full-head bleach. She was very upset and proceeded to tell the stylist that she had bought a home highlighting kit and persuaded her friend to have a go, as it didn't look too difficult. The result was not at all as she expected! After carrying out all the pre-service tests and examinations, the stylist then proceeded to weave out sections of hair, to break up the colour and colour them to match her natural base, but with some added warmth to counteract the effects of the bleach (and prevent the colour from having a green cast). The result was good and Cheryl was very pleased with the result and decided she would leave colouring to the experts from now on.

There are several reasons why highlights or lowlights may need to be corrected. The most common reasons are stated below.

Problem	Caused by	Remedy
High/low lights give the effect of a full-head colour	Too many highlights have been coloured; more likely to occur on fine hair.	Weave out sections of hair and apply a colour to match the client's natural base, giving the illusion of a highlighted effect.
High/low lights do not show	The wrong choice of colour. High/low lights woven too finely. This is most common on clients with thick, dense hair. Not enough hair was coloured.	The whole highlighting procedure should be carried out. If using bleach/lightening products, take care not to bleach/lighten the hair that has previously been treated.
Patches of colour at the roots	Product seepage from foils.	Weave out sections of the affected hair and apply a colour to match the client's natural base. If the product that bled was bleach, you will need to add a little warmth to the base colour to prevent a green cast appearing.

Seepage of product has caused a patchy result

The affected areas are weaved out and spot coloured

The finished result showing even highlights

Pre-softening the hair

Hair would usually require pre-softening due to its resistant tendencies. The resistance of a client's hair is due to the cuticle scales being flat and smooth, usually found in hair in good condition. Some hair, such as Oriental hair, falls into this category as it has more layers of cuticle scales than either European or African Caribbean hair and therefore doesn't allow the colour to penetrate into the cortex and develop.

You may discover a client's hair is resistant to colour when you assess the final result of a colouring service. The indicators would be:

- The colouring product has not covered the natural hair colour
- The white hair has a translucent appearance, e.g. it has been coloured but has not covered.

White hair that is resistant to colour may be recognized by its 'glassy' appearance. You can overcome this by pre-softening the hair, which lifts the cuticle scales, allowing colour molecules to enter the cortex.

Pre-softening the hair is a relatively quick and simple process. It involves applying neat 10 vol or 3% hydrogen peroxide to the resistant areas, drying the H_2O_2 into the hair and then proceeding with the colouring service. You may find it easier to use cream hydrogen peroxide as it has a thicker consistency and is therefore easier to work with.

For common colouring problems and solutions, see Unit H30.

Whatever colour correction service you have carried out, it is essential that you confirm your client's satisfaction at the end of the service. If you have given your client the correct information, both prior to and during the service, the outcome should be as expected.

After the service

When any colour service is complete it is imperative to give the client the correct advice. This will serve to ensure long-lasting results and client satisfaction. It is also a good retail opportunity.

After-care advice

Once the colour correction service has been completed to the satisfaction of your client, you must advise the client on how to care for his or her hair and maintain the colour. You may also need to advise the client to visit the salon for further services in order to keep the hair in the best condition possible. This is essential if the client's hair shows more than minimal damage in the cortex. If you feel the client's hair could not withstand any further chemical processing, you must inform the client of this and outline the possible consequences, e.g. hair breakage.

During the initial and ongoing consultation you will have determined the condition of your client's hair and given advice on the most suitable products for home use, e.g. shampoo and conditioner. You should ensure your client understands the importance of looking after his or her hair in order to maintain the colour and keep the hair in optimum condition. You should discuss the features and benefits of the shampoo and conditioning products that you have recommended and explain that they have been specifically designed for use after colour or colour correction treatments. This may

You need to advise your client on the most suitable products for home use

include the use of a restructuring treatment that will help to rebuild the internal fibres in the cortex and improve the elasticity of the hair. You must ensure the client understands not only how these products help to maintain her hair in good condition but how and when to use them.

Check it out

List the retail products available for colour correction clients to purchase after the service.

Completion of the record card

On completion of the service it is essential that you complete the client's record card. The information contained on the client record card must be clear to other stylists who may colour the client's hair in the future and include explicit details of the colour correction service.

Disposal of waste

At the end of the colour service, any waste products and materials must be disposed of carefully and in a safe manner. All unused colouring products should be disposed of, following the manufacturer's instructions. If you are in any doubt as to how the products should be disposed of, you should contact the product manufacturer and ask for their advice.

Knowledge check

1. List the factors that must be established during a consultation for a colour correction service.

2. Why is it essential to identify any contra-indications prior to the service?

3. Why is it important to consider the hair's elasticity and porosity when carrying out a colour correction service?

4. State the specific safety considerations (COSHH) relating to the use of powder bleach.

5. State the difference between the reduction and oxidation processes.

6. State all the possible methods that you may consider when removing artificial colour from a client's hair that is too dark.

7. When re-colouring a client's hair after a colour removal service, what should you take into consideration?

8. Complete the following table relating to high/low lighting problems:

Problem	Caused by	Remedy
High/low lights give the effect of a full-head colour	Too much hair has been coloured.	
High/low-lights do not show		The whole highlighting procedure should be carried out. If using bleach/lightening products, take care not to bleach/lighten hair that has previously been treated.
Patches of colour at the roots	Product seepage from foils/packets.	

Style and dress hair to achieve a variety of creative looks

Unit H25

Introduction

There are many different ways that hair can be styled and dressed in a creative way; this includes setting, blow-drying, pin curling, finger waving, and using heated styling equipment. You may also need to use added hair to create volume in the style, increase the length of the client's hair, or to give a variety of colour. By combining some of the above techniques, your styling and dressing will become more exciting and innovative, making you a much-sought-after stylist.

The key terms used in this unit are:

- **Current** – styling which is currently fashionable
- **Emerging** – styling that is up and coming, possibly bordering on avant-garde.

What you will learn

- Preparing the client
- Different styling techniques and the effects that may be produced
- Dressing the hair

Different styling and dressing techniques are used to create innovative looks

You the stylist

Styling and dressing hair gives you a great opportunity to use your creative and artistic flair. Sadly, some hairdressers see this service only as a 'finish' to other services, for example, cutting, colouring, or perming. Styling and dressing hair should be looked upon as an exciting opportunity for you to gain valuable insight into ways in which you can personalise your work to suit the individual and the occasion.

Preparing the client

Preparation for any service is essential; it reflects both your salon's image and also your professional approach towards your work. You will need to consider the tools and equipment you will need to carry out the service. To ensure compliance with health and safety legislation, your tools and equipment should be clean and sterile before use on every client to prevent cross-infection and infestation. Methods of sterilising tools and equipment can be found in Unit G1. Any electrical equipment should be checked prior to use to make sure it is safe and fit for purpose. This will safeguard against accidents and minimise the risk of damage to the equipment. Remember, your responsibilities under the Health and Safety at Work Act 1974 apply throughout your work in the salon, regardless of the service you are carrying out.

You should also be aware of your responsibilities under the COSHH Regulations in relation to using styling and finishing products, as well as your responsibilities under the Electricity at Work Regulations 1989 when you are using electrical equipment.

Check it out

What can you remember about the Electricity at Work Regulations and the COSHH Regulations? What are your responsibilities within these health and safety laws? If you are unsure, look back at Unit G1.

What you will learn

- Personal health and hygiene
- Preparing the client for the service
- Thorough consultation

Personal health and hygiene

Your own standards of health and hygiene are important. If you attend work knowing that you have an infectious or contagious condition, you must consider the consequences of cross-infection to other people at work. Working while you are unwell will have a negative impact on the salon, regardless of whether or not you have infected a client or colleague.

In most hairdressing environments, you are working in close proximity to your clients so your personal hygiene is important. It can be particularly unpleasant for clients to experience your second-hand garlic or onions from lunch. Equally, the smell of stale nicotine on your breath or clothes should be avoided. Basic good personal hygiene rules should be followed at all times to ensure you do not cause offence to your clients or colleagues.

Preparing the client for the service

When your client enters the salon, take a good look at her prior to gowning. You should be looking at the type of clothes she is wearing to give you an indication of her image and whether she is more likely to require conventional styling or something more adventurous. Before you begin the service, you must ensure your client is gowned appropriately and the towel is positioned correctly. Keep checking throughout the service to ensure the gown and towel are still positioned correctly and her clothes are protected from spillages.

Check it out

If you are applying coloured mousse or setting lotion, what should you be wearing to protect your hands and clothes from staining? How should you protect your client from accidental spillages?

Thorough consultation

You must make sure your consultations are thorough so that you can carry out your client's wishes accurately. Use a stylebook where necessary to make sure both you and your client fully understand each other and the outcome of the service. There are several influencing factors that need to be considered prior to styling and dressing:

- the desired look
- the hair texture, length and density
- the haircut, client's facial features and head and face shape
- any hair growth patterns and elasticity.

The desired look

You must take into consideration the desired look; the client may be going somewhere special and have preconceived ideas of how she wishes to look. Alternatively, she may have no ideas but is open to suggestions. You need to understand the potential of your client's hair to ensure the final look is appropriate to her age, personality, and the occasion.

The hair texture, length and density

There are many questions you need to ask yourself with regard to your client's hair to ensure optimum results, for example, will the client's hair length, texture and density allow me to create the style required? If the client's hair is too long, thick and heavy, there is the possibility the style will drop quickly; however, with the correct styling products, this may be avoided. If you feel the hair is unlikely to achieve the desired outcome, use your skill and expertise to suggest styles that are achievable.

The haircut and client's facial features

The client's haircut must be suitable for the style you wish to create and the head and face shape should suit the intended style. Any unusual facial features may be disguised by clever styling and dressing; ignoring these could lead to an unsuitable style and unhappy client.

Hair growth patterns and elasticity

If the client has any hair growth patterns, such as a widow's peak or cowlick, this may affect the way the hair lies and should be taken into consideration during the consultation. Again, with clever styling and dressing, these may be disguised. Ideally, the hair should be styled and dressed to follow the natural fall of the hair, as this will prolong the life of the style and help reduce the possibility of the hair lying awkwardly the next day. The hair's elasticity must be considered because, if it is poor, you cannot guarantee a good result.

In the salon

Zaid, the junior stylist, was asked to carry out a blow-dry on a client with fine, one-length, over-bleached hair. As the client wanted her hair as straight as possible, Zaid was blow-drying the hair with a fair degree of tension. With each section that he blow-dried, the hair was visibly stretching. The finished result was very uneven.

- What do you think has happened to the hair?
- Why should you not overstretch the hair in this way?

Keys to good practice

If in doubt, carry out an elasticity test! The hair should stretch and return to its original length when the pulling force is removed.

It is your responsibility to take all the influencing factors into consideration and, should there be any potential problems, discuss them with the client and agree a course of action prior to the service rather than 'hoping for the best'. This will ensure that your client receives a professional style and dress service and leaves the salon as a satisfied client.

Your salon is trying to portray a professional image, which should be reflected in the high standard of work it carries out. Only your absolute best is good enough. Once you are both happy with the outcome of the consultation, you need to decide on the most appropriate styling and finishing products for your client's hair. By this stage, the client should have been made aware of the cost and duration of the service.

Check it out

Find out the times your salon allows for you to complete your styling, dressing and finishing services. These timings should be commercially viable for your salon.

The client should now be prepared for shampooing. While your assistant is shampooing (using a good-quality shampoo to ensure thorough cleansing), you should utilise this time to ensure you have all the tools and equipment you will need close to hand and everything is clean and sterile. This will enable you to provide an efficient and professional service, as you will not have to keep your client waiting while you find whatever is missing.

Different styling techniques and the effects that may be produced

To create variety and originality in your styling, use a combination of the styling techniques below, and remember that the techniques can be mixed and matched. You should not disregard any ideas at this stage; sometimes the results will amaze you!

In this section you will learn about the different styling techniques, how they work, and the results that can be achieved.

What you will learn

- Setting
- Blow-drying
- Pin curling
- Finger waving
- Use of heated styling equipment
- Added hair

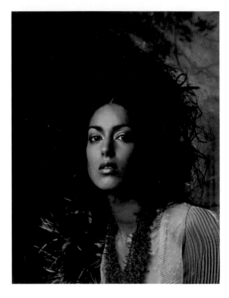

A combination of styling techniques can create amazing results

The results of these styling techniques will cause a physical change within the hair. The change is temporary and will last only until the hair is wet or absorbs moisture from the atmosphere. The temporary changes that take place in the hair are usually classed as either:

- cohesive setting (wet – stretch – dry)
- temporary setting (heat – mould – cool).

Setting

The setting process enables straight hair to be made curly and curly hair made straighter. This is due to the way the hair is structured. As you already know, within the cortex lie a number of polypeptide chains, which run along the length of the hair. The chains are spiral-shaped (called an alpha (α) helix) and have cross-linkages that join them to their neighbouring polypeptide chains. Some of these linkages are permanent and others are temporary.

The hydrogen bonds, which are one of the temporary linkages, are the ones that enable us to set the hair. The hydrogen bonds are not only joined to their neighbouring polypeptide chain, but are also linked within the same polypeptide chain between the coils of the alpha helix. It is these hydrogen bonds that enable the hair to be stretched during setting, giving the hair its elasticity.

Check it out

Which of the above styling techniques are classed as cohesive and which are temporary?

Before the hair is shampooed, the hydrogen bonds hold the coils of the polypeptide chains close together. The hair in this state is known as alpha (α) keratin. Once the hair has been shampooed, many of the hydrogen bonds are broken, allowing the hair to be stretched around the roller or brush (if blow-drying).

Once the hair has been stretched, fully dried and allowed to cool into the new shape, the hair is said to be in beta (β) keratin state. It is essential that the hair is fully dried and allowed to cool before brushing and styling. If the hair is still warm, some of the new shape may be lost.

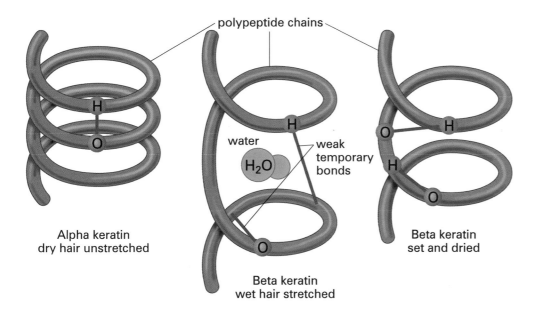

The hair will stay in this new position until the hair is made wet or it absorbs atmospheric moisture. This is due to the hair being hygroscopic – it has the ability to absorb moisture from the atmosphere. Humidity levels (the degree of moisture in the atmosphere) will affect the length of time a set or blow-dry will last. The level of humidity in some salons may be quite high due to the evaporation of water from the hair, towels, and so on. This is also true during damp weather, therefore it is essential that good styling products be used, as this will help to prevent the atmospheric moisture entering the hair as quickly, prolonging the life of your styling.

Some styling products contain plastic resins, which are left as a film on the hair once the hair is dry. This plastic film helps to prevent the atmospheric moisture from being absorbed by the hair.

Temporary setting (heat – mould – cool)

As with cohesive setting, the hydrogen bonds need to be broken. When using heated styling equipment on dry hair, the hair's internal moisture breaks some of the hydrogen bonds; however, it is essential that the equipment be heated sufficiently to turn the internal moisture into steam. As temporary setting utilises the natural moisture that is present in hair, overuse of heated styling equipment will cause the hair to dehydrate.

Tools and equipment for setting

There is a variety of equipment that may be used when setting the hair including rollers, Velcro rollers and Molton Browners (bendy rollers). In addition to conventional setting equipment, this unit will also cover the use of more unconventional items such as pipe-cleaners and matchboxes.

Double rollers may be used to produce spiral curls

For this part of the unit you need to experiment with items that are not normally associated with setting but will alter the shape of the hair. This may include items such as pipe-cleaners, straws, foils, chopsticks, rik-raks, matchboxes, and Toblerone boxes. The shape of the 'former' is the shape you will achieve, for example, if you use a Toblerone box, you will achieve angular curls.

When using items that are made from cardboard, the dry setting method should be used. If the hair is wet, the cardboard will become soggy! You must also ensure the shape of the item will not distort during use, as this would result in an incorrect form.

Many non-conventional items can be found at trade exhibitions, but that does not exclude you from designing your own. You need to consider the potential health and safety risks when choosing non-conventional items. For example:

- Are there any sharp edges that may cause discomfort to the client?
- Will it conduct heat under the dryer and burn the client?
- Is it flammable?
- Will it melt under the dryer?
- Can it be cleaned and sterilised?
- Is it safe to use and fit for purpose?

Check it out

Look at a client who uses straightening irons on a regular basis and test how brittle the hair feels. This is a good indicator of dehydrated hair, not to mention the damage to the cuticle!

Remember

Setting may be carried out on hair that is wet, that is, just shampooed, or hair that is dry. When setting dry hair, heat is required to mould the hair into its new shape.

Using unconventional setting techniques: a step-by-step guide

A fine section of hair and double length of foil is taken. The foil is then pinned at the roots using pin curl clips.

The foil is folded up to the roots and pinned in place. Then the foil is folded from the bottom, backwards and forwards to give a concertina effect.

Secure the foil using pins.

Continue steps 1–3 until all the required hair has been folded. Then heat each 'packet' using straightening irons.

The back of the hair is straightened using straightening irons to add contrast to the finished look.

The finished look.

Check it out

Using a block, try setting the hair using everyday items not usually used for setting. Remember, you must consider the health and safety risks that may be associated with using non-conventional items. For example, a can of hairspray may give a good even round shape, but what are the potential risks when the aerosol goes under the dryer?

Winding techniques

Root to point

Root to point winding is usually carried out on hair that is shoulder-length or longer. The hair is wound on a long thin 'rod', for example, a straw, twig or chopstick, in a spiral manner, working down the 'rod' and taking care not to twist or buckle the hair.

Even curl along the length of the hair

If the hair is wrapped around the rod in this manner, the diameter of the curl stays consistent throughout the length of the hair and produces an even spiral curl formation.

Point to root (croquignole) wind

Most conventional setting is carried out using this method of setting. Depending on the length of the hair, this method of winding will give a looser curl at the root than at the ends, as the hair is wound over the previous hair with each revolution.

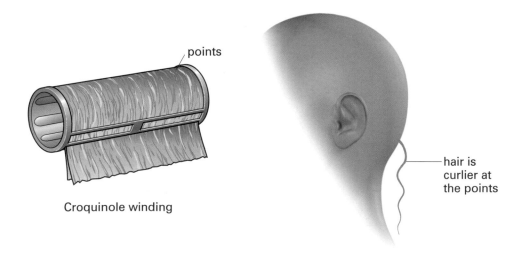

points

Croquinole winding

hair is curlier at the points

The roller size used is determined by the hair texture, density, and the amount of curl required. A general rule would be: the finer the hair, the smaller the roller. A client with fine hair in texture but abundant in mass may find the hair too curly if it is set on rollers that are too small.

Once you have decided on your style, you need to plan how you can achieve this. The direction in which you wind the hair will depend on the intended result (directional setting). You also need to consider the amount of lift required and whether you need to wind on or off base.

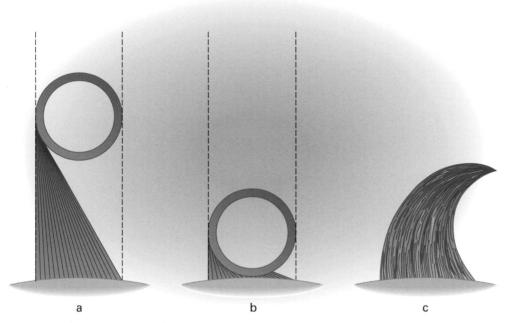

Hair wound to sit on its own base

To achieve normal root lift, the roller must be sitting on its own base. If the hair is dragged forward at an obtuse angle to the scalp, this will give increased lift.

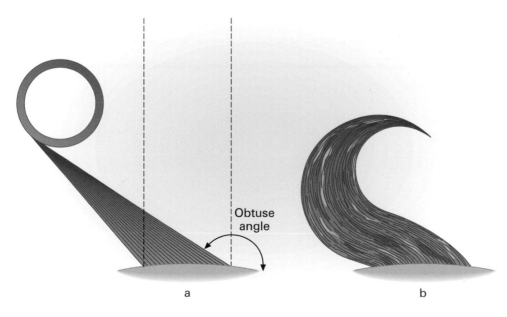

Achieving increased lift

If the obtuse angle is increased (over-directed), the roller will sit off base. The result will give straight roots and curled ends, therefore gaining direction from the root area with some fullness at the ends. This type of setting may be used to create 'flicks' on the ends of the hair or to disguise a high forehead or hair that is receding at the temples.

If the hair is dragged back at an acute angle, the roller will sit off base. Hair with 'dragged' roots would usually be used at the sides and back of the head where the hairstyle requires less volume.

Once your set is complete, your client needs to be placed under the dryer. You must check the position of the setting pins (if used) to ensure they will not cause any client discomfort.

Keys to good practice

If using metal setting pins, make sure they are not in contact with the client's scalp as they conduct heat and could burn the client's skin and scalp.

The length of time the client is under the dryer will vary depending on the length and density of the hair. If the rollers are removed before the hair is completely dry, the set will drop. However, if the client's hair is over-dried, this can cause the hair to become flyaway, making it difficult to dress. In addition, the unnecessary heat will cause the hair to become dry and dehydrated.

When the hair is completely dry, allow the hair to cool before removing rollers and pins, as the hair is still warm and soft at this point and the set may drop. When removing rollers, care should be taken to avoid causing the client any discomfort, especially if you have used a strong styling product that leaves the hair with a 'crispy' feel.

Roller marks should be removed by thorough brushing, which also stimulates the blood flow and sebaceous activity in the scalp. However, some styles do not require brushing. The rollers are removed from the hair and it is teased into shape with the addition of dressing products. Other sets are not brushed but merely combed through with a wide-tooth comb to maintain the curl.

By combining setting on and off base, you can create more personalised and innovative looks.

Blow-drying

Tools and equipment used for blow-drying

You will need:

- hairdryer
- nozzle or diffuser
- fingers
- radial brushes (various sizes available)
- paddle brush
- flat brushes, for example, Denman brushes
- vent brush (for more textured looks).

By now you should have experienced using a variety of different brushes and other equipment and no doubt you will have decided upon those which you find most comfortable to use and give the results you require. However, the industry is always making advances and producing new tools, so do not be afraid to experiment and try out other alternatives.

Drying techniques

By now you should have extensive experience of blow-drying a variety of different styles and determining which method of blow-drying, tools and equipment are most suitable for your client's hair texture. The techniques you learned and mastered during your initial training should now be adapted or modified to meet your clients' ever-increasing demands. Some examples of drying techniques are described below.

Root to point

This type of drying would be used where the main emphasis is shiny hair. To create smooth shiny hair, the hair should always be dried in a root to point direction, with the airflow following the lie of the cuticle.

Point to root

There are many reasons for drying hair in this way, but maximum shine will not be your priority.

When drying hair using a diffuser, the heat is travelling in a point to root direction. The results can vary from a tousled look to very curly.

When blow-drying fine hair that requires volume, you may need to direct the airflow against the lie of the cuticle so the cuticle becomes roughened and 'mattes' the hair together, giving the illusion of body. When 'blasting' hair to create volume, the same principle would be used.

When finger drying short hair, it is sometimes necessary to direct the airflow into the hair to ruffle the cuticle; this will add volume and give a less structured finish to your styling.

Creative blow-drying can produce a variety of different effects from smooth, straight looks to curly, unkempt looks. Your client's requirements should have been discussed at length prior to carrying out the service.

You must consider any influencing factors when preparing for a blow-dry service. Is it possible to create the style the client wishes?

Hair roots

Hair points

Drying from root to point

Pin curling

Pin curls may be used creatively to produce a variety of effects, including flat waves, curl, body and waves. The effects are stunning, especially when used in conjunction with the other styling techniques mentioned in this unit.

Pin curls are not always suitable for frizzy or very long hair; you will achieve the best results using pin curling on medium, textured hair with a little natural movement. Take extra care when pin curling on hair that has been permed, tinted or bleached, as it marks easily and tends to buckle.

Types of pin curl

Barrel curl or stand-up pin curl

Gives the style lift and body. If using barrel curls in conjunction with rollers, you must ensure the diameter of the pin curl is the same as that of the roller.

Half stand barrel curl

Creates springy, loose curls; ideal for use at the sides of the head as the curls move away from the head.

Flat barrel curl

Used to create flat movements that lie close to the head. The flat barrel curl is used when carrying out reverse curling to produce waves.

Flat barrel with the ends on the outside

Used to create styles that require loose uncurled hair ends.

Long stem pin curls

These pin curls are designed to sit 'off base'. They give a flat effect with curl at the ends and may be used to define the style in the nape, at the sides, or the front hairline.

Sculptured curls

Again, these pin curls are designed to sit 'off base'. The hair is combed and moulded into position then either pinned or taped into place. These curls give very soft movement on short hair.

Clockspring curls

A clockspring curl has a closed centre and produces a tight curl on the ends with looser movement at the roots. It is generally used to create a curly effect in the nape of the neck.

You must make sure the heads of the metal pins are not touching the skin, as this may result in burning the client's skin and scalp. If necessary, place a fine mesh of cotton wool underneath the offending pin; this will protect the client from burning.

Keys to good practice

As with any hairdressing technique, the more you practise, the better you will get. For example, mastering pin curling might open up new avenues to creative styling!

Finger waving

Finger waving produces flat waves in the hair; no root lift is achieved using this technique. The hair is moulded into 's'-shaped movements using the fingers and a straight comb. The use of strong styling products is essential when finger waving and the hair must remain wet (but not dripping) throughout the service. When finger waving, you should follow the natural fall of the hair and utilise any natural movement that may be present; this will help to prolong the life of the style.

This type of styling is best carried out on hair that is medium to fine in texture and a reasonable length, especially on the crown. However, if using finger waving in conjunction with another styling technique, good results may be achieved by waving the sides or back, allowing the top area of the style to retain some fullness. Finger waves should be dried under a hood dryer, as the hair should be disturbed as little as possible.

When dressing waved hair, it is not usual to brush through the hair, but to comb it using a wide-tooth comb to encourage the wave formation.

Use of heated styling equipment

Heated styling equipment comes in many different forms, which include:

- tongs
- straightening irons
- crimping irons
- Marcel waving irons
- heated rollers
- hot brush
- flexi curlers (heated bendy rollers).

Before using any type of heated electrical equipment, you should ensure it is fit for purpose and safe to use. You should also know how to use the equipment properly and in a safe manner to prevent accidents from occurring.

Keys to good practice

Ask a senior stylist to show you how to use equipment that is new to you. Under the Electricity at Work Regulations, you should not be using equipment that you have not been trained to use.

Care must be taken when using heated electrical equipment. It is very easy to overheat the hair when using this type of equipment and could lead to damage to the cuticle and dehydration of the hair. The equipment should be in contact with the hair for the minimum time necessary to achieve the desired result. You must ensure that you position your client in a way that enables you to access all areas of the hair without causing unnecessary discomfort or burning of the client.

In the salon

Kath was tonging a client's hair in the salon. It was mid-August and the salon was very warm. The client removed her gown as she was becoming uncomfortably hot. The client was wearing a vest top with narrow shoulder straps. Kath was also becoming very warm and starting to perspire. Suddenly the tongs slipped out of her hands and dropped onto her client's shoulders causing a third-degree burn.

- Was Kath negligible in her duty to her client?
- How could this situation have been avoided?

Remember

Many styling products are flammable, so you must make sure no one is smoking in the near vicinity when you are using such products.

Heated styling equipment should be used on clean, dry hair that does not have excess products on it. Excess products may cause the hair to stick to the heated appliance causing discomfort to the client. It may also coat the appliance, which will then require thorough cleaning, or, at the very least, reduce the effectiveness of the equipment due to heat loss.

When using electrical styling equipment, you must make sure there are no fish hooks. Place the tongs close to the roots and slide the tongs down the length of the hair. This softens the hair prior to styling and also smoothes down the cuticle. The hair is usually easier to manage and it enables you to take the tongs right down to the points of the hair and secure them firmly within the barrel of the tongs.

Types of heating styling equipment and their uses

Equipment	Types	Effects
Tongs	Small barrel Large barrel	Small, tight curls if used on short hair; spiral curls if wound in a spiral manner on long hair. Gives curl and/or movement; may be used for spiral curling on long hair but will give a soft result
Spiral tongs		Spiral curls
Straightening irons	Metal plates	Temporarily straighten the hair
	Ceramic plates	Temporarily straighten the hair; are less damaging to the hair than metal plates and also help to retain moisture
Crimping irons		Give a crimped effect on the hair
Heated rollers	Various sizes	Gives curl, adds lift and volume
Hot brush	Various sizes	Gives curl, adds lift and volume
Flexi curlers	Various sizes	Gives a variety of effects, from large bouncy curls to spiral ones

Keys to good practice

Any electrically heated styling equipment should not be cleaned using water due to the risk of electrocution, but wiped over with spirit.

Positioning of self and client

Client comfort is essential throughout the service. You may need to adjust your client's position to enable you to reach certain areas of the head, for example, when tonging your client's hair in the nape, they should have their head down. This will enable you to get right into the nape area. You should always place a comb underneath the tongs to prevent them touching the skin.

Think about your own posture while you are working. Stooping or stretching will cause unnecessary stress on your body, causing aches and pains. Ideally, you should be standing with your feet at shoulders' width apart and your weight evenly distributed on both feet. Make use of hydraulic chairs, as these may be adjusted to suit the height of both yourself and your client, enabling you to maintain correct posture. Keep your tools and equipment close to hand and positioned in a way that does not require you to over-stretch to reach them.

Throughout the service your work area should be kept clean and tidy. This will help to promote a professional image and should also reduce the risk of cross-infection.

Added hair

Added hair has been around for many years. Its popularity has risen and fallen as fashions have changed. Added hair has been increasing in popularity over the last few years and has seen many younger clients and fashion icons favouring its use. This has had an impact on most age groups and added hair is now instrumental within the styling and dressing service, regardless of the age of the client. Currently there are many different forms of 'added hair' available. They range from clip-on hair swatches through to the more traditional postiche.

Reasons for using added hair

- To add volume to fine hair.
- To add length to the hair.
- To add colour to the hair.
- For special occasions, for example, weddings, graduation ceremonies, parties, etc.
- To cover scarring.

Using added hair to create fashionable styles

You should give considerable thought to the positioning of the added hair and how it may be incorporated most effectively in your styling. You also need to ensure that it blends effectively with the natural hair. The base or fixing of the added hair must be well hidden. More than one colour may be used for added interest or to create a contrast with the natural hair colour.

When using added hair, it is essential that it be secured properly. Your client must feel confident that the added hair will stay in place for the duration it is to be worn. For extra security, when adding a piece that is on a comb attachment, make a cross using two interlocking Kirby grips, then insert the comb underneath the grips.

Many hairdressers shy away from using added hair, especially if it is long. However, once the fear has been conquered, it opens up an exciting area of hairdressing that will enable you to stand out from the crowd. Most of the hairpieces available are made from synthetic fibres and the quality of these pieces is improving all the time. They come in a variety of colours and may be used to match your client's natural hair colour or add contrast.

Acrylic pieces come in a variety of colours and styles but there are limitations to their use. Heated styling equipment must not be used on acrylic pieces, as they will melt. They must only be cleaned in cold water using specialist products specific to acrylic hair. Conventional hairspray should not be used as they cause the fibres to stick together. If cutting is required, a razor should be used as this tapers the ends of the piece giving it a more natural appearance. Do not use your hairdressing scissors – acrylic pieces will blunt your scissors.

Pieces made from real hair have advantages and disadvantages. They may be styled using heated styling equipment. They are usually handmade to the client's specific requirements. They must not be washed, but should either be sent away or left with a reputable hairdresser who specialises in postiche for specialist 'dry cleaning'.

Dressing the hair

During the dressing process, you must continually check the direction, shape, volume and balance of the style. Re-confirm the desired look with your client before dressing to ensure the correct result.

> ### What you will learn
>
> - Styling and finishing products
> - After the service

The direction you dress the hair should be the direction in which it was styled. If you try to dress the hair any other way, you will find it very difficult and unyielding. Continually check the shape, balance and volume as you work through. Check the dressing from every angle – it is important that the final result is superb.

Remember

The free advertising your clients convey to others may also be negative advertising if the quality of your work is not up to standard.

If the finished hair is not quite right, now is the time to address the issue. Do not wait until you have finished. Assess the dressing and make any amendments as soon as possible. Use your knowledge of finishing products and choose the most suitable product for your client's hair and the finished look that is required. The correct product will depend on the desired outcome. Check your finished result to ensure it complements your client's features, for example, does it suit her face shape and facial features? Is it in keeping with her total image?

When you are completely satisfied with the result and you feel it reflects your salon's standard of service, check your client is satisfied with the finished result. When you have her agreement, apply finishing spray to their hair to hold the style in place. If you apply the spray before confirmation and the client is unhappy, it is not always easy to rectify, as the spray will have already 'set'.

Remember

Use a face shield whenever possible when applying finishing spray as this will protect the client's eyes.

Styling and finishing products

Each product manufacturer has its own vast range of styling and finishing products, each with a specific purpose. It is essential that you have a thorough understanding of the whole product range that is available to you so that you can ensure you are using the correct products to maximise the potential of your client's hair. Make sure you follow the manufacturer's instructions regarding the correct use of products and follow their recommendations concerning the most suitable products for specific hair types. Many styling and finishing products contain conditioning agents and UV filters to protect and condition your client's hair.

Mousse

Mousse comes in different strengths depending on the holding power required. It will help to prolong the life of the style by protecting it from humidity. Many also contain UV filters. Care should be taken when using mousse on very fine 'baby hair' as it may be too heavy for the hair and cause the style to drop.

Setting/styling lotions

These are available in different strengths depending on the holding power required. They protect the hair from humidity, prolonging the life of the style. Very lightweight styling lotions are good for very fine hair, as they do not 'drag out' the styling.

Thermo-active sprays

These are used when dry setting the hair with Velcro rollers. These sprays require the addition of heat to enable them to work efficiently. When setting short hair, they may be applied when the set has been completed. On long hair, they are better applied prior to setting to ensure an even distribution along the hair shaft.

Gels

Gels are usually stronger than mousse or styling lotion and are used for sculpting and moulding. Gel may be used on wet or dry hair, but read the manufacturer's instructions to ensure you are using it correctly.

Moisturisers

These are used to help restore lost moisture and improve the strength and elasticity of the hair. It is a good idea to use these after blow-drying if you are to use heated styling equipment, for example, straightening irons, as they help to replace some of the moisture that is lost during the styling process.

Sprays

Sprays may be used during and after dressing to hold the style in place and protect the hair from atmospheric moisture. They come in different strengths depending on the amount of hold needed.

Shine sprays/glosses

These are used after dressing to give the hair maximum shine and UV protection. Care must be taken not to use excess amounts of these products, as this may cause the hair to look lank and greasy. If the client has a problem with static, the use of shine spray will help to reduce this.

Wax/dressing creams

These are used to define the finished style and are particularly good for texturising.

Straightening creams

These are used to defy the effects of humidity on the hair. Straightening creams are not designed to straighten the hair alone. It is the combination of the product and the blow-drying that produces straight results.

A range of styling and finishing products

When using styling and finishing products, it is essential that you are aware of your responsibilities under the COSHH Regulations and have read the manufacturer's instructions on the products' safe usage. When using products, you should be economical with them to ensure you minimise waste and prevent the hair from becoming overloaded.

After the service

Before the client leaves the salon, you must make sure you have given them sound advice on the maintenance of the finished style. You should ensure your client is aware of the effects of humidity (they may go home and have a hot bath before going out), as this will cause the style to drop. Your client should be advised on the correct products to use at home to maintain the condition of the hair and the style that has been achieved. This will ensure the client's hair remains in optimum condition, the styling should last longer, and it shows an accurate reflection of the professional service your salon offers. It also gives you a great opportunity to retail, which will boost the amount of commission that you earn.

Encourage your client to book their next appointment before they leave the salon. The next appointment may not necessarily be a style and dress appointment, but may be a cut or colour service. Once the client has left the salon without an appointment, you cannot guarantee their return. However, a client is more likely to return if another appointment is pending. Even a satisfied client may opt to try another salon; this could result in the loss of a client. Once the client has left the salon, you should tidy your work area to ensure it is clean and tidy, ready for your next client.

You should now be ready to create some wonderful style and dress looks using some of the techniques you have learned throughout this unit. Photograph the work you do and track your progress as your skills develop. The photographs may be used as evidence within your portfolio.

> ### Remember
>
>
> Do not be afraid to try out new ideas or adapt previously learned concepts. Most of all, enjoy using your new-found knowledge and take pleasure in the results you will achieve.

Knowledge check

1. What factors need to be considered before you style and dress the hair?

2. Describe the difference between alpha and beta keratin.

3. What is meant by the term hygroscopic?

4. How are the hydrogen bonds in the cortex broken during temporary setting?

5. When using non-conventional items for setting hair, what factors must you consider?

6. State the reasons for blow-drying the hair from points to roots.

7. State the potential consequences of using excess products when styling hair using electrical styling equipment.

Style and dress long hair

Unit H26

Introduction

Many hairdressers shy away from styling long hair, and tend to leave it for one particular member of staff to deal with. However, there is a large market for hairdressers who have the skills and imagination to create a variety of looks on long hair. There are many different ways long hair may be styled and dressed; this includes rolls, knots, twists, plaits, curls and woven effects. By combining some of the above techniques, you will be able to personalize your styling and dressing service, thus promoting your specialist skills.

What you will learn

- Maintain effective and safe methods of working when styling hair
- Preparing the hair for the service
- Creatively dress long hair
- After the service

You the stylist

You need to be able to work safely whilst performing these services, ensuring compliance with all the applicable health and safety legislation.

John Carne uses many techniques to create this seductive look in his "Hippy Chic" collection

Maintain effective and safe methods of working when styling hair

Preparing the client

When carrying out any service, preparation is essential. You will need to prepare your work area, tools and equipment, and your client. You must ensure your client's clothing is adequately protected throughout the service. As a minimum your client should be wearing a gown and a towel. If your client's hair is to be dried under a hood dryer, the ears should be protected with disposable ear shields, which are designed to protect the ears from the heat. The use of a net may be necessary if the hood dryers in your salon have a fan, as any stray hairs, or those that may come loose during the drying process, may become caught in the fan, causing unnecessary harm to your client.

Preparing your work area

What to do	Why/how?
All the necessary tools and equipment for the service should be ready	Saves time and conveys professional image to the client
Any products needed for the service should be available and ready to use	Regular and effective stocktaking will ensure that all products are available
Work area must be clean and tidy	Prevents accidents occurring, reduces risk of cross-infection and promotes a professional image
Instruct junior staff to prepare the work area correctly	Saves time. Make sure that you clearly communicate what is required – a short list of instructions may be given to junior staff

What to do	Why/how?
Tools and equipment for dressing long hair should be clean, sterilised and fit for the purpose	The appropriate method of sterilisation should be used and equipment should be checked for defects
Electrical equipment should be used in compliance with health and safety legislation	Ensure that junior staff are complying with the safe use of electrical equipment (see Unit G1). This is your responsibility.

Checklist for personal health and hygiene

What to do	Why/how?
Make sure your body and clothes smell clean and fresh	The client will feel more comfortable in your presence. Daily washing and the use of a good deodorant are essential
Make sure your breath smells nice	Use a breath freshener. This will help to combat odours from strong-smelling foods or smoking
Do not work if you are feeling unwell	Infections can be spread in the salon. Keep yourself fit and healthy to ensure that you produce the best work possible
Maintain a good posture while working. Think about whether your client is positioned correctly for your needs as well as their own comfort	This will minimise the risk of injury and fatigue. Make sure you keep your back straight and weight evenly distributed. Having your tools and equipment close to hand will prevent you from overstretching.

Consultation

A thorough and effective consultation must be carried out with the client before commencing the service. The range of looks that are possible with long hair should be discussed so that the client is fully aware of the possibilities. The use of visual aids, such as stylebooks/hair magazines and journals may help to establish your client's exact requirements. This must be confirmed during the consultation procedure and you should check this throughout the service to ensure you are working towards the correct finished look. This will ensure client satisfaction.

Once you have established your client's exact styling requirements, you must consider which products, tools and equipment you should use to achieve the required look. You should also inform the client of the cost of the service and likely duration. All work carried out within this unit should be completed in a commercially viable time.

Preparing the hair for the service

Products

There are vast ranges of products available for styling and dressing long hair. The products you choose to use should be suitable for the hair type and texture you are working with, so you are able to achieve the optimum result. For more information on products that may be used when styling and dressing long hair, refer to Unit H25.

Check it out

You have responsibilities towards your clients and others in the salon under the Electricity at Work Act. Can you remember what your responsibilities are? List the kind of electrical equipment that is used when styling and dressing long hair.

Remember

When dressing long hair, any pins or grips used must not be placed in the mouth or opened with the teeth, as this may lead to permanent damage to your teeth, and portrays an unprofessional image to your client.

Check it out

Find out the time your salon allows for you to complete the styling and dressing of long hair. These timings should be commercially viable for your salon.

Influencing factors

The desired look

This must have been agreed during the consultation. You must ensure you re-confirm the look with the client during the dressing of the hair to ensure client satisfaction. The desired look may be for a specific occasion.

The occasion for which the style is required

There are many occasions when a client may require long hair to be styled and dressed. This may include weddings, balls, parties, etc. It is important that the styling is in keeping with the overall look the client is trying to achieve. If the occasion were a formal ball, then a current or classic look would be more appropriate than an avant-garde style. The clothing the client will be wearing for the occasion must be considered, e.g. the style of the clothing (formal, alluring, etc.). Also, the neckline of the clothing may limit the types of dressing that will be suitable. The age of the client must be considered, as a young client would generally require a trendy hair-up style rather than a more formal one. All of the above will ensure the end result is not only suitable for the client, but exhibits your expert consultation skills.

The client may also require ornamentation in the hair to complement the outfit being worn and the make-up that is used. Ornamentation covers almost anything that may be placed in the hair to give added interest or another dimension to the styling. This may include feathers, chopsticks, flowers, ribbons or items of jewellery. However, you must remember that ornamentation should enhance the overall appearance of the finished look, rather than become the finished look. When using ornamentation, you must consider the health and safety aspects of the item, e.g. is it flammable, excessively heavy, heat conducting, etc.

Ornamentations may be secured into the hair in a number of different ways. They may be attached to pins, grips, combs, hair bands, etc. To ensure ornaments are firmly fixed, you may need to stitch or glue them onto the hair attachment.

It is important when planning possible styles for brides and bridesmaids to consider any head-dresses or other hair accessories that may be worn. You must ensure that the finished style will sit correctly around the head-dress and the elaborate part of the hairstyle will be on show.

Hair growth patterns

Hair growth patterns must be taken into consideration to ensure the best possible result is achieved. You should always try to work with the natural fall of the hair, as it will lie better and the styling will be more durable, and therefore easier, for the client to maintain. The hair growth patterns in the nape area must be checked, as irregular growth patterns may not complement the finished look and you should therefore consider other techniques to mask any such imperfection. A widow's peak may be disguised by covering it with hair from the front hairline, e.g. create a sweeping effect across the front of the dressing.

Hair elasticity

The hair's elasticity must be taken into consideration. Ideally, hair that is to be styled and dressed should be healthy and in optimum condition. Hair with very poor elasticity may be overstretched during the styling process, therefore rendering it likely to break. Hair with poor elasticity is often difficult to sculpt into specific shapes, e.g. barrel curls, as the hair is often quite inflexible.

> ### Check it out
>
> Discuss with friends and/or colleagues items, including non-conventional items, that may be used to enhance long hair styling. Discuss the health and safety issues related to each one. What are the potential hazards?

Head, face shape and features

Your client's head and face shape must be considered prior to starting to style and dress long hair. Clients with round faces will not look their best with their hair all off the face, especially if there is no added height to give the illusion of the 'perfect oval'.

(For more information on head and face shapes, refer to Unit G9.) Facial features, such as a high forehead, large nose and heavy jaw line must also be considered. Failure to consider the above may result in a fantastic style that is marred by the client's imperfections.

Hair texture

The texture of the client's hair should be considered when deciding on the style to be created. Coarse hair may need to be set first to smooth the hair, leaving it more manageable to work with. Products such as waxes and serums will be required to smooth the ends of the hair that would otherwise look dry and brittle. Fine hair has its own set of considerations. The style must be chosen carefully to gain maximum impact, e.g. barrel curls may not appear full enough to create the intended look. Therefore a hairpiece may be needed to give the illusion that the client has more hair than she really has. It may be difficult to hide all the pins and grips used during the dressing, thus not showing your work to its best advantage. Your choice of securing materials must therefore be thought through carefully. Fine pins may be easier to disguise in fine hair, whereas grips may be required in thick, coarse hair to support the weight of the hair.

Hairpeices and creative additions can give the illusion of more hair

Hair length

Very long hair may be difficult to manage if you are dressing the hair in an 'up style'. Equally hair that has been curled may drop very quickly due to the weight of the hair. Plaiting and twisting works well on very long hair and prevents the potential problems stated above. When working with very long hair, try to dress small sections at a time wherever possible, as this will make life easier for you.

With shorter hair, you may need to create the dressing lower down the head, if the hair is too short to reach the crown. Twists work nicely on hair that is shorter, as the ends of the hair are held together in the twist.

Hair density

The amount of hair that you will be working with must be taken into consideration when planning a style. As with long hair, very heavy hair can be difficult to work with, especially if it is to be dressed up. Strong products must be used to give the hair support and manageability. If dressing the hair into a roll, plenty of overlapping grips should be used to ensure the dressing remains secure. You must check the dressing to ensure the amount of hair you are working with hasn't created more volume than you required!

If the hair is sparse, your choice of styling will be limited as an incorrect choice of technique may leave pins and grips exposed and the client looking as if they do not have much hair. Additional pieces may be necessary to give the illusion of plenty of hair.

Styling and dressing techniques

Depending on the finished style requirements, the way the hair is prepared may differ. This may be decided by the style requirements of the client or preference of the stylist. Look at the table opposite to see how to prepare for different dressing techniques.

The hair may be wet set and dried; this will give the hair a firmer and long-lasting curl. However, it is usual practice to dry the hair off a little first as this will reduce the length of time the client is under the dryer and prevent the hair from becoming too bouncy, which will then make the hair difficult to work with. If setting the hair, it should be set in the direction of the intended styling, e.g. if the hair is to be styled into a vertical roll, the rollers should be placed following the finished result. This will prevent breaks in the dressing.

The hair may be washed and blow-dried, then styled using heated electrical appliances, e.g. tongs, heated rollers, straightening irons, etc. Using different heated appliances will produce a variety of results.

The hair can be washed and blow-dried straight and then dressed, but the hair is usually very soft and difficult to manage. This may be helped by the addition of hairspray before styling, as this will make the hair less soft and therefore easier to work with. Many stylists prefer to work with hair that was shampooed the previous day, as that makes it easier to work with. If this is the case, you must ensure you inform the client prior to the service taking place.

The following table gives you a guide as to how the hair should be prepared for each of the dressing techniques and effects in the range.

Rollers positioned for vertical roll

Dressing techniques and effects	Preparing the hair
Rolls	The hair may be blow-dried, set or dry set using Velcro rollers or heated rollers, depending on the amount of curl required
Knots	The hair should be dried straight
Twists	The hair should be dried straight
Plaits	The hair may be dried straight or plaited into wet hair. However, care must be taken if plaiting wet hair as the hair will shrink when dry and this may cause discomfort for the client and the possibility of traction alopecia
Curls	The hair may be wet set, dry set or tonged, depending on the amount of curl required
Woven effects	The hair should be dried straight

Creatively dress long hair

When styling and dressing long hair, it may be useful to have a junior member of staff available to assist you to pass pins and grips, etc. Many stylists like to work with the same junior member of staff when carrying out this type of work as they become accustomed to the needs of the stylist. This type of relationship usually develops over a period of time. The advantage of working with the same member of staff is that it should reduce the time you take to complete the task and also give the junior stylist a good insight into styling and dressing long hair.

Check it out

List the tools and equipment that may be used for styling and dressing hair. Find out how to use them. If you are unsure, ask your tutor or trainer to demonstrate for you.

Keys to good practice

When dressing up long hair it is essential that you maintain even tension throughout to ensure optimum results. If the tension is not maintained, the result will be uneven. Working with small amounts of hair may help you to maintain even tension.

Rolls

Rolls may be used anywhere on the head depending on the effect to be achieved. The most common form of roll used is a vertical roll or French pleat. The methods used for each will be the same.

1. The hair being sectioned

2. The hair being combed across and interlocking grips up the middle of the head

3. Brush the left side to the middle and twist the hair upwards

4. The pleat being made

5. Pinning the hair into place

6. Backcomb the ends of the hair (either tucked in for a more formal look or fanned out and possibly tonged to create a barrel curls look).

The front area may then be swept, twisted, plaited, etc., as requested by the client. If your client requests a woven effect, this should be done before the roll.

Plaits

Plaits can be used in a variety of ways to produce a number of different effects. As there are numerous different plaits to choose from, the scope is almost endless. They may be used in conjunction with other techniques or on their own.

Scalp plaiting creates a very visual effect and adds texture to the styling. However, to gain maximum effect, your sections should be accurate and of the required width, whether the plaits are intended to be straight or curved. Plaiting off the scalp may be used to create a wide range of effects and, again, will add texture to your styling.

Whichever plaiting technique you choose, it is essential that your tension remains even throughout, thus maintaining the uniformity of the plait.

The ends of the plaits may be secured in several different ways, for example, using suitable bands, threads, ribbons, hair, etc. Ornamentation, such as beads may then be added. Coloured ribbon, thread or hair may be woven into the plait to create a greater impact.

Twists and knots

When creating twists, your sectioning should be accurate and the required width, whether the twists are intended to be straight or curved. The tightness of the twist will depend on the effect you are creating and your client's wishes. When securing the twist, the hairgrip should be hidden (unless the client specifies otherwise). This may be done by holding the grip in the same direction as the twist, hooking a few hairs at the end of the twist, and then turning the grip until it slides through the twist.

Knots may be used to finish a twist or they may be used independently to create a number of different effects.

Ensure your tension remains even throughout, or the plait could 'kink'

Curls and woven effects: a step-by-step guide

The hair is sectioned off from ear to ear. The back section is smoothed into a high ponytail at the crown.

A 1-inch thick, horizontal section is taken from the front hairline.

The section is weaved. Hold the woven-out hair securely and allow the remaining hair to fall.

A square-shaped section is taken from the front hairline and drawn back towards the ponytail.

The hair is pinned into the ponytail.

Continue as steps 2–5 until the side is complete. The hair will have a checkered appearance. Repeat on the other side of the parting.

A section is then taken from the ponytail and combed forward to cover the elastic and is secured with a grip.

Then clip the hair piece over the grip.

Using the original section of hair, barrel curl the hair back onto its base and grip into position.

Still using the same section of hair, another barrel curl is made in the same direction and gripped into place.

The ends of the hair are tonged to create a curled effect. Continue with the remaining hair until the style is complete.

The finished look.

Curls

In addition to dressing the hair up into curls, the curls may be left loose and gently teased out into tendrils. You must remember to use products to separate the curls, e.g. wax, serum, dressing creams, etc.

An "up-do" using loose curls

Check it out

If you are unsure how to carry out any of the above techniques, ask your tutor or trainer to demonstrate them to you.

Added hair

Added hair has increased in popularity over the last few years and has seen many younger clients and fashion icons favouring its use. This has had an impact on most age groups and added hair is now instrumental within the styling and dressing service, regardless of the age of the client. Currently there are many different forms of 'added hair' available. They range from clip-on hair swatches through to more traditional postiche.

Reasons for use
- To add volume to fine hair
- To add length to the hair
- To add colour to the hair
- For special occasions, e.g. weddings, graduation ceremonies, parties, etc.

You should give considerable thought to the positioning of the added hair and how it may be incorporated most effectively in your styling. You must consider the shape you want to create and work around this shape to decide the most appropriate position for the added hair. You also need to make sure that it blends effectively with the natural hair. The base or fixing of the added hair must be well hidden. More than one colour may be used for added interest, to complement the outfit or to create a contrast with the natural hair colour.

When using added hair it is essential that it be secured properly. Your client must feel confident that the added hair will stay in place for the duration it is to be worn. For extra security, when adding a piece that is on a comb attachment, make a cross using two interlocking kirby grips, and then insert the comb underneath the grips. For more information on added hair, refer to Unit H24.

Securing added hair

When dressing long hair, any pins, grips or bands used should be hidden, unless it is a style requirement for them to be on show. When using fine hair-pins, to ensure they remain firmly in the hair, bend the ends of the pins back on themselves to form a fishhook. This will prevent them from working loose and falling out.

Using backcombing and back brushing

Backcombing may be used for several reasons during the dressing of hair. The method you use will depend on the result you wish to achieve. Backcombing may be carried out as a means of supporting the root area of the hair when creating lift and volume. Comb a mesh of hair up from the scalp, holding the ends firmly in one hand, and comb down the hair from points to roots. Some of the hairs within the mesh will be pushed downwards towards the root area, producing a supporting pad of hair at the roots. This type of backcombing should be done close to the roots, on the underneath of the section using the fine teeth of the comb, as it is not intended to be seen.

Backcombing along the whole length of the hair is sometimes carried out if plenty of volume is required, e.g. fine hair. It may also be used if the hair is too soft to work with, as it raises the cuticles so the surface of the hair is roughened. 'Teasing' the hair is the name given to gentle backcombing done on the top of the section to blend the hair during dressing.

Back brushing is carried out in much the same way, except using a brush, rather than a comb. It is more suitable for long hair as it doesn't create too much lift. This may be done on the top or underneath the section, depending on the desired results.

Many stylists prefer to add volume to the hair during dressing by the use of hair pads. These may be bought or made to match the client's hair colour, thus making them easy to disguise.

Avoiding damage to the hair

Care must be taken as physical damage to the cuticles or tearing of the hair may occur through excessive backcombing/brushing, using poor-quality tools or by using an incorrect technique. It is essential that you use techniques that will minimize the amount of damage caused to long hair. Pins, grips and bands must be placed with care to avoid tearing the hair. If using bands to create a ponytail as a base for further dressing, the bands must be of the covered variety. To further ensure no damage occurs, place a grip at either side of the band, hold the ponytail firmly in your hand, insert one of the grips into the ponytail and then wrap the band around the hair until it feels firm, then insert the other grip through the ponytail. Failure to use the correct securing equipment may result in trichorrhexis nodosa (see page 55).

The effects of heat and humidity on the hair

As hair is hygroscopic (it will absorb moisture from the atmosphere), it is essential to use hair products that will help to prolong the style. Most styling and finishing products contain plastic polymers that coat the hair and help to prevent the absorption of atmospheric moisture. They also contain UV filters to protect the hair from the harmful effects of the sun. You must advise your client of the effects of having a hot bath or entering a damp environment after styling and dressing the hair, as this will ultimately cause the dressing to drop. For more information regarding the effects of humidity on the hair, see Unit H25.

Excessive use of heat may cause the hair to become dehydrated, as it will cause some of the natural moisture to be lost. It may cause damage to the cuticles, if electrically heated appliances are left in contact with the hair for too long. In addition, it may cause scalp burns if used too close to the skin or without due care.

Throughout the dressing service you should be continually checking the progress of the dressing with the client. This gives the client the opportunity to express her opinions and any necessary alterations may be made on an ongoing basis.

On completing the look, you must ensure the shape and balance of the finished style is correct; using the mirrors in the salon will help you to do this. There may be areas of the dressing that require modification, e.g. the style doesn't balance. You must also check the volume of the finished style is as the client intended. Check this in relation to the client's features, e.g. does it accentuate the client's large nose or make the head look too big in proportion to the size of the body?

You must ensure that the total dressed look is a true reflection of the client's wishes and your professionalism. Only when you are completely happy with the result should you confirm the client's satisfaction with the finished look. Any finishing products should now be applied to the hair to ensure it remains in the intended style for the maximum length of time.

Finishing products should be used to maximise the life of the style

After the service

Before the client leaves the salon, you must make sure you have given her sound advice on the maintenance of the finished style. You should ensure your client is aware of the effects of humidity (for example, she may go home and have a hot bath before going out), as this will cause the style to drop. Your client should be advised on the correct products to use at home to maintain the condition of the hair and the style that has been achieved. This will ensure the client's hair remains in optimum condition; the styling should last longer and give an accurate reflection of the professional service your salon offers. It also gives you a great opportunity to retail, which will boost the amount of commission that you earn.

You must advise your client on how to remove pins, ornamentation, added hair and backcombing. Failure to do this may result in the client dragging pins, etc. from the hair thus causing unnecessary damage. Added hair should be removed carefully to prevent damage to the client's hair and also to minimise unnecessary wear and tear on the hairpiece (especially if it belongs to the salon and the client has it on loan!) Backcombing should be removed from the hair by gently combing the hair using a wide-tooth comb, starting at the ends of the hair and working gradually up the length of the hair to the roots. This way, any knotting in the hair will not become intensified, thus causing additional problems later.

If you have clients who regularly wear their hair in tight braids, twists or ponytails, you must be vigilant for signs of traction alopecia; this will be more evident at the point of tension (see page 53).

Clients with braids and/or twists are likely to show signs of traction alopecia around the hairline, whereas clients who regularly wear their hair in a ponytail may show signs around the base of the ponytail. You must inform your client immediately it becomes evident and advise them to remove all tension from the hair, until it grows back. Even then, extreme care must be taken to prevent a recurrence.

You must ensure your clients are aware of the potential effects on the hair, skin and scalp of wearing their hair up over a long period of time. The potential effects are:

- Traction alopecia (caused by excess tension on the hair in the follicle)
- Hair breakage (especially if uncovered bands are used)
- Hair becoming knotted, matted and tangled
- Headaches or scalp sensitivity caused by muscle trauma
- Infestations (in severe cases this may include cockroaches!).

Encourage your client to book her next appointment before she leaves the salon. The next appointment may not necessarily be a style and dress appointment, but may be a cut or colour service. Once the client has left the salon without an appointment, you cannot guarantee her return. However, a client is more likely to return if another appointment is pending. Even a satisfied client may opt to try another salon; this could result in the loss of a client.

Once the client has left the salon, you should tidy your work area to ensure it is clean and tidy, ready for your next client.

Knowledge check

1.   *In what ways can ornamentation be secured into the hair?*

2.   *State the different ways the hair should be prepared for the following style and dress services:*
      • *Curls*
      • *Knots*
      • *Twists*
      • *Plaits*
      • *Rolls*
      • *Woven effects.*

3.   *State the reasons for using added hair when styling and dressing long hair.*

4.   *Why do you use backcombing when dressing long hair?*

5.   *What are the potential effects of using excessive heat when styling the hair?*

6.   *State the potential effects on the hair, skin and scalp of wearing hair up for long periods of time.*

Design and create a range of facial hair shapes

Unit H20

Introduction

Beard and moustache shapes create a personalised look for each client

This unit is concerned with the trimming and re-designing of beards and moustaches. There are three different types of looks that you need to be aware of:

1   **Traditional** – This type of look has been established and popular over a long period of time.
2   **Current** – A current look is one that is fashionable at the time. It is likely to be seen on the high street.
3   **Emerging** – This type of look is a forerunner of fashion and may in time become a current look if it becomes commercially acceptable.

While undertaking the cutting of beards and moustaches, you will use several of the cutting techniques that you have already learnt, for example, scissor-over-comb, clipper-over-comb and free hand. You will need a high level of skill in all three of these cutting techniques in order to create the looks required by men. You must consider that you are using your cutting tools near to the face and the risk of cutting the skin is greater.

What you will learn
• Preparing the client • Creating the look • After the service

You the stylist

The ability to concentrate and your manual dexterity will be vital in assisting you to produce a variety of looks. This unit will help you to appreciate the tremendous versatility in the designs of beards and moustaches.

Preparing the client

This section covers everything that is important when preparing the client for any facial hair cutting services. Being thoroughly prepared reflects your own professionalism and the salon's image, and is an essential part of the process.

What you will learn	

- Thorough consultation
- Influencing factors
- Personal hygiene
- Personal protective equipment
- Preparing the facial hair for the cutting service

Thorough consultation

The initial consultation plays a crucial part in determining the final outcome (see also Unit G9). As the stylist, it is your responsibility to determine the client's requirements and advise the client accordingly. The use of visual aids to assist you in this task may be necessary, for example, a stylebook or picture from a magazine. If you feel confident enough, drawing the style you are thinking of creating could be beneficial. During your consultation there are several factors that you must consider and these are known as influencing factors.

Influencing factors

Although influencing factors have been greatly covered in Unit G9, there are several points that are purely relevant to cutting facial hair.

Head and face shape

When designing a look for a beard or moustache, the client's personal preferences must be considered as well as their head and face shape. The size of the beard or moustache should correspond with the facial features. The rule of thumb is a larger, thicker beard or moustache for heavy or large facial features, and a smaller design for fine, smooth facial features. You must also consider the following points:

- The size of the mouth, for example, a small mouth should have a narrow, short moustache.

- The size of the nose, for example, a prominent nose should have a large or thick moustache.

- The face shape, for example, a square face should have a curved beard or moustache. A round face should have a square-edged design.

Any unusual features can be cleverly disguised with the use of a beard or moustache, particularly any facial scarring.

Hair growth patterns

You should be looking all over the facial hair for any deviance in the way the hair grows. This can play a vital part in the finished outcome. For example, if a client has a whorl in the growth pattern, it will affect the finished shape.

Nape whorls

Whorls can look untidy as they begin to grow out, which makes the design harder for the client to maintain. There may be some areas of baldness in the facial hair, which can affect your choice of design. For example, if the client required a full beard and moustache but no hair grew at the sides of the mouth, you would suggest a moustache without the beard connected.

Hairstyle

The way the client wears his hair will have an effect on the look and design of the facial hair. Although there are no set rules on what can or cannot be worn well together, it would be beneficial for the client to have a design that complemented the hairstyle. If the client has little or no hair then a large, thick beard and moustache can look out of place. Alternatively, if a client has thick long hair then a fine, small moustache can also look misplaced. As the stylist, you should work with your client to find a design that suits both his personal preference and the overall look.

Adverse skin conditions

It is imperative that on the initial consultation you look carefully for any suspected infections or infestations as these may prevent you from continuing with the service (see Unit G9 for more on this topic).

Keys to good practice

If a client has heavy facial hair growth at the start, you must be extra vigilant. Take time to comb through the hair, parting it and looking at the skin. It can be difficult to spot a cold sore on a lip if the client has a thick moustache.

If you begin a service and then discover something that you suspect to be infectious, you should inform the client and give any advice you feel is necessary. You may have to finish the service you are carrying out, but be sure to thoroughly sterilise any tools and equipment you have used to prevent the risk of cross-infection. (Refer to Unit G1 for the correct methods of sterilisation.)

Hair density

The thickness of the facial hair will affect the choice of style and cutting technique used. For example, if a client has very dense facial hair then a fine, narrow moustache may not be possible. You also need to consider that if the hair is thicker then you may have to use the clippers to cut the beard or moustache, as a scissor-over-comb technique may take too long.

Keys to good practice

As clippers remove more hair and move through the hair more easily, they are not only quicker to use, but also a more comfortable option for the client. Trying to comb through thick hair when using a scissor-over-comb technique can cause discomfort to the client.

Facial piercing

It is essential that you discover all facial piercings and ask the client to remove them before you carry out any facial hair cutting. It will not only hinder the close scissor or

Check it out

Take a look at men with facial hair, both in the media and in public, and note the hairstyle that is worn with it. Do you notice any patterns or trends? If you are looking at magazines, you could cut out the pictures to make a stylebook. Alternatively, you could invest in a digital camera and take some photographs of your own work to produce a stylebook.

clipper work that needs to be done, but, more importantly, if you were to catch the piercing, it could tear the skin. If your client does have any facial piercing, take note of when it was carried out and if it looks inflamed or infected. It may be that if it is relatively new, the skin may still be inflamed, in which case you would advise the client to leave the treatment and re-book at a later date.

Sterilisation

Sterilisation of tools and equipment is essential to prevent the spread of infection or infestation. There are several methods that you can use in the salon, all of which have been covered in great detail in Unit G1.

> ### Keys to good practice
>
> If you are using a razor with a fixed blade in your work in the salon, you must sterilise the blade between clients. It may be necessary to have a couple of razors to enable you to have a ready supply of sterilised razors to use. Alternatively, change to a razor with disposable blades, which will allow you to dispose of the blade safely after each use.

Check it out

List the tools and equipment that you use in the cutting and designing of facial hair and write next to each one the method of sterilisation that you currently use in the salon. You should check that what you are using is sufficient by looking at Unit G1. Could your methods be adapted to improve your sterilisation routine?

Personal hygiene

As with all hairdressing services, you are working in close proximity to your client. You must ensure that your body and breath are fresh. Regular washing and bathing is essential as is the use of a good deodorant to prevent body odour. After a cigarette or lunch break, make sure that your breath smells fresh by either brushing your teeth or using a breath freshener. A client may take offence at strong odours and it is very unpleasant for them. Your own health is important when you are working in the salon. If you do not feel one hundred per cent, the quality of your work may reflect this. Also, if you are infectious or contagious, you may spread germs to your clients and colleagues.

Personal protective equipment

The personal protective equipment that you use when cutting facial hair is essential to provide protection to the client from small, sharp hair cuttings. The facial hair is often coarser and can cause infection by entering the skin. Removing loose hair as you progress through the cut will help to prevent this and taking special care at the end to ensure all hair is correctly removed is also beneficial. Care needs to be taken to ensure that hair cuttings do not fall onto the client's clothing by correctly gowning him. The gown should also be checked regularly to ensure it has not slipped and is still providing a high level of protection. You can place small, round cotton wool pads over the client's eyes to protect them. This will also help to keep their eyes closed, but remember to let the client look, when needed, for an opinion on the length or shape of the beard, or moustache.

Preparing the facial hair for the cutting service

You should thoroughly detangle the facial hair before you begin the cut and it may be necessary to cleanse the facial hair as well. While you are carrying out the initial consultation, you should be combing the beard or moustache looking for any adverse skin conditions. If your client is returning home from work, the hair may contain dirt or debris. Removing grease, dirt or dandruff from the facial hair will prevent any damage to your cutting tools. It will also show your professionalism by preparing the hair correctly for the cutting service.

Cleansing the facial hair can be done using a variety of methods. If you are shampooing the client's hair then it can be carried out during this process. Alternatively, you may ask the client to wash their face, or if it is only a small moustache, then a facial cleansing wipe could be used.

If you are carrying out a complete re-design of the facial hair, drawing an outline on the facial hair growth will assist you, as you will be able to follow a guideline. On lighter hair, you could use an eyebrow pencil; alternatively, on very dark hair you could use a white pencil. Remember to remove any leftover pencil on completion of the cut.

Creating the look

In this section you will find all the information that will assist you in carrying out facial hair cutting. You will need to be aware of the cutting tools available for use and the various techniques you can adopt to achieve a variety of looks. There are several safety considerations that you must consider; remember that you are working in close proximity to the skin on the face and extra care will need to be taken. You will need to research and find a variety of designs of beards and moustaches for you to use on clients in the salon. Being aware of the trends and designs of facial hair is paramount to your success.

What you will learn
• Cutting tools and their uses
• Cutting techniques used in facial hair cutting
• Types of beards and moustaches
• Procedure for facial hair cutting
• Safety considerations

Cutting tools and their uses

Of all the cutting tools available for use on the hair, there are only two that we use on facial hair. These are scissors and clippers.

Scissors

The scissors that you use on a client need to be extremely sharp and great care must be taken when cutting hair on the face. Scissors can be used to trim or re-design either a beard or a moustache. They can be used for both scissor-over-comb work to reduce the bulk of the beard or moustache or for free hand work when outlining.

Keys to good practice
When you are using a pair of scissors, they are just an extension to your hand and should feel very comfortable to hold. If not, they can become clumsy to use, causing carelessness and possible cutting of the client's skin. If you are not happy with the scissors you are using then change them for a different pair that feel more comfortable.

Clippers

When using clippers on facial hair, the smaller, trimmer clippers are more commonly used. They are particularly good for removing the hair on the outline of the beard or moustache as they cut very close to the skin. This will assist anyone who is not confident enough to use a razor to shave off the excess hair.

Hygiene spray for clippers

However, the traditional clippers may also be used, but as they are larger and more bulky, it is much harder to work in finer detail.

Clippers are used to remove bulk from a beard or moustache, especially if the facial hair is thick or very long. It will save time to use clipper-over-comb, as this technique will remove the hair at a quicker rate. Both types of clippers work in the same way with a set of two serrated-edge blades, one of which moves rapidly over the other. It is an essential requirement that after each use you thoroughly clean the clippers, using a small brush to remove any loose hair cuttings. The blades should also be oiled regularly to prevent them from seizing up. Manufacturers of clippers provide the brush and oil for maintenance and a hygiene spray can be purchased in order to disinfect.

| **Remember** | |

Clippers are electrical and should be used in line with the Electricity at Work Regulations. Refer to Unit G1 to remind yourself of these responsibilities.

Cutting techniques used in facial hair cutting

There are three cutting techniques that you will be using when cutting beards and moustaches and they are: scissor-over-comb, clipper-over-comb and free hand.

Scissor-over-comb

The scissor-over-comb technique will allow you to carry out fine graduation on short beards and moustaches. When using this technique, you place the comb into the hair against the skin and by moving the comb away from the face, cutting the hair that protrudes through the teeth of the comb, you will cut the hair to the required length.

Scissor-over-comb technique

> **Remember**
>
> Any scissor-over-comb work that you carry out requires a great deal of skill and accuracy. Caution needs to be taken, as you will be working around the soft tissue of the face, for example, the lip area.

Clipper-over-comb

This technique produces the same effect as scissor-over-comb but cuts the hair at a much quicker rate, making it ideal to use if you are busy in the salon. Generally, you would use the smaller, trimmer clippers, not only to allow you to work more freely in the confines of the facial curves, but also to produce finer gradation. As previously stated, if as a barber stylist you are not yet confident enough to use a razor to shave off excess facial hair, then trimmers will cut very close to the skin. Clipper-over-comb work is carried out in the same way as scissor-over-comb. The comb is placed against the skin and moved away from the face, with the hair protruding through the teeth of the comb being cut by the clippers.

Clippers have a lever on the side that allows you to open or close the blades at varying degrees. If you are working on coarse, dense hair then it is beneficial to open the blade out to allow the clippers to cut through the hair without dragging, causing discomfort to the client. Alternatively, if you are cutting fine hair, or wish to cut close to the skin, then closing the blades will ease cutting the hair.

Types of beards and moustaches

Beards and moustaches have been worn in various forms for centuries. They can signify religious beliefs or just serve as a fashion statement. In recent times, facial hair has once again grown in popularity, with many celebrities wearing goatees or sideburns in a range of shapes and designs.

Clipper-over-comb technique

Moustaches

| Emerging | Current | Traditional |

Beards

| Emerging | Current | Traditional |

Procedure for facial hair cutting

Whether you are carrying out a complete re-design or just a trim on the facial hair, it is crucial for you as the barber stylist to know where to begin the cut and how. The type of beard or moustache you are working on will determine the cutting techniques you use. For example, if it is a fine, narrow moustache then scissor work will suffice; however, if you are cutting a coarse, dense beard then using the clippers is preferable.

Before you begin, you must be aware of what you are trying to achieve and how to reach that point. Always ask the client, 'When did you last have your beard or moustache cut?' This will give you a good indication of how much hair needs to be removed. If you consider that the hair grows on average 1 to 2 cm per month, this will allow you to determine how much the hair has grown since the last cut.

It is usual to remove the bulk first and then to outline the shape of the beard or moustache afterwards. By removing the bulk of hair it will allow you to see clearly the outline shape. While carrying out the cutting service, remove any loose hair cuttings as you go along, not only for your client's comfort, but also to allow you to see a clear picture of your design. Even if your client's eyes are closed and covered, ask them to look as you go along to ensure you are achieving a design they are happy with. When you are satisfied with the finished look, you must remove the hair that is left outside the outline. You may use the trimmer clippers for this, or alternatively, shave off the hair with a razor.

The table below shows the types of problems that you may encounter and how to overcome them. It can be used as a quick reference guide.

Types of problem	Possible remedy
Cutting the skin	Administer first aid immediately
Bald patch in the facial hair	Style in a way to avoid exposure of the bald area
Adverse skin conditions	If infectious, do not carry out the service and advise to seek medical attention
Unusual growth patterns in the facial hair	Avoid styling in a way that will look uneven when growing out
Uneven result on completion	Use a pencil to draw the outline and re-style to even out the design

Check it out

Before you begin the service, you should be aware of your salon's expected service times for the cutting of facial hair. The service time may differ from salon to salon and can vary by as much as fifteen minutes. Find out the expected service times in your salon for several facial hair cutting services, include a full beard and moustache trim, a moustache trim, and a complete re-design.

Trimming facial hair: a step-by-step guide

Before the cut.

The facial hair is disentangled using a comb.

Clipper-over-comb is carried out to remove bulk.

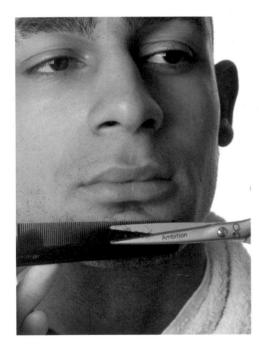

Scissor-over-comb is used to produce fine gradation.

The facial hair shape is outlined with taper clippers.

The finished look.

Safety considerations

Extreme caution must be taken at all times when using sharp implements next to the client's skin. Your concentration must never falter and you should not be distracted from your work. If your hand is hovering over a client's face holding a pair of scissors or a razor and you are looking away to talk to someone else, this will prove to be a very uncomfortable experience for the client. If you do cut a client's skin, you must follow strict health and safety procedures when dealing with the incident.

Procedure for dealing with a cut

- Use a steri-wipe to clean over the area; if doing this yourself, you must be wearing gloves to prevent the risk of cross-infection. This will remove any loose hair cuttings and prevent them from entering the skin.
- Applying pressure to the cut will stem the flow of blood.
- You should continue with the service only when the cut has stopped bleeding.
- When you continue with the service, give the client a clean tissue to keep wiping around the area to prevent any hair from entering the skin.

The tools you are using against the skin need to be clean and sterile for each use. Never re-use a razor on another client's skin, as there is a high risk of cross-infection. Using clean, sterile tools will also prove your ability to the client and demonstrate your high level of professionalism.

> **Check it out**
>
> There are strict laws concerning the use of sharps in the salon that you need to be fully aware of. Be aware of what your responsibilities are.

In the salon

Janine had a regular client who came into the salon for a haircut and a moustache trim every three to five weeks. One day when he came into the salon for his trim, she noticed a fresh scar on his nose during the initial consultation. Laughingly, she asked him, 'What have you been up to, then?' Janine half-expected a tale about a football injury. The reply he gave was not what she was expecting at all. He explained that a couple of days after his last appointment, which had been three weeks ago, his nose became red, swollen and sore. By the third day, there was a boil forming on his nose, which was proving to be extremely painful. He explained that he went to see the nurse at his doctor's surgery and during treatment the nurse pulled out a small, sharp hair from the skin. It was obvious that it had entered the skin during the moustache trim he had had previously. Once the hair had been removed, the boil took another week to clear up, which is why the scar still looked so fresh.

Janine was horrified to think that it was her fault – if she had taken more care to remove all the hair cuttings from her client's face then this would not have happened. She was extremely apologetic to the client and offered the service this time for free. The client was happy to accept her offer and, although he had been through a bad experience, was happy to return to the salon again.

- Why do you think the hair entering the skin caused this type of reaction?
- What measures could you take to prevent this from happening to any of your clients?
- Why do you think Janine offered him a free service this time?

After the service

This section looks at completing the service with your client by offering after-care advice and recommending when he should return. It is essential to complete the service as professionally as you have carried it out to provide the client with an all-round first-class service.

What you will learn
• After-care advice and recommended intervals between cuts • Exfoliating the skin • Disposal of waste materials

After-care advice and recommended intervals between cuts

Clients will have a preferred time interval between the cuttings of their facial hair. However, you should be advising three to five weeks, which usually falls in line with their haircut. In between visits to the salon, the client will have to maintain the look by removing hair outside of the outline, usually carried out by shaving. You may need to give advice on this, for example, how often and in which areas.

Ensuring that your client is fully informed about how to look after the design of his facial hair is important. If the client cannot take care of the design at home then you may find that when he returns to the salon he has changed the shape completely, or even shaved off his beard or moustache. Even though the client may have been happy when leaving the salon, unless the maintenance of the look has been fully explained, dealing with the design at home may prove difficult and leave the client feeling frustrated. If this happens, the chances of the client returning to you will be greatly reduced.

Exfoliating the skin

It is important to advise your client about the benefits of exfoliating the skin. Nowadays there is much less stigma attached to men using facial products. This is evident by the number of products available on the market. You have a responsibility as the barber stylist to educate your clients and inform them of how to look after their skin.

Exfoliation of the skin is essential to remove the dead skin cells from the top layer of the epidermis. It will not only improve the texture of the skin, but will also help to prevent in-growing hairs from forming. The action of exfoliating also stimulates the circulation, which provides the much-needed blood supply and nourishment for the skin.

There are many different product manufacturers who supply various forms of exfoliating products.

Exfoliating products

They can be bought in the form of cleansing grains that are mixed with water to form a paste, or alternatively, a ready-mixed granular paste. The other type of exfoliator for the skin is fruit acid peels. All skin types benefit from exfoliating, but you must be sure to recommend the most suitable one and inform your clients of the importance of following the manufacturer's instructions.

Keys to good practice

Granular paste exfoliants are more abrasive and should not be recommended for use on fine or ageing skin. You could, however, recommend fruit acid peels, which remove the dead skin cells but do so less harshly by a process of dissolving.

The action of exfoliating not only brightens the skin, but will also make it more receptive to moisturising products, helping the skin to hold its elasticity and youthful glow. If you are selling the benefits of regular exfoliating in this way, how can the client resist buying the product?

Disposal of waste materials

Disposal of waste should always be carried out in line with any health and safety legislation. The most likely waste to be disposed of after facial hair cutting would be:

- hair cuttings
- used razor blade
- eye pads
- empty product containers.

Each of these must be disposed of safely and hygienically following salon procedure.

Check it out

Looking at the list of disposable items, write down the key points about how each should be disposed of correctly (see Unit G1 for more information). Compare your salon's procedures for disposal of waste to current health and safety legislation.

In the salon

At Waheed's salon, the staff were complaining that, as they were all so busy carrying out services on clients, there was not enough time to clean up properly. He decided to give them a helping hand and employed a cleaner for a few hours per week. Shirley had been cleaning at the salon for a couple of weeks and all was going well. The staff were much happier as they did not feel under as much pressure, knowing that Shirley would do the jobs they did not have time for.

One Friday evening, after a busy day at the salon, Shirley was getting on with the cleaning and Waheed was cashing up. Suddenly Shirley screamed and Waheed looked up to see her holding her hand with blood running out of a wound. He rushed over and immediately administered first aid. Shirley told him she had been pulling some rubbish out of the small pedal bin to put into the large bin bag for disposal. She could see only some tissues and did not notice that there was a used razor blade in the bin. On closer inspection, Waheed could see that the wound was quite deep and would need further medical attention. He locked up the salon and took Shirley straight to hospital.

The next day in the salon, Waheed called an emergency staff meeting to discuss the incident and find out how it could have happened. It appeared that the salon assistant had thrown the used blade into the bin and was oblivious to the hazard she had created. In fact, it was the salon's fault for not educating her in the use of a sharps box and its importance.

- By cutting herself on a used razor blade, what risks has Shirley been exposed to?
- Who do you think was negligent: Waheed, Shirley, or all the staff?
- How could this incident have been avoided?

Knowledge check

1. Why is it important to protect clients from hair clippings?

2. What safety considerations must be taken into account when cutting facial hair?

3. What important factors must be given consideration prior to cutting facial hair?

4. What effects might continual close clipper work have on dark skin?

5. What three methods of cutting are used when cutting facial hair?

6. How might you establish guidelines for a new look?

7. If a client has a facial piercing what should you do before proceeding with the service?

8. Why should you recommend exfoliation of the skin?

Provide shaving services

Unit H19

Introduction

This unit is about providing a professional shaving service to clients. In order to deliver a service professionally, a good knowledge of the tools for use is required along with a high level of skill when using an open blade razor. With the widespread use of safety razors and electric razors, the service of shaving in the salon has declined. However, since most men require daily shaving to feel clean and look presentable, there is a great demand for this service. As a stylist offering shaving services, you should be making every effort to attract clients into the salon.

What you will learn
• Preparing the client • Shaving tools and equipment • Creating the look • After the service

Daily shaving is a popular request

You the stylist

When carrying out shaving, you are removing the visible part of the hair over the face and neck with minimum irritation to the skin. Shaving can take place over the whole face or just in certain areas to tidy up the outline of the beard or moustache. There are factors that must be considered during the shave, such as the texture of hair, skin sensitivity and direction of growth, each of which will affect the way in which shaving is carried out. You must also consider your own position and that of the client during the service, as ease of access to the areas to be shaved is important to ensure accuracy.

Preparing the client

This section looks at everything that is important when preparing the client for the shaving service. Being prepared and ready with everything to hand reflects not only your own level of professionalism, but also that of the salon. It will also serve to save you time and increases your client's confidence in your ability.

What you will learn
• Thorough consultation • Influencing factors • Safe working practices • Preparation of self and client

Thorough consultation

Determining your client's requirements accurately is essential in order to provide a service that the client is happy with. You must be able to communicate well with your client, not only to extract the right information from him, but also to ensure he fully understands your perceptions of this. It is during this initial process that you will determine the service to be provided, for example, will the client need a beard trim before a full face shave or is just the outlining of the beard required?

You must appear confident and knowledgeable in order for the client to feel confident in your ability. Remember that you are using an open blade directly on the face and a high level of trust between yourself and the client is required. Discuss your client's shave in detail, ensuring that he is made aware of the full process and knows what to expect at each stage.

Keys to good practice

- During the shave, most clients will close their eyes and relax, knowing that moving or talking could result in cutting the skin. However, it is always wise to have discussed this during consultation and make it known to the client that, although you may continue to communicate, the client needs to remain still.
- You need to inform the client of the expected length of the service and this should fall within the expected service times for your salon. Remember that these will differ according to the type of service required, for example, full or partial shave.

Influencing factors

Influencing factors are all the points that must be considered during the consultation. They may affect the service you provide or even prevent you from continuing.

Hair growth patterns

The way in which the hair grows over the neck or face must be looked at in great detail prior to commencing the shave. Once you have applied the lather, you can no longer see the pattern of growth, therefore it must be considered initially. You should look for deviance in patterns, for example, whorls or bald patches, as again this will affect the shave. The razor should be used over the hair in the pattern of growth to prevent any discomfort or skin irritation. Shaving over the hair against the pattern of growth is advised only on a client with coarse, stubborn hair, as it causes irritation and in-growing hairs.

Adverse skin conditions

Skin and scalp disorders may prevent you from carrying out the service and should be given careful consideration. If the client is suffering from an infection or infestation, you must not continue with the service, as there is a high risk of cross-infection. It is crucial that these are found on initial consultation and not during the service.

Unusual features

Looking for unusual features is important as they may affect the shaving process. Care should be taken in sensitive areas such as over the Adam's apple; if it is larger than average, extra care will be needed. Dimples in the cheeks or chin will also need to be catered for by stretching the skin to pull out the fold, allowing you access with the razor. Look at the area below the lower lip to see if the bottom lip rolls over the skin, hiding any hair in this area. This is a sensitive area and you should take extra care when shaving there.

Check it out

List the types of skin and scalp disorders likely to affect the shaving service and state the reasons why they might prevent you from continuing with the shave.

Client's wishes

During the consultation, you will have determined your client's wishes and will know if they affect the service in any way. For example, the client may have long or thick sideburns that he does not want shaving, or a beard or moustache that he requires outlining. You may need to advise the client on another option if you feel what they require is not suitable, but remember to do this with tact and professionalism.

Facial piercing

Any piercing worn in the face must be removed prior to the shaving service being carried out. It will hinder the use of the razor over the skin and could lead to a severe cut. If your client does have any facial piercing, take note of when it was carried out and if it looks inflamed or infected. It may be that if it is relatively new, the skin may still be inflamed, in which case you would advise the client to leave the treatment and re-book at a later date.

Safe working practices

While working in the salon, it is a requirement of law that you comply with health and safety legislation. The tools you use must always be sterilised and fit for purpose. The methods of sterilisation you use will depend upon what is available in the salon; however, it may be that you have other options to consider.

Keys to good practice

- If you are using a razor with a fixed blade in your work in the salon, you must sterilise the blade between clients. It may be necessary to have a couple of razors to enable you to have a ready supply of sterilised razors to use. Alternatively, change to a razor with disposable blades, which will allow you to dispose of the blade safely after each use.
- You also need to consider your responsibilities under the Electricity at Work Regulations. Do you visually check any electrical equipment before use? Is all the electrical equipment tested regularly for faults? You must be sure that both you and the staff for whom you have responsibility, are complying with the safe use of electrical equipment.

Preparation of self and client

Preparing yourself for the shaving service is crucial to presenting a professional approach. You must use the correct personal protective equipment. Wearing an apron and gloves will not only protect your clothes from spillage, but your hands from becoming irritated through regular use of detergent. You should be wearing gloves when applying lather and during the shave. Your client should be gowned correctly following salon policy.

The positioning of the client prior to commencing the service is important. You must adjust your chair for both your own comfort and that of the client. The client needs to feel comfortable and relaxed and you need to adopt good posture whilst working to prevent fatigue. If either you or the client moves to find a comfortable position during the shave, this could result in an accident, causing injury. Ensuring that all your equipment and products are close at hand and fit for purpose is also important. Regular stock checks will avoid the problem of running out of products and equipment.

Keys to good practice

Preparing the client for the shave may involve some facial hair trimming prior to lathering and care must be taken to prevent any loose hair cuttings from falling onto the client's clothing.

Check it out

List the tools and equipment that you use in the salon while shaving and write next to each one the method of sterilisation that you currently use. You should check that what you are using is sufficient by looking Unit G1. Could your methods be adapted to improve your sterilisation routine?

Check it out

Go to your local council offices and look up any local by-laws that affect the work you do in the salon, particularly regarding the use of razors. You have a duty to follow these, and remember, if you move to another salon in a different area, the relevant by-laws may change.

Remember

Wearing gloves during the shaving service will help to reduce the risk of cross-infection. If you were to cut the client's skin, you may become exposed to body fluids, which can lead to you contracting very serious illnesses such as hepatitis or HIV.

Shaving tools and equipment

This section covers the process of the shaving service. You will need to be aware of the types of razors for use, the different techniques employed during the shave, and how to use them safely. Your greatest concern when shaving is damage to the skin and this can be prevented only by taking care while performing the shave and by using sterile, sharp tools. Your success in shaving will become apparent through attention to detail and experience.

What you will learn 💡

- Tools and equipment
- Lathering techniques

Tools and equipment

Several of the tools you use during the shaving process will already be familiar to you in your haircutting work, such as the clippers and razor. Although you will have gained plenty of experience with clippers, using the razor with an open blade is likely to be less familiar. You must use it with great care and give it the respect it demands.

Clippers

Before you commence the shave, you need to assess the length of the facial hair. If it is too long then you must remove some. Clippers may be used to remove a dense growth of facial hair. Cutting close to the skin, leaving only short facial hair, will help you enormously in your task. However, care must be taken to ensure the skin is not irritated by close clipper work, as this could lead to damage to the skin during the shaving process.

Open blade razor

A safety razor

There are two types of razor that may be used during shaving: safety razors, which contain disposable blades, and fixed blade razors that do not. Whichever one you use, it is imperative for the blade to be extremely sharp, as a blunt edge will cause grazing or even cutting of the skin. The use of open blade razors is governed not only by government regulation, but also local by-laws. Some local areas prevent the use of fixed blade razors and will permit use only of razors with disposable blades.

Check it out 🔍

Look up the rules for the use of open blade razors at your nearest council offices. These may be found in local by-laws.

When using a razor with a detachable blade, a new one must be used for each client to prevent the risk of cross-infection. It should be disposed of immediately after use. With fixed blade razors, the blade is not removable so you must sterilise the razor between clients and sharpen the blade when it becomes dull.

> ## Keys to good practice
>
> Before the shave, let the client see you fitting the new blade or removing the fixed blade razor from the steriliser. This will prove your professionalism to the client and serve to increase his confidence in your skills.

> ## Remember
>
> If your salon does not have a sharps box then you are not abiding by the rules of safe disposal of used sharps. There is a high risk of cross-infection or injury when disposing of used sharps and the correct use of a sharps box is essential.

Types of fixed blade razor

There are two types of fixed blade razors: hollow ground and solid ground. Both are made of tempered steel (steel that has been hardened) with the solid ground being of a soft temper (less hard). The shape of the razor differs in that the hollow ground has a concave body, which gives the appearance of the sides hollowed out, whilst the solid ground has a full body.

The hollow ground is the more favoured of the two, as it is easier to feel any resistance from the beard during shaving, letting you know when sharpening is required. However, it is not suitable for use when razor cutting hair. The solid ground blade is favoured by more experienced practitioners. Due to the bulk of the blade, it is also suitable for use when cutting hair.

Hone and strop

Both of these tools are used in the process of sharpening the blade of the razor. A razor's edge contains very fine teeth that are not visible to the naked eye. When these teeth become damaged, the edge needs to be re-sharpened by honing and stropping.

> ## Keys to good practice
>
> As both these techniques require precision, it is best to practise on an old razor until you have perfected the skill.

Honing

Honing is also known as 'setting' and is carried out on a rectangular block of abrasive material. As the razor is made of steel, the hone must be made of a stronger substance. Hones come in three different varieties: natural, synthetic and combination. The type the barber stylist uses will be dependent on personal choice.

Natural hones

Natural hones, such as Water or Belgium, are cut out of rock formations and originate from Germany and Belgium. These types of hone will cut the edge at a slower pace and need to be lubricated with either water or lather to facilitate the movement of the razor. They both produce a very sharp cutting edge.

Synthetic hones

The Carborundum hone is the most common type of synthetic hone. Lubricating before use will aid the action of the razor over the hone. It will produce a quick and sharp edge to the razor, but great care must be taken not to over-hone, as this will damage the edge of the blade.

Keys to good practice

During honing, the edge of the razor should be tested regularly to prevent over-honing. This can be carried out by carefully drawing the razor's edge over a moistened thumbnail and feeling for any signs of snagging, which would indicate a dull edge.

Combination hones

This type of hone is double-sided; one side is made of synthetic and the other side is natural. Its benefits are that if your razor is badly damaged and needs extreme honing then the synthetic side will produce the results. Alternatively, the natural side will allow fine honing if the razor just needs a slight sharpen.

It is important during your training to become familiar with all types of hone, allowing you to make a choice as to which one you prefer to use. Honing should be carried out in a figure of eight motion, taking the blade across the hone and turning over as you reach the end. You must follow the manufacturer's instructions on use of a lubricant. The illustration below shows the action of honing a razor:

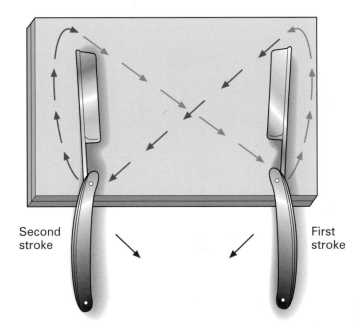

Second stroke

First stroke

Honing a razor

Stropping

Stropping a razor is carried out to produce what is known as a 'whetted' edge. This means that the edge of the razor is not only extremely sharp, but that the fine teeth are both aligned and clean. There are two types of strop: the hanging strop and the French or German strop. The most commonly used is the hanging strop, which often has a canvas side and a leather side. The leather side can be made of cowhide, horsehide, or imitation leather, with the horsehide being the most expensive and best quality. The French or German strop is again a combination strop and is less commonly used.

A German strop

With the blade facing away from you, move the razor's edge along and across the strop, ensuring you cover the whole length of the blade.

Keys to good practice

- When using the strop, never move the razor with the blade facing forward, as the edge will cut into the surface and damage both the strop and the razor.
- The best-quality strops will be already broken in when purchased. However, if the strop requires breaking in then you should follow the manufacturer's instructions. Most strops are broken in by rubbing with a dry pumice stone, massaging a stiff lather on the strop, and finished by rubbing a glass bottle over the strop until a smooth surface is achieved.

Correct stropping and honing will serve to lengthen the life of the razor and protect the client from damaging the skin, as it provides a fresh, clean cutting edge. You must, however, remember to sterilise the razor after stropping and honing to prevent the spread of bacteria.

Lathering tools

A bowl and lather brush

Most lather is applied to the face using a bowl and lather brush. There are, however, lather dispensers that serve not only to dispense the right amount of lather, but also to pre-heat the lather, making it more comfortable for the client.

Sponges

Sponges are used during a sponge shave. They are soaked in hot water and drawn over the face just before the blade to open the follicle and lift the hair, allowing coarse hair to be more easily removed.

Remember

Sponge shaving must be carried out only following a second over-shave on a coarse beard. Care should be taken as damage may be caused to the skin by using such an aggressive technique.

Keys to good practice

Remember to sterilise the lathering brush and sponges after each client.

Lathering techniques

It is necessary before lathering the face to apply hot towels, as lather should be applied to warm skin. This will serve to:

- soften the hair
- cleanse the face
- open the follicle and lift the hair
- prepare the skin for the lather.

A few towels used one at a time over the face will suffice and the lather should be applied directly following the removal of the last towel. This will ensure the lather is applied to a warm face. Towels can be heated via a warming cabinet or by running under hot water and ringing out thoroughly. The towels should be moist and warm but never dripping wet or very hot.

Keys to good practice

Hot towels should never be used on a client with sensitive or irritated skin, as they could cause further irritation, which would prevent you from shaving the face.

Traditionally, lather was made up beforehand from soap and applied with a brush. However, we now have the benefit of various foams and gels available for use. These can be applied by the traditional brush method but, as a time saver, you can apply using a gloved hand. The brush serves to lift the hairs ready for shaving when brushed over the skin, so you must emulate this action when massaging the lather over the face.

To save time, you can apply lather by hand, wearing a glove

Lather should be applied quickly, taking care not to cover the nose and mouth, or getting it into the ears or eyes. Most lathers contain conditioners and a lubricant to help the razor glide over the surface of the skin. However, while you are carrying out the shave, if you feel the lather drying, you must re-apply to prevent any damage to the skin.

Keys to good practice

Never cover with lather any areas you will not be shaving. You need to leave these exposed to give you a clear indication of any outlines or contra-indicated areas, for example, a raised mole.

In the salon

Stella was having a very busy day in the salon and, as it reached late afternoon, she was feeling tired and anxious. Like any other busy day, she soldiered on without complaining. Her next client was a full face shave so she carried out her consultation and then began the service. As she applied the hot towels, she forgot to ask the client if the towels felt comfortable. As the client was a regular and trusted Stella, he did not raise any objection when the towels felt uncomfortably hot. On removing the last towel, Stella did not pay enough attention to detail and carried on lathering the client's face. What she had not noticed was that on the sensitive area around the lip, the skin had blistered slightly and she had now covered it with lather.

The client felt relief at the towels being removed and the lather had somewhat cooled the face so he did not raise any objections. As Stella was shaving over the blistered area, the client felt sharp pain and stopped Stella, asking her to check if he was cut. Stella was surprised, as she had not felt the skin pull anywhere and felt sure everything was okay. Just to reassure the client, she wiped off the lather to take a look. When the skin was exposed, she could see that there were several small blisters around the lip and that she had taken the top off a few. Stella explained to the client what had happened and he said he felt the towels were uncomfortably hot at the time and this must have caused the blistering. Stella was extremely apologetic and offered to finish the rest of the shave free of charge. However, the client had lost trust in her professionalism and decided to leave.

- What should Stella have done when she felt tired and anxious?
- Not checking with the client regarding the heat of the towels was Stella's first mistake, but what was her second?
- Do you think the client was justified in leaving the salon?

Creating the look

The practice of shaving the skin with an open blade requires a great deal of skill and accuracy. The shaving strokes need to be fluent and methodical and this will only be achieved through practice. It is a good idea to begin by practising shaving on fine facial hair that is less stubborn to remove. You should also consider that mature skin, having lost its elasticity, drags more easily and requires greater tensioning. Therefore, practise first on younger clients. Once you become more experienced and build up your confidence, you will find the skill becomes much easier to carry out. You will become more aware of the influencing factors and what problems may arise and how to overcome them. For example, continued use of close shaving on dark skin can cause darkening and thickening of the skin. With experience, you will recognise the signs and advise remedial action accordingly.

Backhand and forehand shaving

The razor may be held in the forehand or backhand position. Whilst working in forehand, the razor is used working towards yourself and when using backhand, the razor is drawn away from you. You should follow a methodical pattern throughout the shave to ensure that your work is accurate. Look at the example below and use it as a guide.

Position during the shave

During the shave, if you are right-handed, you must stand on the right of the client and if you are left-handed, you must stand to the left. This will ensure smooth operating. You should begin with the side closest to you and work over to the side of the face furthest away to allow you ease of access to the lathered face.

Skin tensioning

While carrying out the shave, you must keep tension on the skin in the area you are drawing the blade across. The hand you use to pull the skin with should be kept dry and free from lather to prevent slipping. Tensioning the skin will help to prevent cuts, allowing the razor to glide over the skin with ease. The older we are, the less elasticity our skin has, therefore more tension is required as the skin will be more likely to fold.

Shaving techniques: a step-by-step guide

Before the shave.

A hot towel is applied.

The lather is applied.

The face is fully lathered ready for the shave.

Begin the 1st stroke from the ear sweeping across the face, while the skin is tensioned with the free hand.

Keeping good tension, this stroke is continued down the face and across the cheek.

Shaving is continued down the neck area.

Again, tensioning the skin, sweep across the chin area.

Once the shave is completed, the excess lather is removed by patting the face with a damp towel. Never rub the skin.

A cool towel is then applied.

After-shave balm is applied.

The finished look – the client has also had his moustache length reduced.

Keys to good practice

During the shaving process you will need to remove the lather from the blade. To prevent any damage to the blade or cutting of skin, you must wipe the blade away from yourself and the client. Keep the blade flat and wipe with the blade drawn away.

A second over-shave may be required if the hair was not removed first time. This is carried out by shaving against the grain of the beard and should be done only on coarse, stubborn hair and never on fine or sensitive skin. Second over-shaving can cause irritation to the skin and in-growing hairs so should be done only if completely necessary.

Sponge shaving

Sponge shaving is carried out only on a coarse, stubborn beard when a second over-shave was not enough. It involves dipping a sterilised sponge in hot water and wiping over the skin directly before the razor is drawn over. This will serve to open the follicle and lift the hair, allowing the blade to remove any stubborn hairs. Great care must be taken, as shaving so closely can damage the skin or cause in-growing hairs. This type of aggressive shaving should never be carried out unless absolutely necessary and never on fine or sensitive skin.

Shaving outlines

You will need to thoroughly assess the look the client wants and take great care not to shave into the shape required. Tensioning is still required and shaving outlines calls for you to be both precise and dexterous in your work, as a large degree of accuracy is needed. When shaving the outline of facial hair or a neckline, care should be taken not to apply too much lather. Blocking your view of the outline could lead to an unsatisfactory result.

Cooling the skin

The final stage of the shaving process is to cool the skin. If a client is proceeding to a facial massage, this is not required; therefore you must be sure of your client's requirements. Once all the lather has been removed with a damp towel or sponge, you must pat dry the face, taking care not to drag or pull the skin, as it may feel sensitive. You can now apply a cool towel but be sure to ask the client how cool they would like the towel to be. Some clients prefer only a cool towel and others prefer the fresh feel of a cold towel. The towel is applied in the same way the hot towels were applied at the beginning and this serves to cool the skin and close the follicles.

You may also apply talcum powder to dry off the face and prevent chapping. Nowadays there are various products available other than aftershave, such as balms and moisturisers, that will both moisturise and soothe the skin, helping to prevent irritation following a shave. These are ideal to use if the client does not like the feel of aftershave on the skin.

There is a wide range of products available to moisturise and soothe the skin following the shaving service

Problem solving

There are several problems that you may encounter during the shaving service, the most obvious being cutting the skin. However, no matter how serious the cut is, you must not feel overawed and, with the correct training, you should feel in control at all times.

The table on page 325 shows the kinds of problems that you may experience, along with the cause and action or remedy you may use.

Problem	Possible cause	Possible action/remedy
Cuts to the skin	Incorrect skin tensioning; using a razor with a dull edge	Stop shaving, administer first aid and continue only if bleeding stops. If necessary administer first aid
Uneven skin surface	Dimples; acne; moles; scar tissue	Take greater care and omit areas of concern
Patchy shave result	Dull edge on blade; uneven pressure applied whilst shaving	Strop and hone blade or change disposable blade; ensure steady pressure is used all over the face
Folliculitis	Inflammation of the hair follicle; in-growing hair	Do not proceed with shave and advise client to seek medical advice
Shave is not close enough	Coarse facial hair; lather has dried out; poor tensioning of skin; holding razor incorrectly	Carry out a second over-shave and possibly a sponge shave; re-apply lather as required; ensure good tensioning whilst shaving and check the angle of razor
Discomfort during shave	Blade has a dull edge; shaving dry skin; shaving against the hair growth pattern	Strop and hone blade or change disposable blade; lather efficiently; always shave with the grain of the beard unless second over-shave
Shaving rash	Blade has a dull edge; shaving dry skin; shaving against the hair growth pattern; shaving too close	Strop and hone blade or change disposable blade; lather efficiently; always shave with the grain of the beard unless second over-shave; stop shaving

After the service

This section looks at the disposal of waste after the service and advice you may give to the client about intervals between shaves, and products to use at home. It is essential to complete the service as professionally as you have carried it out to provide the client with an all-round first-class service.

What you will learn

- Disposal of waste
- Recommended intervals
- After-care advice

Disposal of waste

Following a shave service, you will have some waste materials that need to be disposed of in line with both legislation and the salon's procedures. It is imperative to dispose of used razor blades in a sharps bin; if your salon does not have one, you are in breach of government legislation. A sharps bin should be clearly labelled to identify its purpose and should be stored safely with the lid closed at all times. If you have lather that you have not used, it should be washed down the sink and not re-used on another client; this will prevent the risk of cross-infection. Used towels should be placed in a covered towel bin and any used tissue also placed in a covered litter bin. Failing to adhere to strict rules on safe disposal of waste not only leaves you open to the risk of prosecution and legal action, but also shows unprofessionalism in your work.

Recommended intervals

The time between shaving services will vary for each client. If the client has a dense growth then it is likely that he will require shaving more often. If the facial hair is fine and sparse then less frequent services will be required. In the same way, a client with dark facial hair will require more regular shaving than a client with lighter hair, as the dark growth will be more noticeable. In either case, you should recommend to the client what you feel is adequate, as they will be able to judge themselves from the apparent visible growth.

After-care advice

The advice you give to the client should take into account any problems that may arise at home; for example, shaving rash or in-growing hairs. In-growing hairs can happen when the hair grows back on itself and continues to grow under the skin; this is more likely to occur on curly hair. Exfoliating should be advised to help alleviate this problem. However, if this does not suffice then the skin will have to be broken with a sterile needle to release the trapped hair. Shaving rash can occur when the skin is irritated and should be treated with sensitivity. Moisturising the skin will help to prevent discomfort and the use of strong astringents such as aftershave should be avoided.

Retailing products for home use will not only improve your profile but also extend the service you provide into the client's home. You can increase your revenue while ensuring your clients are using reputable, good-quality products. Advise the client on their correct use and explain all the benefits of buying your products.

You may also be required to give your client advice on how to maintain the look at home. If you have shaved a new shape into the facial hair then it is important that the client understands how to shave the outline to maintain the look. Demonstrate how this is done and question the client to check their understanding. Remember that the client is a walking advertisement for your salon – he may leave the salon with a professional finish, but will it still look so good in a few weeks? This should have also been discussed at the initial consultation to ensure the look is achievable for the client at home.

Knowledge check

1. Why is it important to wear gloves during the shaving service?

2. What safety considerations should be taken into account during the shaving service?

3. Why is it important to keep your work area clean and tidy?

4. Why must fixed blade razors be honed and stropped?

5. Why is it necessary to apply a warm towel to the face before lathering?

6. Why must tension be applied to the skin during the shaving process?

7. When might it be necessary to carry out a sponge shave?

8. What effect will a cool towel have on the face after the shaving process?

9. What action should you take if you cut the skin during shaving?

10. How should used blades be disposed of safely?

Style hair using thermal techniques

Unit H33

Introduction

Throughout this unit you will be looking at how to style African Caribbean hair using a variety of thermal techniques. You will need to be aware of the different characteristics of hair and how these affect your choice of thermal styling technique. You must also consider the risk of using hot tools on the client's hair and the likelihood of them feeling some heat near the scalp. There are several thermal styling techniques that you will have to become familiar with and they are: curling, waving, straightening and blending the hair. Thermal styling is a method of using heat to mould the hair into a new shape temporarily. Hair contains weak hydrogen bonds that are easily breakable – the heat you apply will break the bonds and allow you to mould hair into a variety of shapes and styles.

Using heat to mould hair into a new shape

What you will learn
• Preparing the client
• Preparing the hair for thermal styling
• Creating a variety of fashion looks using thermal styling techniques
• After the service

You the stylist

As you become more confident in thermal styling, develop your skills by mixing and matching techniques to create individual and personalised styling for your clients.

Preparing the client

This section looks at everything that is important when preparing the client for thermal styling. You will need to take into account the health and safety considerations that apply when using thermal styling tools and equipment. The most obvious of these is the risk of burning the client; therefore you must remain alert to this hazard at all times.

What you will learn
• Thorough consultation
• Checking for contra-indications
• Personal health and hygiene
• Personal protective equipment
• Preparing your work area

Thorough consultation

Your initial consultation with your client is a major factor in determining the finished outcome (see Unit G9 for more detailed information). It is essential that at this stage you get it right to allow you to style the client's hair using the correct method. Choosing the incorrect thermal styling technique at this stage can lead to burning of the client's hair, skin or scalp. This could lead to irreversible damage. You must begin by talking to your client about their requirements. This is best carried out before the gown is placed on the client to enable you to see the way the client dresses, as this may influence the styling technique you choose. A client may have a picture of the look they require or your salon may have some stylebooks. This will help to give a clearer picture of the client's requirements. It also allows you as the stylist to show your ideas and to advise on what is realistically achievable. During the consultation, be sure to inform your client of any discomfort that they may feel during the service.

> **Remember**
>
> The important point that you must make is for the client not to make any sudden movements, as this could cause burning. If the client is experienced at having thermal styling treatments then this should not be a problem. However, it may be the first time and you must be sure you have explained thoroughly the implications of using hot tools.

Checking for contra-indications

An essential part of your consultation will be checking for any contra-indications. These are the factors that might prevent you from continuing with the service or change the techniques you use.

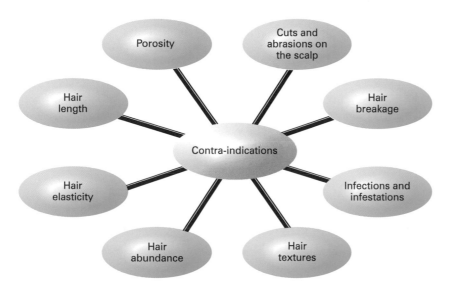

In the salon

Monique was having a very busy day in the salon. Her next client was a friend and she asked the assistant to gown her friend and prepare the hair for styling to save her time. Monique had styled her friend's hair many times and knew what her requirements were, so she skipped the consultation again to save some time. The client was having her hair pressed and as Monique was about a third of the way up the back of the head she was sure that she had spotted some lice eggs. On further inspection she could see a louse and found herself in the unfortunate position of having to inform her client that she could not continue. Her friend had forgotten to mention that a couple of weeks ago her two children had been infested and did not realise she had caught them herself. Monique would now be held up even longer as she would have to sterilise all the tools and equipment she had used on her client. In an attempt to save time by skipping over a crucial part of the consultation, she had in fact slowed herself down even more.

- What does this say about Monique's judgement in this case?
- Should you be allowing yourself to risk your professionalism in this way?
- Why is it important that Monique sterilises her tools and equipment immediately?

It is your responsibility as the stylist to determine if the client's hair is suitable for the service. If the hair is porous, broken or highly bleached, then you must advise against thermal styling. This is due to the extreme heat used on the hair, which can cause the hair to become dehydrated, porous and brittle. You can advise on a course of conditioning treatments to improve the condition of the hair, which may allow thermal styling in the future.

Personal health and hygiene

As the stylist, it is important for your own personal health and hygiene to be of a high standard to ensure you maintain a high level of professionalism. You will be working in close proximity with your client and you need to smell fresh and clean to avoid offence. Make sure your breath is fresh, especially after lunch or a cigarette break. Clients and colleagues may be offended by unpleasant odours; therefore it is essential you maintain good levels of personal hygiene. Ensure that your hands and nails are clean and presentable as they are constantly on show. If you wear make-up, touch it up throughout the day to ensure you always look your best.

Personal protective equipment

It is an essential requirement when thermally styling hair that your client is adequately protected, not only from the heated appliances that you are using, but also from any products that you are using on the hair.

Your client must be wearing a protective gown and a towel around the shoulders. If you accidentally over-saturate the hair with product, the gown and towel will help to protect the client's clothing. When you are thermally styling, many of the products that you are using are cream- and oil-based; therefore, if they were to be spilled onto your client's clothing, they would cause staining and there is always the possibility that stains cannot be removed. You would then be liable for the cost of any cleaning or replacement of your client's clothing. It is much safer and more professional to make sure your client is adequately protected with a gown at all times. During thermal styling the equipment that you use is extremely hot. Thermal heat pads are available to protect your fingers and hands from the heat.

Preparing your work area

It is vital that you have all the necessary products, tools and equipment ready for the start of the service and they are positioned to ensure everything is within easy reach; this will prevent you from over-stretching and possibly pulling a muscle. It also enables you to provide an efficient service. Being organised in this way will show your client that you are a professional and help to instil confidence in your ability as a stylist. It does not create a good impression if you have to keep leaving your client whilst you find something essential to the service.

Remember

You own health is very important when you are working in the salon. If you do not feel one hundred per cent, the quality of your work may reflect this. If you are suffering from an infectious illness, you run the risk of infecting your clients and colleagues.

Check it out

- Does your salon have a specific policy for gowning clients?
- Do you feel the salon should have its own gowning policy?

Remember

Keep checking throughout the service that the client is still appropriately protected and make any adjustments necessary to ensure the client's skin and/or clothing is covered.

Using thermal heat pads

Remember

If using an oven to heat your styling tools, this should be switched on early enough to ensure the tools have heated to the correct temperature by the time they are needed.

Below are the items you should have ready on your trolley prior to the service.

Electric pressing comb

Curling irons of various sizes

Tail comb and wide-tooth comb

Electric or gas heater

White tissue paper

Sectioning clips

Protective cream/oil

The tools and equipment you use should always be maintained correctly and checked before use for any faults. For example, thermal irons should be kept clean and well oiled at the joints as this will help to prolong their working life. All tools and equipment must be fit for purpose to prevent the risk of harm or injury to yourself or your client.

If you are using electrical equipment, it should be used following the requirements of the Electricity at Work Regulations (see Unit G1). This applies to the thermal styling tools you use and also the electric oven.

You must consider the regulations regarding the use of products (for example, COSHH) and ensure you are fulfilling any legal requirements on storage, handling, usage and disposal. Read the manufacturer's instructions if you have any doubt about a product's ability. The manufacturers have tried and tested their products in a variety of different ways and their instructions will ensure optimum results.

In addition, you must be aware of the potential problems that may occur during the thermal styling process.

<table>
<tr><th>Problems</th><th>Cause</th><th>Remedy</th></tr>
<tr><td>Burning the skin or scalp</td><td>Lack of due care; not placing vulcanite comb underneath irons to protect the skin, especially around the ears; not positioning the client correctly when using tools around the ears and neck</td><td>Apply cold water immediately. If serious, seek medical advice</td></tr>
<tr><td>Overly dehydrated or damaged hair</td><td>Tools are too hot for the hair; not using protective products on the hair prior to thermal styling; hair in poor condition before service commenced</td><td>A course of intensive conditioning treatments; no further heat or chemical treatments until the hair's condition has improved</td></tr>
<tr><td>Cicatricial alopecia</td><td>Cicatricial alopecia caused by scarring from a heat burn</td><td>No treatment available, permanent scarring</td></tr>
<tr><td>Indentations</td><td>Incorrect use of thermal styling tools or incorrect sectioning techniques</td><td>Re-style the hair using the tools correctly and sectioning accurately</td></tr>
<tr><td>Traction alopecia</td><td>Traction alopecia caused by excessive tension when pressing the hair</td><td>Cease applying tension to the hair and it should grow back</td></tr>
</table>

When using thermal styling tools, the temperature of the tools should be tested prior to each use. Placing the thermal styling tool onto a piece of white tissue will show if the tools are the correct temperature. If the tools are too hot, the tissue will discolour and scorch.

Test your thermal styling tools on white tissue before commencing the service

Keys to good practice

The practice of testing the temperature of thermal styling tools on the ends of the hair should not be undertaken whilst you are learning these new skills. Many experienced African Caribbean stylists use this method in the salon. However, this practice should be discouraged, as the risk of burning the hair is high.

Check it out

- How often are stock checks carried out in your salon?
- What systems are in place for reporting low levels of stock?

Stock levels must be checked regularly in order to prevent the embarrassment of running out of a particular product and it is not always possible to substitute one product for another. This would create an unprofessional image, as the finished result might not be satisfactory.

Your work area must remain clean and tidy at all times. This will not only look good to your clients, but will prevent the risk of cross-infection. If you regularly clean and sterilise your tools, there will be less chance of any bacteria being spread. Your combs should be kept in a chemical jar to prevent the growth of bacteria and brushes can be sterilised in an ultra-violet cabinet. The heated equipment that is used during pressing should always be wiped over immediately after use. This will prevent build-up of product and carbon on the equipment, which will affect its efficiency. Should product build-up occur, you must use the product manufacturer's recommended cleaning aids.

Check it out

Does your salon have a specific policy for storing, handling and cleaning thermal styling equipment?

Preparing the hair for thermal styling

This section looks at preparing the hair and the tools and equipment you would use for thermal styling. It is also important that you understand the effects this type of styling will have on the hair structure. As with all hairdressing services, problems may occur and you need to know how to overcome them. With practice and dedication, you can develop skills that will allow you to create a variety of effects on hair. However, in order to create wonderful looks, it is vital that you understand the underlying principles relating to thermal styling.

What you will learn

- The science of thermal styling
- Thermal styling on white hair
- Influencing factors

The science of thermal styling

When you are thermal styling or pressing the hair, the internal structure is undergoing some changes of which you need to be aware. As you already know, within the cortex lie a number of polypeptide chains, which run along the length of the hair. The chains are spiral-shaped (called an alpha (α) helix) and have cross-linkages that join them to their neighbouring polypeptide chains. Some of these linkages are permanent and others are temporary. The hydrogen bonds, which are one of the temporary linkages, are the ones that enable us to style the hair. The hydrogen bonds are not only joined to their neighbouring polypeptide chain, but are also connected to the same polypeptide chain between the coils of the alpha helix. It is these hydrogen bonds that enable the hair to be stretched during styling, giving the hair its elasticity.

The hair in its natural state – alpha keratin

Prior to styling, when the hair is in its natural state, this is known as alpha (α) keratin. Once the hair has been styled using thermal styling equipment, many of the hydrogen bonds are broken, allowing the hair to be stretched into a new shape. Once the hair has been heated, moulded and allowed to cool into this new shape, the hair is said to be in beta (β) keratin state. It is essential that the hair be allowed to cool before styling and finishing, as if the hair is still warm, some of the new shape may be lost.

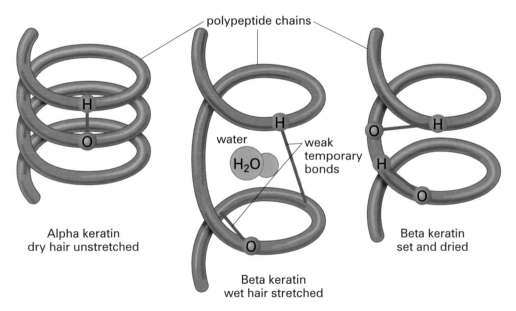

Alpha and beta keratin

The hair will stay in this new position until the hair is made wet or it absorbs atmospheric moisture. This is because the hair is hygroscopic – it has the ability to absorb moisture from the atmosphere. Humidity levels (the degree of moisture in the atmosphere) will affect the length of time the style will last. The level of humidity in some salons may be quite high due to the evaporation of water from the hair, towels, and so on. This is also true during damp weather; therefore it is essential that good styling products are used as this will help to prevent the atmospheric moisture entering the hair as quickly, prolonging the life of your styling.

When using heated styling equipment on dry hair, the hair's internal moisture breaks some of the hydrogen bonds; however, you must heat the equipment sufficiently to turn the internal moisture into steam. This breaks the hydrogen bonds and allows us to shape hair into a variety of styles.

As temporary setting utilises the natural moisture that is present in hair, overuse of heated styling equipment will cause the hair to dehydrate. Leaving the hair to cool down before dressing is important. If you disturb the hair before it has cooled and set into the new shape then you will have undone the work you have achieved.

Keys to good practice

If you are forcing moisture out of the hair with heat styling, you must replace this moisture by using moisturising and conditioning products on the hair.

Check it out

What factors about a client's hair do you think might influence the thermal styling process? Make a list of these and state how you think each may affect the process

The hydrogen bonds within the hair structure are easily broken by moisture. If you have styled a client's hair and they enter a moist atmosphere, then the style will easily 'drop' out. You must advise your clients of this to enable them to prolong the life of the style.

Styling products

There are a variety of styling products that you can use to help you overcome the effects of humidity on hair.

The thermal styling products used coat the hair shaft and help prevent any moisture from being absorbed. Some of the products contain moisture-repellent ingredients that repel any moisture. Any product that you put on the client's hair will usually have an effect for a few days but will gradually wear off. The client can maintain the style at home by adding more products to the hair; this will help to extend the life of the style. It is important to remember that despite the amount of product used to combat the effects of the hair's hygroscopic nature, some moisture will penetrate the hair shaft, affecting the style. If the client is caught in a rain shower or sweats heavily then you cannot guarantee the style will hold.

Thermal styling on white hair

When you are thermal styling on white hair, there are several factors that you must consider:

1   Take care not to discolour the hair through scorching or over-heating. You should always test the temperature of the tools you are using before using them on the hair. Think of the way hot tools will scorch white tissue paper – the effects on white hair will be exactly the same.

2   Take care not to discolour the hair with product usage. If you apply excessive amounts of styling/moisturising products to the hair then you run the risk of staining any white hair. Ensure that you apply only the correct amount of product and always follow manufacturer's instructions.

3   The texture of white hair must be taken into consideration. White hair tends to be coarser and more resistant so take care not to apply too much heat to combat this. It will lead only to irreparable damage.

4   Watch out for discoloration due to prolonged use of heated appliances. When you are thermally styling white hair, although you are aware of the amount of heat you are using at the time, over a longer period, continued heat application may cause damage to the hair. If this occurs, you should be advising your client to give the hair a rest from heat and trying alternative styling methods.

If you take note of the above points then thermally styling white hair should not present any problems to you.

Influencing factors

There are several influencing factors that you need to consider when styling hair using thermal styling tools. Each of the factors may present problems to you during the process if you have not taken time to consider their relevance.

The haircut and length

You will need to consider the client's haircut, as you must ensure the styling technique you choose is suitable for the length and style of the client's hair. For example, if the client's hair is excessive in length, you would not choose to create a head of barrel curls but would perhaps choose spiral curls.

Shorter hair is ideal for barrel curls. When pressing, if the hair is too short, there is a greater risk of burning and it may just not be possible.

Barrel curls suit shorter lengths

The hair re-growth of chemically relaxed hair

You will need to ensure there is enough re-growth for you to work with. You should be able to judge your level of skill with the pressing comb and know your limitations. Care must be taken when pressing short hair, especially around the front hairline, as the hair tends to be finer and the likelihood of burning the client becomes greater. Another important factor to consider is if the hair has been chemically relaxed then it will be more fragile than the root area that you are pressing. Take care not to overlap as breakage may occur on the previously relaxed hair.

Hair elasticity

You will need to carry out an elasticity test on the hair (see Unit G9). Hair with poor elasticity is usually due to internal damage, in which case you must reconsider the hair's suitability for thermal styling. If the hair is chemically treated then it is most likely that the elasticity will be poor. The addition of heat is likely to further weaken the hair's condition, and may cause breakage.

Hair density

The amount of hair a client has will determine the size of the sections you take. Your sections will need to be finer if the hair is thicker. This will allow better penetration of heat through the hair and will ensure an even result. For example, if you are tonging the hair, make sure that the section you take is no larger than the barrel of the tongs. Alternatively, if you are crimping, take a finer section to ensure a good indentation is left in the hair.

Remember

If you feel the hair's elasticity is too poor for thermal styling, recommend conditioning treatments until such a time as the hair's condition improves sufficiently to carry out the desired service.

Ensure that the sections you take are appropriate to the hair's density

Hair texture

The texture of the hair is the thickness of each individual strand of hair. In hairdressing the different textures are known as fine, medium or coarse. The finer the hair, the less heat it will require to style. Alternatively, the coarser it is, the more heat will be needed. An example of this is when you are pressing the hair; if it is coarse, it will require hard pressing and if it is fine, a softer press.

Curl pattern

Our genes will predetermine the curl pattern of our hair. There are several types of curl pattern ranging from tight curly to wavy and they will affect the techniques that you carry out. For example, a client with curly hair will require more tension and heat to straighten the hair than a client with wavy hair. You will need to consider the implications on the hair's condition of using more heat and tension. Over the whole of the head there can be several different curl patterns and you should be looking at all the different areas to assess how resistant the curl formation will be.

Types of curl patterns

Head and face shape

As with all hair styling, this is an influencing factor that cannot be overlooked. You must ensure that the finished look will suit the client's head and face shape. This is carried out at the initial consultation and you will by now be familiar with the many different face shapes and which styles are best suited to them (you learnt about this in Unit G9).

Check it out

What effect will extremes of heat and tension have on the hair?

Creating a variety of fashion looks using thermal styling techniques

What you will learn

- Hair pressing
- Styling the hair using curling irons

There are several different techniques that you need to perfect within this unit. Below is a table showing each of the techniques, with examples of the tools used and the effects they produce.

Technique	Tools used	Effect produced
Soft or hard pressing	A pressing comb can be heated in a stove or electrically	Straightening; hair can be prepared by blow-drying (or wrap-drying) to smooth out first
Curling	Tongs or irons can be heated in a stove or electrically	Barrel curls, flicks or smoothed hair
Crimping	Crimping irons	Zigzag indentations
Smoothing	Flat irons	Flattens and smoothes the hair

You need to be familiar with each of the techniques and be able to decide which one is correct for your client's hair. This will depend on the client's requirements, the hair's condition, and its texture. You should have determined the outcome of the service during the consultation.

Before starting work with the thermal styling equipment, the hair should be shampooed, conditioned, blow-dried or wrap dried. A wide-tooth comb attachment may be used when blow-drying the hair straight; this helps to prepare the hair for subsequent treatments as it smoothes and disentangles the hair, making it much easier to work with. You also need to make your client aware of the need for correct positioning whilst the treatment is being carried out. Working on the hair in confined areas, such as in the nape or around the ear, will require you to move the client's head to an appropriate position. You must then keep the head positioned where it is to prevent any contact between the hot tools and the skin.

Keys to good practice

Check with your client that they are comfortable throughout the process. Do not exert too much pressure when moving their head into the correct position, as this can cause discomfort or even injury to the client.

Styling hair using thermal techniques: a step-by-step guide

Hair before styling, previously shampooed, conditioned and blow-dried.

Thermal styling product is applied to protect the hair from the heat.

The hair is sectioned into straight sections ready for curling.

The heat of the thermal tongs is tested on white tissue paper.

The section of hair is smoothed before curling.

The ends are tucked smoothly into the curling tongs to avoid fish hooks.

Finger protectors are used to create the flicked-up effect.

Large tongs are used on the crown section to create height.

Sections of hair are spiral curled.

Tongs are loosened to remove the hair. The finished look.

Hair pressing

This technique uses a hot comb to straighten and smooth the hair. It is a good technique to use on a client with a re-growth requiring relaxing, or on a full head to be straightened. Pressing combs can be heated electrically or by the use of a hot oven. The advantage of electrical combs is that they are thermostatically controlled. Some electrical combs have a temperature dial so you can select the correct temperature for your client's hair (for example, a client with fine, tinted or bleached hair would need a lower temperature to achieve the desired result). This means that they will not overheat, causing burning and damage to the hair. If you are using a pressing comb that you heat in an oven then, as the operator, you must determine if the comb is at the right temperature. You need to use a piece of white tissue paper, press the comb against it and look for signs of scorching or burning. This tells you whether or not the comb is too hot. If you put the pressing comb into the hair and it is too hot then it will burn the hair, causing irreparable damage.

Using the pressing comb with an oven takes a lot of practice and with experience you will find it much easier to judge. You must, however, always remain alert to the hazard of burning the hair or skin.

> **Remember**
>
> Checking the temperature of your tools at the start of the service is not enough. Your thermal styling tools should be checked each time they are removed from the oven.

> **Keys to good practice**
>
> The teeth of the comb and the back of the comb have two different functions when pressing hair. The teeth of the comb separate the hair, allowing the comb to glide through the hair more easily. Combs have different-sized teeth, with different spacing between them. As a general rule, the smaller the teeth and the more tension you use, the straighter the results. Most importantly, it is the back of the comb that actually straightens the hair.

You must keep your tension even while pressing to ensure that your finished result is of an even straightness. The pressure and angle that you hold the comb at must also remain even throughout, for the same reason.

The effects of pressing oils and creams are shown below.

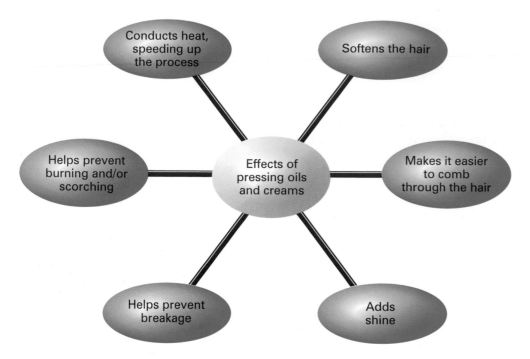

These products should be used sparingly before pressing, as overuse may cause the hair to smoke, which may be a little disconcerting to the client!

Sectioning guide when pressing hair

The texture and density of the hair must be taken into consideration when sectioning the hair for pressing. A general guide is shown in the table below.

Hair type	Size of section
Fine, sparse	2–3 cm
Medium	1.5–2.5 cm
Coarse, dense	1–2 cm

There will always be exceptions to every rule, but practice and experience will enable you to make these decisions based on your knowledge of African Caribbean hair.

Styling the hair using curling irons

Curling irons or tongs are available with different-sized barrels, weights and styles and give a variety of different effects, from large curls through to waves in the hair. They may be heated electrically or by using a gas or electric oven.

Remember

When placing the irons in the heater, make sure they are in correctly as a serious burn could result if they fell out onto somebody.

Conventional curling irons

These are available in different sizes and weights and get much hotter than electrically heated irons; this makes them more versatile, as they may be used on all African Caribbean hair types. Great care must be taken when using the irons as they may easily burn the hair and skin.

Electrically heated irons

These are the safer option, as they do not get as hot as the conventional irons. They are thermostatically controlled; therefore the risk of burning the hair or skin is less. They are available as cordless appliances that are heated on a base unit, alleviating the problem of the flex wearing away due to continued use. However, this makes them less durable as they may not be hot enough for very coarse hair.

The temperature of the irons should be tested in the same way as the pressing comb; that is, by placing the barrel onto white tissue paper for five seconds. If the tissue discolours or burns, the irons are too hot and will need to be placed onto a cooling pad until they reach the required temperature.

The temperature of the irons is dependent on the hair texture and condition. As a general rule, coarse hair can withstand more heat, but if the hair is fine or has been lightened or tinted, the temperature should be lower. Hair in poor condition may break if thermal styling is carried out; therefore it is important to test the hair's elasticity prior to the service. If the hair shows signs of damage, thermal styling should not be carried out, as once the hair has been scorched, the damage is irreversible.

Holding the irons

Holding the irons correctly will ensure you have control of them when working. Hold the irons in the right hand (not too close to the joint to avoid the heat), place the first three fingers on the lower handle, with the little finger on top. The thumb gives support and balance whilst using the irons.

> ### Remember
>
> Switch off the irons at the socket when you have finished using them – this will help to prolong their working life and prevent accidents.

Holding irons correctly

Practise opening and closing the barrel using your fingers to control the movement; this should produce a clicking sound as the barrel closes.

Now practise turning the irons: move your hand forwards, towards your body. This is the technique you will use to create curls. You will need to learn both of these techniques, as the two combined will enable you to create movement in the hair.

In the salon

Danielle was very busy one Saturday afternoon tonging her client's hair. The client was a regular client to the salon and Danielle usually carried out the client's styling services. She looked up and noticed her brother and some of his friends outside the salon. They were behaving really badly and she was worried. When she turned back to her client and opened the tongs to remove them from the client's hair, she discovered that the client's hair had stuck to the tongs.

- What caused this problem?
- What should Danielle have done differently?

When first using curling irons, practise with cold irons until you have mastered the art of turning or rolling them.

Creating barrel curls

Barrel curls are usually used on short or medium-length hair to create lift, curl and movement. The hair should be prepared prior to curling. The size of irons you use will depend on the texture and length of the hair and the amount of curl you wish to achieve.

The irons should be placed about 1 cm from the scalp. You must ensure you apply a little tension here to prepare the base. After sliding the irons along the hair shaft, make sure the ends are tucked in properly to prevent fish hooks, then wind the hair down so the irons sit on their own base. As with roller setting, you can curl the hair to add volume or to minimise it when necessary.

Curling to add volume

Comb the section of hair at an obtuse angle to the base (over-directed); place the irons approximately 1 cm from the scalp. Begin to wrap the hair around the barrel of

Remember

The angle at which you comb the hair will determine the direction of the curl.

Curling to add volume

Remember

Place a vulcanite comb between the irons and the scalp to prevent burning the client's scalp.

the irons. Hold the hair in this position for a few seconds to form a strong base. Then rotate the irons until they reach the root area. The curl will sit off base. This method of curling will create maximum lift and volume.

Curling to reduce volume

Comb the section of hair at an acute angle to the base (dragging the roots); place the irons approximately 1 cm from the scalp. Begin to wrap the hair around the barrel of the irons; you should not need to hold this position, as a strong base is not required. Rotate the irons to complete the curl. Again, the curl will sit off base. This method of curling will produce very little curl or volume and is generally used to blend the hair between the style lines or when the finished result requires just the ends to curl, for example, a bob.

Spiral curling

Spiral curling is carried out on longer hair. The hair should be cleansed and prepared for the service; and the correct products used following the manufacturer's instructions. The hair should be sectioned off before you start to curl the hair, as this will help you to work in a methodical manner. The hair should then be divided into vertical sub-sections for you to curl.

Place the irons into the section, close to the root (about 1 cm away), then open and close the irons whilst you turn them and feed the hair into the irons. You must ensure the ends are tucked in properly to prevent fish hooks.

Using irons to wave the hair

Waving the hair using irons

This procedure would usually be carried out on hair that has been chemically relaxed. This effect may also be achieved using waving irons. The hair should be prepared as for thermal pressing.

The irons should be placed into the hair about 1 cm from the roots, with the rod at the top. As you close the irons, comb the hair to the left and move the irons to the right, then turn the irons towards you for half a turn. Allow the hair to heat then open the irons and move them down the section of hair a little until the groove of the irons is slightly below the wave you have just produced and turn the irons upwards. Allow the hair to heat then continue until you have completed the waving.

Flat irons and crimping irons

Both of these types of irons, although producing a different look, are used on the hair in a similar way. To prepare the hair, you would always shampoo, condition, blow-dry or wrap dry first. Starting in the nape and working up the head, small sections are taken and the irons are used along the length of the hair from root to point. The flat irons are taken along the hair length in order to straighten and smooth the hair. The finished look should be even and without indentations.

The crimping irons are placed along the hair length at even intervals to produce the crimped look. It is important to apply the crimping irons evenly otherwise the finished result will have an uneven crimp.

Both an even and a uneven crimp can be seen

<table>
<tr><td>

Check it out

What are your salon's expected service times for the thermal styling techniques you carry out? Are the senior staff times different from those for the junior staff?

</td></tr>
</table>

After the service

After the service is complete, ensure you fill in/update the client's record card. You should give the client any necessary advice and ensure that you dispose of any waste materials as soon as possible.

What you will learn

- Completing client records
- Confirmation of the finished look
- After-care advice
- Disposal of waste

Completing client records

You should record details of the treatment and also the information extracted from the client during consultation; for example, hair colourants used, whether they are professional or home colours, how she cares for her hair between visits, and so on. A record card provides you with essential information about the client. This information is vital to you the stylist and will influence any decisions you make about their hair treatments.

Confirmation of the finished look

When you have finished styling the hair, you will need to check the balance, overall shape and volume of the finished style, and confirm with the client that they like the end result. Always look in the mirror and check the overall balance from every angle around the head, as this is what everyone will see of your client's look. Show the client the back, making sure that she can actually see through the back mirror. A good rule of thumb is if you can see the back or sides through the mirrors then your client will also.

After-care advice

It is an essential part of the service to provide your client with after-care advice. Not only is it a fantastic selling opportunity, but it also presents a professional image. You must have thorough product knowledge and ensure that you always have the full product range in stock. The products that you use on your clients whilst carrying out the service should always be offered to the client to buy and use at home. This will help the client to maintain the style with the correct products.

Spending a little time offering the client some advice on how to style and maintain the look will be time well spent. It will show the client that you are interested in how they look after their hair, which ultimately reflects on your salon.

Get to know the full range of products in your salon

Disposal of waste

Any waste produced by the service, for example, used tissue, should be removed and your work area cleaned in preparation for your next client. You must dispose of any waste in line with your salon's policy and following the requirements of law. However, if you are using products correctly and following the manufacturer's instructions, then there should be no need for waste. Product wastage can be costly for the salon and should be discouraged.

When using thermal styling techniques, remember you can mix and match the techniques to create individual and personalised styling for your clients. Keep your camera handy so you can photograph the work you produce; this may be used as evidence in your portfolio.

Check it out

Are you fully aware of all the salon's rules regarding disposal of waste? Is your salon environmentally friendly and adopting a recycling of waste policy? For example, is there a paper recycling collection point in your area? Maybe this is something that you could recommend.

Knowledge check

1. *What responsibilities do stylists have when using styling and finishing products as stated under the Control of Substances Hazardous to Health Regulations?*

2. *During thermal styling, why should white hair be treated differently?*

3. *What remedial action could you take if the following problems occurred during a thermal styling service:*
    a *Burning the skin or scalp*
    b *The hair has become overly dehydrated or damaged during the treatment.*

4. *Why should thermal styling tools be kept free of excess oils and dirt?*

5. *What is meant by the term hygroscopic, and why is this important when thermally styling hair?*

6. *Why is it essential that you consider the elasticity of the hair prior to thermal styling?*

7. *Following thermal styling, what are the benefits of giving the client effective after-care advice?*

Provide corrective relaxing services

Unit H31

Introduction

This unit is primarily concerned with providing specialist, relaxing services to rectify a range of relaxing problems. There are three key stages to the process of correction. Firstly, it will be necessary to thoroughly analyse the hair and determine the problem. Next, plan and agree a course of action with the client. Finally, use corrective relaxing techniques to solve any problems.

Relaxing and colouring hair adds vibrance to any client's look

What you will learn
• Preparing the client
• The relaxing process
• After the service

You the stylist

As the stylist providing the corrective service, it is your responsibility to analyse the problem and agree a course of action that you feel will be to the client's best advantage. It may not always be possible to remedy the problem with one salon visit. You may decide to offer your client a course of treatment over a period of time, covering several appointments. The corrective relaxing service you provide may not necessarily be on a client whom you have previously treated. Therefore, it is important to ascertain your client's previous history regarding their relaxing treatments during a thorough consultation.

Preparing the client

This section contains all the information relating to the preparation of yourself and the client for the corrective relaxing service:

• Thorough consultation
• Checking for contra-indications
• Preparation of work area
• Personal health and hygiene
• Personal protective equipment.

Ensuring that you are fully prepared for the service is an essential part of the treatment, from making sure that you have the correct products in stock to having all the necessary tools and equipment to hand.

Thorough consultation

A detailed and thorough consultation is essential in order to ascertain the action you will use to correct your client's relaxing problem. During the consultation you must ask specific questions about the client's hair to determine the previous history of treatments. The client's previous chemical history should be available on her record card and you should refer to this if it is available, as this will indicate which products,

Remember	
Lye relaxers are not compatible with no-lye relaxers and vice versa.	

including relaxing products, have been used, the development time of the process and any reactions that may have occurred. This information is essential. If, for example, the client had a calcium-based relaxer (no-lye) last time, this may cause problems if a sodium-based relaxer were to be used in the next treatment.

This may be difficult to ascertain if the client is new to your salon, therefore it would be advantageous to carry out a strand test to ensure the products are suitable. You will need to ask investigative questions to discover as much information as possible.

If the hair has been coloured using a high-lift tint or bleach, you should not recommend a relaxing service, due to the likely poor condition of the hair. If you carry out the service on hair in this state, it may lead to damage and/or breakage of the hair. Hair that has been coloured may be relaxed, but only if the hair is in good enough condition. This may be determined by carrying out both a porosity test and an elasticity test (see page 46). You may also choose to carry out an incompatibility test if you have any doubt as to the colourants on your client's hair. Failure to carry out these tests may lead to the deterioration of the hair condition and possible breakage.

During your consultation, you should also check the hair and scalp for contra-indications. Any cuts and/or abrasions on the scalp would prevent the treatment from being carried out because the relaxing product might enter the open wound, causing the client discomfort and with the potential to cause infection.

Keys to good practice

You should record the client's responses on a consultation sheet or record card in order to be sure that you have extracted the right information.
This will also serve to be useful if there are any repercussions following the corrective treatment you are providing.

CLIENT CONSULATION SHEET

Client's name:

Client's address:

Stylist's name: Date:

When was your hair last relaxed?

Which product was used?

When did you last shampoo your hair?

Have you ever experienced any of the following problems during a chemical relaxing process?

• Scalp irritation

• Hair breakage

• Unsatisfactory result

If scalp irratation has been experienced, is it the complete scalp or isolated areas?

Have you had permanent colour on your hair?   Yes / no
If so, when?

Have you had your hair permed?   Yes / no
If so, when?

Has your hair been thermally styled with a thermal comb or tong?   Yes / no
If so, how long ago?

When was your last conditioning treatment?

A client consultation sheet

You must accurately determine the problem by using suitable techniques and should be looking at:

- **The nature and extent of the relaxing problem, which includes:**
  - Under-processed ends
  - Under-processed roots
  - Mid-length under-processing.
- **The condition of your client's hair, skin and scalp**
  - Is the hair strong enough to withstand a relaxing treatment?
  - Does the client have a sensitive scalp?
  - Are there cuts and abrasions or any other contra-indications?
- **The extent of processed hair and natural hair**
  - This may affect the sequence of application
  - This would determine the strength of relaxer to use
  - This will have an effect on the processing time.

The techniques you should use include questioning, observation and testing.

At this point, you need to question your client to establish what they consider their relaxing problem to be and what kind of result they would like to see at the end of the service. You will need to ask your client both factual and feeling questions, e.g. 'Do you *feel* there's too much curl in the hair?' (For more information on this and other methods of communication, refer to Unit G9.)

You must listen carefully to everything the client has to say, to make sure you do not miss any detail that might affect the outcome of the corrective relaxing treatment. Once you completely understand the nature of the problem, you can then move on to complete any necessary tests and checks for contra-indications. Once you are satisfied that you have thoroughly explored not only your client's exact requirements, but also the hair's potential to achieve what is required, you must summarise and discuss this with your client to check their understanding. The course of action you may take will be either:

- To remove the curl in the hair
- To reduce the amount of curl in the hair.

Be as specific as possible and inform the client of the likelihood of achieving the degree of straightness required, and the cost, duration and expected outcome of the service. You should ensure your client is totally aware of the nature of the service that you need to perform, the products that will be used and the anticipated outcome of the service. You must then record your client's agreement. Finally, you should make your client aware of any restrictions the service you are to carry out will place on further hairdressing services. For example, if the hair will be left fragile and sensitised, then thermal styling may have to be avoided due to the extreme amount of heat used on the hair, which may lead to breakage.

Checking for contra-indications

It is important to ascertain any contra-indications prior to a corrective relaxing service to prevent any serious problems arising. For example, if you accidentally overlooked a skin disorder and applied the relaxing treatment, a serious reaction could occur, causing burns or even scarring.

The table below shows the contra-indications that you should be looking for and discussing with your client.

Contra-indication	How to assess the problem
Skin sensitivities	Ask the client during consultation and look at previous record card or consultation sheet information. Thoroughly check the scalp as an excessively dry scalp may indicate some sensitivity. Hair that has recently been plaited/braided or had hair extensions, may also be quite sensitive.
Previous history of allergic reaction to relaxing products	Ask the client during consultation and look at previous record card or consultation sheet information.
Known allergies	Ask the client during consultation and record any known allergies.
Skin disorders	Thoroughly check the skin and scalp prior to commencing the relaxing service. Check the scalp for skin disorders such as eczema or psoriasis; broken skin would contra-indicate the service. You should also be looking for any signs of infection.
Incompatible products	Certain products are deemed incompatible with a relaxing service; this includes high-lift tint, bleach and incompatible relaxers and colourants with metallic salts. Remember, if in doubt, TEST!
Medical advice or instructions	Ask the client during the consultation about any medical problems they have and/or medication they are taking which could prove problematic. If necessary, ask for notification from their GP.

All of the above will need to be considered, as they will have an effect on both whether you proceed with the corrective relaxing treatment and also the type of products for the protection and relaxing you will use. For example, if a client has skin sensitivity then the use of a no-lye relaxer would be advised, along with barrier cream and a protective base for the scalp.

Before you begin, you must check that your client has not recently shampooed their hair (a minimum of five days should suffice); the scalp needs sebum to be present, as this acts as a barrier to protect the scalp. Remember to advise your client of this when they book the service. You must also make sure your clients do not overload their hair with products prior to the service, as this too may act as a barrier. Advise your clients accordingly when they book their appointments.

It is not advisable to relax hair immediately after removing scalp plaits/braids or hair extensions, as the hair is likely to be severely dehydrated and would benefit from conditioning treatments beforehand. The scalp may also be quite sensitive.

You must also ensure that you leave sufficient time between the relaxing treatment and the corrective relaxing service, e.g. two weeks, as this will give the hair and scalp time to recover from the process and will also minimise the damage caused to the hair and scalp.

It is imperative that any information regarding tests be recorded on either a record card or consultation sheet. This can be used to show to a client your professionalism and also to refer back to if a problem does arise.

> **Check it out**
>
> Why do you think a porosity and elasticity test are required before relaxing the hair? Write a short description of how each of the tests is carried out and the potential consequences of not carrying out the tests.
>
> To help you, look at the step-by-step pictures in this unit to see how a porosity and elasticity test are carried out.

Preparation of work area

In order to minimise disruption to the smooth running of the salon, you must prepare your work area in anticipation of the service you are to carry out.

Checklist for preparing your work area

What to do	Why/how?
All the necessary tools and equipment for the service should be ready	Saves time and conveys professional image to the client
Any products needed for the service should be available and ready to use	Regular and effective stocktaking will ensure that all products are available
Work area must be clean and tidy	Prevents accidents occurring, reduces risk of cross-infection and portrays a professional image
Instruct junior staff to prepare the work area correctly	Saves time. Make sure that you clearly communicate what is required – a short list of instructions may be given to junior staff
Tools and equipment should be clean, sterilised and fit for the purpose	The appropriate method of sterilisation should be used and equipment should be checked for defects
Electrical equipment should be used in compliance with health and safety legislation	Ensure that junior staff are complying with the safe use of electrical equipment (see Unit G1). This is your responsibility.

Keys to good practice

Leaving your junior staff to prepare for you does not mean that your responsibilities are any less important; you must also remain alert to any potential hazards or risks arising, and act accordingly.

Personal health and hygiene

While in the salon you are working in close proximity to your clients and other staff members; it is therefore important to present a professional image at all times.

Checklist for personal health and hygiene

What to do	Why/how?
Make sure your body and clothes smell clean and fresh	The client will feel more comfortable in your presence. Daily washing and the use of a good deodorant are essential.
Make sure you breath smells nice	Use a breath freshener. This will help to combat odours from strong-smelling foods or smoking.
Do not work if you are feeling unwell	Infections can be spread in the salon. Keep yourself fit and healthy to ensure that you produce the best work possible.
Maintain a good posture while working. Think about whether your client is positioned correctly for your needs as well as for their own comfort	This will minimise the risk of injury and fatigue. Make sure you keep your back straight and balance evenly distributed. Having your tools and equipment close to hand will prevent you from over-stretching.

Personal protective equipment

Relaxing treatments require the use of chemicals that can be harsh if used incorrectly. Therefore, it is an essential requirement when relaxing a client's hair that you use a gown, plastic cape and towel to protect the client and their clothing from the chemicals you are using. Care should be taken to ensure that adequate protection is provided throughout the service and that if the gown or towel slips it is replaced immediately to prevent any accidents. You must also be wearing both gloves and an apron in order to protect your skin and clothing from the chemicals you are using. Be aware that prolonged use of strong chemicals can cause allergy, sensitivity and contact dermatitis which makes the risk of not using personal protective equipment too great. It is also a requirement of law that, as a manager or salon owner, you provide personal protective equipment for the staff working in the salon to use when needed.

In the salon

During the completion of a corrective relaxing treatment, Louise hadn't noticed that her client's gown had loosened, exposing her shirt at the back. Unfortunately during the application of the treatment Louise had splashed a little relaxer onto the gown and while it was developing, Cara, the client, had moved and the relaxer had smeared onto her shirt at the back. It was only on completion of the relaxer, when Louise took off Cara's gown, that she spotted that her shirt was stained. On further investigation, Louise realised what had happened and explained to Cara that unfortunately relaxing product wouldn't wash out. Cara was very distressed about her shirt being ruined and became upset. Not wanting to lose either the client or damage the salon's good name, Louise offered to pay for the shirt to be replaced. Cara accepted Louise's offer and, although she wasn't happy about the situation, felt that Louise's goodwill gesture was enough to appease the situation and for her to remain a client at the salon.

- How could this situation have been avoided?
- Do you think Louise was right to offer to pay for Cara's shirt to be replaced?
- If Louise hadn't mentioned the staining and had let Cara go home to find the stain later, what do you think might have happened?
- If you were Cara, would you return to the salon again?

The relaxing process

This section is concerned with the types of corrective relaxing problems that can occur and how to correct them. You will need to understand the science of the relaxing process and the effects that the chemicals used have on the hair structure. You must also be aware of the types of problems that may arise and how to correct them, plus the relaxing techniques used during the process. (This will be demonstrated in the step-by-step photographs.)

A good working knowledge of the products and equipment used when relaxing is also required, as this will ensure you are working professionally and allow you to achieve the best results possible. This section will cover:

- Hair relaxing science
- Products, equipment and their use
- Relaxing problems.

Hair relaxing science

During the process of chemical relaxing, a product is applied to the hair that will penetrate the cuticle and work on the internal structure of the hair shaft. (Unit G9 contains more information on the hair structure.) Within the cortex there are bonds, known as disulphide bonds or bridges, and a percentage of these will need to be broken and reformed into lanthionine bonds during the relaxing process.

Hair in its natural state. prior to relaxing

The relaxer has been applied. Some of the disulphide bonds are broken by hydrolysis, making cysteine (HS) and sulphenic acid (SOH).

Relaxed hair now contains one amino acid lanthionine (S)

The science of relaxing hair

When the relaxer is applied to the hair, it penetrates the cuticle into the cortex and starts to break down the disulphide bonds. The relaxing product carries water into the hair and this breaks the disulphide bonds. This process is known as hydrolysis. The water molecule splits in two, and one part of hydrogen is added to one of the sulphur atoms, making cysteine (HS), while the rest of the water (HO) is added to the other sulphur atom, making sulphenic acid (SO-H).

As the hair straightens, the cysteine (HS) and the sulphenic acid react together to form the amino acid called lanthionine. Lanthionine has only one sulphur atom; therefore the spare sulphur atom combines with the water to form a more stable substance that may be removed from the hair by thorough rinsing. This is a continuous process and does not require neutralising in the conventional way; however, the relaxing product must be thoroughly rinsed from the hair and a neutralising shampoo used to return the hair back to its acidic pH.

Remember that this is a simplified version of the complex process that actually takes place, but this information should be sufficient to enable you to understand the science of hair relaxing.

The disulphide bonds are strong and only with the aid of chemicals can they be broken; however, if too many are broken during the relaxing process then this will result in irreparable damage or even breakage of the hair. This makes the timing of the process crucial. If the chemical relaxer is left on too long, this may result in breakage. Alternatively, if it is not left on for long enough, it may result in unsatisfactory relaxing of the curl.

Remember

Once hair has been chemically relaxed it is impossible to perm. This is because perming causes the disulphide bonds to be broken and reformed. However, following relaxing, there are no longer enough disulphide bonds to work on within the hair's structure. Not only will it produce an unsatisfactory result but also the hair will be left dry and brittle, with a high chance of breakage occurring.

Keys to good practice

Additional heat should never be used when developing cream relaxers. Additional heat might not only cause irritation to the scalp but also over-processing and breakage of the hair. However, the temperature of the room in which you are working must be taken into consideration; if the room is warm this may speed up the process. By the same principle, if the room is cold, development may take a little longer.

Products, equipment and their use

Remember

When applying the relaxer at the roots, remember not to apply it directly to the scalp. Prolonged contact will cause the client discomfort.

Do not 'mix and match' relaxing products; stick to one range

Products

Before, during and after relaxing, you must be aware of the correct products to use in order to achieve the best results and maintain the hair's condition. Any products that you use during the relaxing process are governed by the regulations relating to COSHH. You have a duty to store, handle, use and dispose of chemicals in line with manufacturer's instructions, salon procedures and policies, and local bylaws. You must also be aware of using products economically and the consequences on the salon's finances of overusing products. Wastage of products is as good as throwing money away and you have a duty to ensure that not only yourself, but any staff you are responsible for, are using products economically.

There are not only various types of chemical relaxers but also different types of pre- and post-relaxing treatments. You must have an understanding of their role in the process and their benefits of use. Product manufacturers will supply a full range of all the necessary products to use and it is important that you follow their recommendations. Never use a relaxing cream from one manufacturer with a neutralising shampoo from another manufacturer. You must remember that they are all scientifically developed for use as a complete range. They are developed to complement each other and be used solely in conjunction with the rest of the products in the range. If you were to mix and match products, this could result in an unsatisfactory result or scalp sensitivity.

Check it out

Although you may feel you are completely familiar with the products that you use in your salon, take the time out to read the manufacturer's instructions carefully. You may find information or tips that you had previously missed.

Pre-relaxer treatments

A pre-relaxer should be used on the hair prior to the application of relaxing cream if the hair is dry or porous. A pre-relaxer will coat the cuticle with a polymer film, which will act as a barrier to the relaxing cream, therefore slowing down the development process. This action will allow you more control over the development time and will help to prevent over-processing. They contain protein products and help to protect the hair from over-processing. They also allow the relaxer to penetrate the hair at a more even rate, thus producing an even result.

The pre-relaxer may also be applied as a protective measure to the hair that has previously been relaxed.

Protective base

Application of pre-relaxer treatment

Applying the protective base

You should apply a protective base to the scalp before the application of the relaxing cream. They are usually petroleum-based and offer protection to the scalp from irritation, which is especially useful if you are using a lye relaxer, which may cause scalp irritation. They are light to the touch and will spread easily over the scalp as they are designed to melt at body temperature. Due to their lightness they are easily removed from the scalp when the relaxing cream is rinsed and shampooed. While applying the base, you must be careful not to allow it to get on the hair that is to be relaxed, as this will cause a barrier and prevent the relaxer from penetrating the hair, thus giving an unsatisfactory result.

Keys to good practice

If you are applying a relaxer to a new or existing client and you are unsure of the level of sensitivity on the scalp, then the use of a protective base is highly recommended.

Barrier cream

Barrier cream is a product used for protective purposes. When applied to the skin it will create a barrier between the skin and the harsh chemicals used in hairdressing. However, care must be taken not to apply any to the hair, as it will also create a barrier to the chemicals you are using on the hair, thus causing an unsatisfactory result.

Barrier cream should be applied to the skin and scalp to prevent any product from touching the areas and causing skin irritation. You should pay particular attention to the ears, the soft skin behind the ears and the back of the neck. It is recommended for use if the client has any known sensitivities, or if the client is new and you are not aware of their previous history.

Lye and no-lye chemical relaxers

Most relaxing creams have a high alkaline pH; between 9 and 14 on the pH scale. Due to their high alkalinity they are potentially dangerous to use on the hair and scalp. Therefore, it is crucial to always follow the manufacturer's instructions during use. All relaxing creams contain hydroxide; however, lye relaxers are sodium-based and no-lye can be either calcium-, potassium-, lithium- or guanidine-based.

Lye relaxers are more likely to:

- Cause irritation to the scalp
- Penetrate the cuticle more quickly
- Dry out the hair less than no-lye relaxers
- Leave more moisture within the hair.

No-lye relaxers are more likely to:

- Cause less irritation to the scalp
- Penetrate the cuticle more slowly
- Cause the hair to dry out and become more fragile
- Leave the hair requiring regular conditioning treatments.

Lye and no-lye relaxing products

As mentioned above, lye relaxers are sodium hydroxide-based and have a pH of between 9 and 14. They are available in three strengths to allow you to choose the correct one for your client's hair type and texture. The strongest is **super relaxer** for strong, coarse, resistant hair. The middle strength is **regular relaxer** for normal hair and the weakest is **mild relaxer** for fine, weaker or colour-treated hair.

The recommended development time for each of the above strengths will vary from one manufacturer to another. Therefore it is essential that you read the manufacturer's instructions carefully before use. You should check the development of the relaxer every 3 minutes until the desired result has been achieved. Failure to do this may lead to hair breakage, over-processing and client dissatisfaction.

During development you may find that one area has reached the desired result and the rest of the hair has not. In this instance you must immediately remove the products from the areas that are ready, without disturbing the hair that is still processing.

Neutralising shampoo

Once the relaxer has processed for the correct amount of time and the desired result has been achieved, the hair must be thoroughly rinsed and a neutralising shampoo used to stop the action of the alkali. When rinsing the hair, you must make sure the water isn't too hot as this may lead to the scalp becoming sensitive. If the water is too cold, the product may not be fully removed, therefore causing damage to the hair and scalp. The water pressure should aid removal of the relaxing products. The hair should be shampooed gently and care taken to avoid tangling or breaking the hair. This should be carried out at a backwash basin to prevent the relaxer from entering the eyes.

Remember

If the client feels any sensitivity on the scalp when you are using chemical relaxer, it should be rinsed off immediately and the process stopped. This will prevent any burns or irritation to the skin or scalp.

Neutralising shampoo

The neutralising shampoo has an acidic pH and not only prevents the relaxer from continuing to develop any further, but also closes the cuticle scales and returns the hair back to its natural acidic pH of 4.5 – 5.5. This is an important part of the process of relaxing and should never be omitted, as the hair may become over-processed causing dryness and breakage. Some manufacturers produce neutralising shampoos that change colour to indicate that the neutralising is complete.

Post-relaxing treatments

Post-relaxing treatments restore the hair's moisture

A post-relaxing treatment should also be used to both moisturise the hair and help return it to its natural acidic pH of 4.5 – 5.5. The treatment should be used to compensate for the harshness of the relaxer and replace some of the natural oils and moisture lost during the relaxing process. They come in the form of cream or liquid conditioners. Not all manufacturers produce post-relaxing treatments; however, some produce different formulas depending on the hair texture.

Check it out

Find out which pre- and post-relaxing treatments are available in your salon, and how and when they should be used.

Equipment

The use of a tint bowl during the service is required to hold the relaxing cream during application. A tint brush is used for applying the product, particularly in areas where you need to apply precisely when correcting relaxing problems, e.g. spotting in certain areas along the hair length.

A non-metallic tail comb can also be used to apply the relaxing cream directly from the tint bowl onto the root area. It must be non-metallic to prevent any reaction between the metal and the chemicals you are using, which could have a detrimental effect on the hair and the result. Some stylists prefer to use a wide-tooth comb, especially if the result requires some movement left in the hair. Others may apply the relaxing product using their fingers; however, great care must be taken if using this method to ensure an accurate application with no overlapping of previously treated hair. You may already have a preferred way of applying the relaxing product and smoothing the hair, but if not, try the above methods and see which one you prefer.

You will need to section the hair off during application to allow you to work both methodically and also to prevent the product touching unwanted areas. Using sectioning clips will help.

Development strand test

This may be carried out in several ways. You may choose to use cotton wool to wipe off the relaxing cream and check if the curl appears sufficiently relaxed, or you may prefer to use the back of your comb to remove some of the relaxing product and check its development.

The relaxing process: dealing with under-processed ends

Hair before relaxing treatment – showing re-growth of natural hair, and under-processed ends.

Fingers were run along the hair shaft to test the porosity.

The hair shaft was stretched gently to test the elasticity.

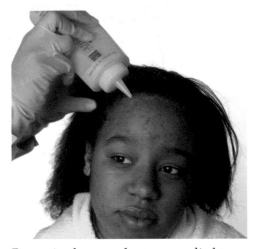

Protective base product was applied to skin and scalp.

Pre-relaxer treatment is applied to hair to even out the porosity and to protect the hair.

Relaxer is applied to re-growth area.

Once re-growth application has been applied, relaxer is applied to the under-processed ends. Be careful not to overlap onto the mid-lengths.

The relaxer is thoroughly rinsed from the hair.

The hair is gently shampooed using a neutralising shampoo to ensure all the relaxer is removed.

Wet hair before it is styled.

The finished look.

Relaxing problems

Problem	Possible causes	Prevention	Remedy
Mid-length under-processing	1 Incorrect strength of relaxer used on previous application of relaxer.	1 Ensure the correct strength of product is used.	Test the hair; if the condition allows:
	2 Incorrect timing on previous relaxer.	2 Ensure the relaxing service is correctly timed.	• Protect the roots and ends with pre-relaxer treatment.
	3 On previous application the relaxer not taken up to demarcation line.	3 Ensure you apply the relaxing product up to the demarcation line. Tip: After the pre-perm treatment has been applied, both the look and the feel of the hair alters, therefore the demarcation line is easier to identify.	• Choose correct strength of relaxer (possibly a weaker strength as the hair has already been chemically processed).
	Incorrect sequence of application on virgin head application.*	See * overleaf	• Apply the relaxer to the under-processed areas only, taking care not to overlap. • Process until desired result is achieved. • Shampoo the hair with the correct neutralising shampoo and apply a post-relaxer conditioner. • Advise the client on home care routine.
Under-processed roots	1 Incorrect strength of relaxer used on previous application.	1 Ensure the correct strength of product is used.	Test the hair; if the condition allows: Protect the mid-lengths and ends with pre-relaxer treatment.
	2 Incorrect timing on previous relaxer.	2 Ensure the relaxing service is correctly timed.	Choose correct strength of relaxer (possibly a weaker strength as the hair has already been chemically processed).

Problem	Possible causes	Prevention	Remedy
	3 Failed to check development.	3 Check development properly. Apply the relaxer to the under-processed areas only, taking care not to overlap.	Apply the relaxer to the
	4 Poor application (sections taken were too large)	4 Ensure sections are the correct size to ensure no parts are missed.	Process until desired result is achieved. Shampoo the hair with the correct neutralising shampoo and apply a post-relaxer conditioner. Advise the client on home care routine.

* The correct sequence of application for a virgin head application would be to apply the relaxer to the mid-lengths and ends first. When processing has begun, apply to the root area. The root area will develop more quickly due to the heat from the body.

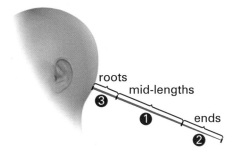

Apply relaxer to mid-lengths❶, then ends ❷, and lastly to the roots as this area will process more quickly due to the heat from the body.

Virgin head application

Keys to good practice

When commencing the corrective relaxing service, you should begin your application on the part of the hair that will require the most development. This is usually the curliest or most resistant part of the hair. If the client had an uneven result from the last relaxing service, it is essential that you examine all areas of the head before starting your application, as the curliest/most resistant part of the head may not always be where you would expect. The nape area may not be most resistant, but quite fragile due to lack of moisture.

Ensuring client comfort

Throughout the service you must keep checking to make sure your client is not experiencing any discomfort from the relaxing products. If your client does experience discomfort, the relaxing product must be removed immediately, rinsing the hair with cool water. Throughout this remedial procedure, you must reassure your client by using effective communication, explaining what you are doing and why. Your tone of voice should be calm and reassuring. If the products are not removed soon enough, the scalp may appear inflamed and be sore; in this case, it may be wise to refer your client to their GP. Failure to do so may result in chemical burns to the scalp and possibly cicatricial alopecia.

Confirming client satisfaction

When you have completed the service, you must check the result is satisfactory to your client and confirm the result is as anticipated. It is essential that your client is satisfied with the results achieved, to ensure further visits to the salon.

After the service

At the end of the service, any waste produced, e.g. unused relaxer, must be disposed of immediately according to the manufacturer's instructions.

Your corrective relaxing service should be completed within a commercially viable time for the salon where you work.

You must ensure your client's records are accurate, up to date and easy to read. This information will assist the salon when the client returns for their next appointment. In addition, it will ensure that you are complying with your responsibilities under the Data Protection Act.

After-care advice

This is an excellent opportunity for you to retail. You must ensure you give your clients sound after-care advice to enable them to treat their hair correctly in between visits. You must inform them of the correct products to use at home to maintain the condition of their hair and, if necessary, recommend further salon services.

Check it out

Which health and safety legislation covers the disposal of waste? Think about this carefully, as there may be more than one!

Check it out

What are your salon's expected service times for a corrective relaxing service?

In the salon

Marcia, a 13-year-old client, came into the salon with her Mum, three weeks after having her hair relaxed. Her hair was very dry, brittle and matted and she wanted to complain about the relaxing service. Keisha, the stylist, examined her hair and questioned her regarding the home care routine she had been advised to carry out (shampooing and conditioning her hair weekly and applying a moisturising product every other day). She replied that she didn't have time to do this in the morning before going to school and she had too much homework to do in the evening.

Keisha advised Marcia to have a deep conditioning treatment that day and she then reiterated the importance of caring for her hair now that it had been chemically treated. Keisha then suggested that Marcia visited the salon at least every month to check she was continuing with the maintenance programme. Three weeks later when Marcia visited the salon, her hair was much better and she told Keisha that she had been getting up 15 minutes earlier every day to ensure her hair remained healthy.

- How did Keisha demonstrate her professional skills in this situation?

Knowledge check

1. Why is it important to establish any contra-indications to the corrective relaxing service?

2. What contra-indications should you check for?

3. Which tests should you carry out prior to the relaxing service, and why?

4. What is the purpose of a pre-relaxer treatment?

5. Why should you not perm hair that has been previously relaxed?

6. State the reasons for using a neutralising shampoo?

7. What are the different ways in which a developmental strand test may be carried out?

8. State the three possible causes of under-processed ends following a relaxing treatment.

Create complex styles using African Caribbean styling techniques

Unit H35

Introduction

Use plaiting and styling techniques to add excitement to a client's look

This unit is about creating complex and innovative hairstyles using a variety of traditional African Caribbean plaiting and twisting techniques. You must be able to achieve the looks in a variety of ways, both full head and partial, and including both classic and sculptured designs. There are a number of different types of plaits and twists, some of which you may already be familiar with and others that you may know by another name. By studying the step-by-step photographs in this unit, you will develop a greater understanding of how to achieve some of the looks.

What you will learn
• Preparing for the service
• Creating the look
• Looks and styles
• Twisting techniques
• Plaiting techniques
• After the service

You the stylist

Before you begin to create complex styles using African Caribbean styling techniques, you need to know about the correct products to use and how and why you will need to use them. It is also essential that you understand the importance of any influencing factors and the effect they may have on your client's chosen look. In order to plait and twist the hair with skill, you will need to be dexterous, creative and conscious that the styling technique may take several hours to complete; patience is therefore the key to this unit. These skills will be developed over time, through practice and commitment.

Preparing for the service

In this section you will find all the information regarding the preparation of the client, yourself and your work area when carrying out plaiting and twisting techniques on a client.

What you will learn

- Thorough consultation and influencing factors
- Preparing the work area
- Personal standards of health and hygiene
- Personal protective equipment
- Preparing the hair.

Thorough consultation and influencing factors

While completing your consultation you will be assessing the client's hair for the suitability of the chosen style. Looking at style books and discussing any pictures brought in by your client will be important in ascertaining your client's exact requirements. You should then be able to select the appropriate products and tools required for you to carry out the requested service. You may need to consider the use of added hair or ornamentation to achieve the look required. This should be discussed and any implications for cost and length of service made clear to your client. The consultation you complete with the client must also take into account any influencing factors such as:

- The desired look
- Hair elasticity
- Head and face shape
- Hair texture
- Hair length
- Hair density
- Alopecia

The desired look

This should be thoroughly discussed with your client prior to starting the service. The use of visual aids, e.g. stylebooks and/or other examples in the salon may assist your clients in making their choice. You must be both honest and realistic when discussing styling possibilities with your client. If you know you can't achieve your client's choice of style, you must explain the reasons why and suggest a more suitable option.

You should also discuss the direction of the twist/plaits. If your client has any strong hair growth patterns, this may influence the direction of the twists/plaits. Twists/plaits should follow the hair growth patterns as this will encourage the hair to lie flat to the scalp and therefore reduce the amount of tension placed at the root area.

Hair elasticity

This must be considered, as hair with poor elasticity may break if too much tension is applied. Hair that has recently had plaiting and or extensions, particularly with tension, for fairly long periods of time is unlikely to have good elasticity.

Remember

Hair that has been chemically treated may have poorer elasticity

---

Head and face shape

The style you wish to create must flatter your client's head and face shape. Refer to Unit G9 for more information on head and face shapes.

Hair texture

The texture of the hair must be considered for several reasons:

- If the hair is very curly, it may require drying with a comb attachment on the hairdryer to elongate the curl prior to plaiting. This will stretch out the curl, leaving the hair easier to work with.
- The texture and curl pattern may vary across the head, e.g. the hair at the frontal region is sometimes finer and therefore may have a tendency to break. It may be advisable to perform off-scalp plaiting in this area and avoid unnecessary tension. You may also choose to use added hair to give the illusion of thicker hair.
- The hair in the nape area often has a tighter curl and is more dehydrated and brittle.
- Hair that is in transition, e.g. part of the hair has been relaxed, while the remainder is natural, needs to be treated with care as the hair shaft has two different textures. At the point where the textures meet the hair may be prone to breakage.

Remember

The length of time the braids or twists should remain in the hair will be dependent on:
- the type of braid or twist
- the hair's texture
- the client's ability to maintain the style

Hair length

The length of the hair you will be working with should be considered. You must make sure the hair is long enough to achieve the desired results. The length may also influence your decision regarding the use of added hair.

Hair density

The density of the hair will affect the size of the sections you take when plaiting or twisting the hair. It must also be considered if you are proposing to use added hair.

Alopecia

Traction alopecia is more prevalent among clients who wear their hair braided. This is due to the amount of tension used when braiding the hair. It usually occurs around the frontal and temporal areas of the scalp, due to the stylist starting the braids with too much tension.

It is important that you can identify the first signs of traction alopecia and begin a programme of correction before the condition deteriorates further. The first indications of traction alopecia include:

- Thinning of the hair, usually in the frontal and temporal regions
- A sore and tender scalp.

Traction alopecia may also occur in clients with hair extensions as a result of adding too much extension material, in proportion to the amount of natural hair within a section. The extension material becomes too heavy for the natural hair to support, thus putting undue stress on the natural hair.

Wearing the braids for too long may also cause traction alopecia. You should advise your clients to have their twists or braids removed after 6 weeks (if not before) and allow their hair and scalp to recover before re-braiding the hair.

Keys to good practice

If you have clients with traction alopecia it is your responsibility to:

- Question your clients on their styling techniques to ascertain why the condition has happened.
- Make notes on the client's record card of their responses and note all affected areas.
- Make the client aware of all the affected areas and the potential consequences of ignoring the condition.
- Ensure all tension is removed from the hair and treatments are applied to the hair and scalp.
- Re-educate your clients so that the condition will not recur in the future.
- If necessary, refer the client to a trichologist.

In the most severe cases, traction alopecia may never improve, due to the trauma caused to the follicle and surrounding tissue. This may ultimately result in cicatricial alopecia.

In the event that you identify any adverse hair, skin or scalp conditions that may contra-indicate this service, it may be necessary to refer your clients to others for further treatment before you are able to carry out creating complex styling. Refer to Unit G9 for more information on hair, skin and scalp conditions (including other types of alopecia).

Each of the influencing factors should be thoroughly explored and any areas for concern identified. For example, if a client is suffering from traction alopecia, then plaiting and twisting the hair and all the tension this places on the hair follicle is not advised.

In summary, when carrying out plaiting and twisting services it is essential that you have an understanding of the effects of these techniques on the hair. This will enable you to recognise any serious conditions such as alopecia and give advice accordingly.

Check it out

Write a short description on the influencing factors that would affect any plaiting and twisting services.

Preparing the work area

Checklist for preparing your work area

What to do	Why/how?
All the necessary tools and equipment for the service should be ready	Saves time and conveys professional image to the client
Any products needed for the service should be available and ready to use	Regular and effective stocktaking will ensure that all products are available
Work area must be clean and tidy	Prevents accidents occurring, reduces risk of cross-infection and portrays a professional image
Instruct junior staff to prepare the work area correctly	Saves time. Make sure that you clearly communicate what is required – a short list of instructions may be given to junior staff
Tools and equipment should be clean, sterilised and fit for the purpose	The appropriate method of sterilisation should be used and equipment should be checked for defects
Electrical equipment should be used in compliance with health and safety legislation	Ensure that junior staff are complying with the safe use of electrical equipment (see Unit G1). This is your responsibility.

Personal standards of health and hygiene

Checklist for personal health and hygiene

What to do	Why/how?
Make sure your body and clothes smell clean and fresh	The client will feel more comfortable in your presence. Daily washing and the use of a good deodorant are essential.
Make sure your breath smells nice	Use a breath freshener. This will help to combat odours from strong-smelling foods or smoking.
Do not work if you are feeling unwell	Infections can be spread in the salon. Keep yourself fit and healthy to ensure that you produce the best work possible.
Maintain a good posture while working. Think about whether your client is positioned correctly for your needs as well as their own comfort.	This will minimise the risk of injury and fatigue. Make sure you keep your back straight and balance evenly distributed. Having your tools and equipment close to hand will prevent you from over-stretching.

Check it out

Think about the methods of sterilisation you currently use in the salon. Are they the most suitable options? Look at Unit G1 and consider the various methods available to use: then decide if you need to change to a more suitable or economical method.

Personal protective equipment

The use of personal protective equipment benefits both you and your client. It is used to protect clothes and skin from the effects of any products that you are using and also to prevent the client from becoming covered in hair. The use of a gown and towel during plaiting and twisting services will protect your client both from stains from products being used and from hair. It is crucial that you use clean gowns and towels for each client to prevent cross-infection. Both items need to be boil-washed to ensure their cleanliness. You also need protection from products and hair and this can be achieved by wearing an apron.

Preparing the hair

It is essential to prepare the hair thoroughly prior to commencing the plaiting or twisting services. Depending on the look to be achieved you may have to shampoo, condition, blow-dry or wrap dry the hair to thoroughly disentangle the hair and loosen the curl. Loosening the curl will enable you to achieve smoother results. This may be performed using the comb attachment on the hair dryer.

However, before any plaiting or twisting takes place you should moisturise the hair and scalp with a dressing oil. You may also need to apply a wax, gel or oil for dressing purposes as you continue with your styling. This, however, depends on the look you are creating. Accurate sectioning before you begin is essential and, as you continue with your styling, you must make sure your sections are neat and even. This will determine the direction of the plait/twist and create a strong base for the plait to ensure optimum results. It also reduces the risk of trauma to the scalp, if hair from one section is braided or twisted into another.

Remember

When using electrical equipment, you must consider your responsibilities under the Electricity at Work Regulations 1989.

Creating the look

Once you are fully prepared and understand your client's requirements, you are ready to begin the service. As you are working towards the completion of the style you must be aware of how the style is to be achieved and which techniques, products and equipment you are using and why.

> **What you will learn**
>
> - Correct positioning of self and client
> - Products
> - Tools and equipment

Correct positioning of self and client

Plaiting and twisting is a service that can take a long time to complete. Therefore, it is important that you remain aware of your personal stance and the positioning of the client's head throughout the service. These factors can have a dramatic effect on the outcome, as they can affect the angle of the plait and/or twist. For your own safety you must stand and be working over your client in a position that allows you freedom of movement. Your position should not cause you any undue stretching or leaning, which may lead to fatigue, harm or injury.

As well as considering your own comfort, you must also think about the needs of your client. It is vital that the client's head is positioned to allow you to reach areas and achieve the degree of tension needed. However, you should not expect your client to feel discomfort during the service. You should check that your client is able to move his or her head into the position you require. Any prolonged bending of the head is likely to cause your client pain and discomfort.

> **Keys to good practice**
>
> As you will be concentrating and involved in what you are doing, it is easy to forget the needs of your client. To prevent this, ask a junior member of staff to check the client's welfare regularly and make sure that he or she is not experiencing any discomfort.

> **Remember**
>
> As a stylist working in a salon you cannot afford to ignore the potential long-term effects of incorrect posture. It may lead to repetitive strain injury, which could bring about an early end to your career as a hairdresser.

Products

Your salon may be loyal to only one product manufacturer. However, this is not always the best option – you could be missing an opportunity to use a styling product that is more suited to the needs of your clients. You can keep up to date with what is available on the market by:

- Visiting the wholesaler and looking at other products
- Talking to manufacturers' representatives visiting the salon
- Looking through trade publications
- Attending trade events, e.g. competitions, trade fairs
- Using websites.

However you choose to stay up to date is your own personal choice but it is vitally important that you develop your product range in line with the needs of your clients.

> **Check it out**
>
> Take the time out to read the manufacturer's instructions on the styling and finishing products you use. You may find that you are misusing or wasting products by overuse which is not cost-effective.

Failure to do so may result in you being left behind by the competition and your clients may choose to visit a salon with a more varied product range.

Features and benefits of products

Although there are a variety of products that you may use when plaiting and twisting, it is essential that you understand their particular features and benefits.

Product	Features	Benefits
Gel	Gel is used to aid the styling process by holding the hair in place.	Use of gel aids the styling process and holds the style in place for longer. It is also useful for keeping stray hairs smooth and tidy.
Wax	Using wax will help to soften the hair and make it more pliable. However, avoid overuse on fine hair.	Wax will moisturise and help prevent damage to hair that is under stress. Helps to hold the style.
Spray	Sprays are used to hold the hair in place both during and after styling.	Spray will help to maintain the style for longer and hold the hair in place while carrying out the service.
Sheen spray	Gives sheen to the hair.	Adds moisture to the hair and helps prevent dehydration.
Oil	Oil is used to moisturise the hair and scalp. It is especially effective on dry, coarse hair.	It will help to prevent the hair from becoming dehydrated and damaged.
Braid spray	Gives shine to the hair and scalp.	Helps prevent flaky and dry scalp, adds moisture to the hair, thus preventing dehydration.

All of the products should contain ingredients to protect the hair from the effects of humidity, by coating the hair with a protective film. They should also contain conditioning/moisturising agents to nourish and lubricate the hair and scalp. All products should be used economically to prevent unnecessary wastage and overloading the hair and scalp.

> **Remember**
>
> COSHH legislation governs any products that you use in the salon. Under these regulations you have a duty to store, handle, use and dispose of products according to salon policies, local by-laws and manufacturers' instructions.

Tools and equipment

Tools and equipment	Uses
Blow-dryer with comb attachment	Used to loosen the curl before plaiting or twisting the hair, and aid disentangling.
Wide-tooth comb	Used to disentangle the hair prior to plaiting and twisting.
Tail comb	Used for sectioning the hair to ensure even sections. May be used to help with the removal of plaits.
Sectioning clips	Used to effectively secure any hair not being styled and to keep sections visible.
Hackle	Used to disentangle added hair prior to use. May also be used to blend different colours of hair together.
Drawing brushes	Used to hold the disentangled hair until needed. They enable you to select a small amount of hair at a time without disturbing the rest.
Hair grips and pins	Used to secure the hair in place.
Scissors	To cut the added hair to the required length.

Looks and styles

Classic look

A classic look is one that is timeless and has been popular for a long period of time, e.g. cane row.

Sculptured look

Sculptured looks are designed using patterns within the style to achieve movement and different textures within the style, for example, a Godess braiding.

Full head

A full head style means that all the hair has been plaited or twisted to achieve the final look.

Partial head

A partial head style is a style where not all of the hair is included in the plaiting or twisting, e.g. flat twists with areas of the hair left unplaited or twisted. In these areas the hair may be left natural, thermally styled or shaved.

Added hair

The use of added hair when twisting and/or plaiting may be for several reasons:

- To add volume to the hair
- To give the style another dimension
- To add colour
- To extend the length of the style.

Types of added hair

There are many different types of added hair that may be used when creating styles using plaiting or twisting techniques. These include both natural and synthetic fibres that are available in a variety of lengths, textures and colours. The added hair may be purchased on a weft or as a bundle.

Nylon synthetic hair – this is the cheapest option to use. However, you must make sure that the quality of the hair is good as poor-quality nylon synthetic hair has been known to break the hair.

Kanekalon – this is a much better option, as the quality of the synthetic fibre is very good. Many stylists prefer to use kanekalon as it feels softer, tangles less and does not damage the natural hair.

Human hair – this is the most expensive option for added hair. The quality may vary quite considerably. You must ensure you use a reputable wholesaler who can guarantee the quality of the hair. This may be a good option if you have clients who are known to have allergies to synthetic products.

Lin – this is a wool fibre with a matte finish. It is sometimes used for Senegalese twists.

Yak – this is often used when adding hair, as it is relatively inexpensive. It is a natural fibre and when mixed with small quantities of human hair it loses the artificial shine.

How to divide and separate added hair

Experienced stylists will divide and separate added hair by picking it from the bundle as they work through the plaiting or twisting service. However, you may find it beneficial to prepare the hair prior to use. This necessitates the use of a hackle and drawing brushes. The hackle is basically steel prongs protruding from a wooden board. It is used to disentangle the hair and blend colours by drawing the hair through the steel prongs. The drawing brushes are wooden boards with short bristles coming out from the board. The pre-hackled hair is placed on top of one of the drawing brushes, and another drawing brush placed on top to hold the hair in place. This enables you to draw off small amounts of hair at a time without disturbing the remaining hair, which is held in between the drawing brushes. The hair may be cut to the desired length before, or after, using.

How much hair should be added

The amount of added hair you use will depend on several factors. If the hair is very fine and you are using added hair to give the hair a thicker appearance, you must ensure the amount of hair you use will not put undue stress on the natural hair, as this may result in traction alopecia. It may be necessary to use only five or six strands of added hair.

Methods of securing the added hair

There are several different methods that may be used to secure added hair. The added hair may be:

- Fed into the style during plaiting
- Knotted onto a strand of the natural hair, then introduced into the plait or twist
- Twisted around the natural hair and tied with a matching coloured thread.

When adding hair to a Senegalese twist, you should:

1 Section the hair accordingly.
2 Take a sub-section and split into two equal parts.
3 Take the required length of hair to be added and place between the two equal parts.
4 Each of the two parts of the hair (with the added hair) should be rolled between the fingertips to blend the natural and added hair together.
5 You should now be ready to begin the Senegalese twist, as demonstrated by your tutor/trainer.

It is important to follow this process when adding hair to a Senegalese twist as this will help you maintain even tension throughout.

Braid extensions can help create an elegant, glamorous look

Check it out

Watch your tutor/trainer use added hair to create a number of different styles and note:

- The amount of added hair used
- The texture and density of the natural hair
- The results that are achieved.

The amount of hair that you add must be in proportion to the desired result. However, you must ensure that your finished result is balanced and well proportioned.

Twisting techniques

Flat twist with knots

Twisting the hair is achieved by using the fingers or a comb to twist the hair into strands. This can be done either by on-the-scalp techniques, such as flat twists, or off-the-scalp as with two-stem twists. You must be able to twist the hair both clockwise and anti-clockwise, as the need arises. This may be due the style requirements or to ensure you are working with the client's natural hair growth pattern. You must also be able to create a uniform twist, keeping it in the centre of the section. This may be achieved in a number of ways. The base of the twist should be started in the centre. Make sure that you are 'picking up' even amounts of hair on both sides. Also ensure that you use the correct posture, as failure to stand in the correct position may cause the twist to sit off centre.

Two-stem twists

This type of twist is carried out off the head and helps to keep the hair looking tidy and well groomed. The use of a gel to assist with the twisting process is required; however, overuse can leave the hair feeling dry. Therefore, adding pomade to the mixture will help to prevent this.

Method

1. Prepare the hair for twisting by shampooing, conditioning and towel drying.
2. Begin by taking a small horizontal section in the nape and securing the rest of the hair out of the way with clips.
3. Taking sections between 0.5 and 1 cm in width, apply the product along the length of the hair.
4. Divide the section into two and begin by twisting the left over the right or vice versa so that they are wrapped around each other.
5. Continue with this all the way up the head, ensuring you use a brickwork pattern to prevent gaps appearing in the design.
6. Once the whole head has been twisted, the hair must be styled and dried.
7. Arrange the twists in a way to allow them to lie naturally.
8. Apply finishing spray.
9. Dry the hair by use of added heat but without disturbing the style, for example, using a clymazone on a natural dry setting.

Check it out

Ask your tutor/trainer to demonstrate the following techniques:

(a) Tree plaiting on and off the scalp
This technique involves plaiting which leaves stems of hair protruding down the length of the plait at regular and even intervals. May be carried out both on and off the scalp.

(b) Fishtail plait
A four-strand plait that is achieved by crossing four pieces of hair over each other to create a herringbone look.

(c) Goddess braiding
This type of plait involves plaiting the hair into three to five extra large cane rows that are swept up onto the head and the loose ends styled on the top of the head.

Corkscrew twists

This is a method of twisting sections of natural curl in the hair by using products and fingers to achieve corkscrew-look, finger-sized sections.

Senegalese twists

A Senegalese twist consists of two stems of hair that are individually twisted in the same direction, then crossed over. This creates a rope effect.

Check it out

Ask your tutor/trainer to demonstrate the following techniques:

(a) Comb twists on and off the scalp

(b) Twists created in the hair using a comb.

Check it out

Search the internet (using search engines such as Google or Ask Jeeves) to find examples of the various plaits and twists covered in this unit. Ask your tutor/trainer to demonstrate the looks.

Creative use of twisting techniques can enhance your client's personality

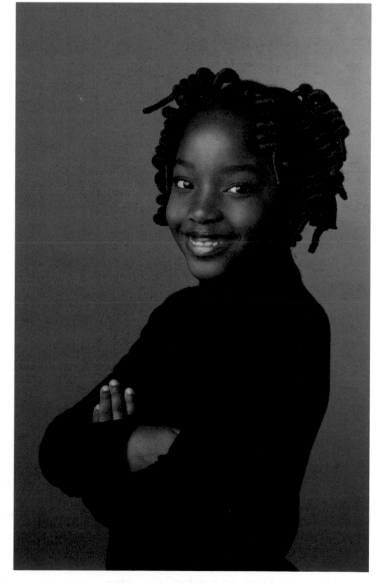

Twisting techniques: a step-by-step guide

Before the service.

Starting from the front hairline, a flat twist is created going back behind the ear.

Continue until the front and side are complete.

Working around the back of the head, flat twists are created from right to left.

Continue up the back of the head until complete.

A knot is then formed with the end of each twist.

The knot is secured.

Right-hand side complete showing secured knots.

The remaining hair is then styled using heated styling equipment.

The finished look.

Plaiting techniques

Plaiting the hair is a method of dividing the hair into sections and placing them over or under each other to achieve a variety of looks. As these techniques involve 'picking up' hair at the base, it is essential that the hair you pick up comes from underneath the area where you are plaiting. The picked up hair must never come from another subsection or further down the plait, as this will create unnecessary tension on the roots of the hair, which may lead to breakage. Your plaiting should be carried out without undue tension being applied; however, the tension you use must remain even throughout the service if you are to create an even result.

The techniques you will use include on-the-scalp plaiting, e.g. tree plaiting on the scalp, off-the-scalp plaiting or a combination of both.

Potential effects of wearing added hair over a long period of time

The length of time that your client can wear added hair will be dependent on the type of braids and/or twists. If your client fails to follow your instructions, this may result in:

* the natural hair becoming dehydrated
* hair breakage
* traction alopecia
* the hair becoming matted
* the scalp becoming very dry and flaky.

If your client suffers from any of the above consequences, it is likely to have a negative impact on your professional reputation and that of the business.

Finishing off the plait or twist

There are several different ways in which the plait or twist may be finished, for example:

* Using the singeing method, apply heat to the ends of the hair, then rub the ends with your fingers to seal them.
* Using covered elastics. These must be bands for professional use to prevent hair breakage.

Carry out plaiting with even tension, to create an even result

- Knotting the ends of the hair and cutting off loose ends close to the knot.
- Tying the ends of the hair with leftover added hair.
- Using a braid sealer. This cuts and seals the ends of the hair at the same time.
- The ends may be dipped into hot water at the backwash. The hair must be long enough to reach the water. Remember this method is suitable only for added hair – not natural hair!

Care must be taken when using the singeing method of finishing plaits and twists, especially when using added hair, as some types of added hair are highly flammable. Always read the manufacturer's instructions to ensure that you are using added hair safely and correctly.

Plaiting techniques: a step-by-step guide

Hair in its natural state before the plaiting service.

Shampooed and conditioned hair before blow-drying.

The comb attachment is used to help loosen the natural curl while blow drying the hair.

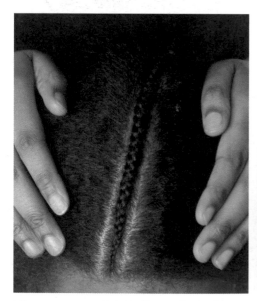

The cane row plait is directed, on the scalp, from the front hairline to the crown, leaving the ends free.

Cane row plaiting to alternate sections is continued (for photographic purposes the remaining sections were twisted to show plaits).

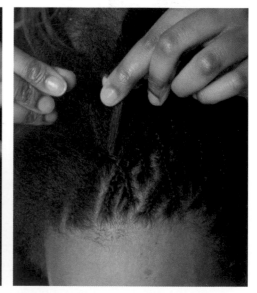

The remaining sections are used to cane row diagonally, creating the criss-cross effect.

From the nape, a small section of hair is taken and split into two. Starting at the roots, one strand is crossed over the other and continued down to the ends of the hair.

Two-stem twists completed to halfway up the back of the head.

The free ends from the cane row are styled using off-the-scalp plaiting technique.

The finished look.

After the service

Once you have achieved the finished look it is important that you complete the service professionally by ensuring the client is happy and understands how to maintain the look. You must advise the client on the products required to moisturise and nourish the hair and scalp. This also keeps the style in place longer. You must explain not only how to care for the style but the importance of correctly removing the plaits or twists. Whether you advise a salon visit for this or advise on how to remove them at home depends on the complexity of the finished look and the client's requirements.

Check it out

List the different plaiting and twisting services that are available within your salon and find out the length of time given for each different styling technique.

Confirmation of the finished look

On completion of the style you have created it is imperative that you check with your client to confirm their satisfaction. Discussing the finished look is all part of the professional service you are offering. You must show the client the new style from every angle using a back mirror, checking that they are happy with the finished effect. This will ensure your client does not leave the salon feeling disappointed with the finished look. It also gives your client an opportunity to discuss the outcome of the service and for you as a stylist to gain feedback on your work. This will help you to continually develop and improve your skills. The work you produce should be of a high standard that will enhance not only your own professional image, but also that of the salon.

Your work should be completed within a time that is deemed commercially viable for your salon.

After-care and home advice

You have a responsibility to your client to make sure that he or she fully understands how to maintain the style and take care of his or her hair at home. Your clients are a walking advertisement for your salon; therefore you must ensure the work that you carry out reflects the kind of image you want to portray. Giving your client expert advice on how to look after and maintain his or her hair will not only help him or her to feel confident about how he or she looks, but will also enhance your reputation as a professional hairdresser.

Your client will reflect the image you want to portray for your salon

> **Keys to good practice**
>
> If a client shows signs of traction alopecia, you must advise immediate removal of all plaits or twists. The hair must be given time to recover and no stress placed on the hair until it has grown back and is healthy once more.

The table below gives guidance on how to maintain the look and includes advice on shampooing and conditioning the hair.

Technique	Maintenance	Shampooing and conditioning
Plaiting	A light oil may be applied to the scalp to moisturise it. A light oil-based spray may be used on the plaits to add shine and prevent the hair drying out.	Use products specifically made for plaited hair, following the manufacturer's instructions. If shampooing the hair, apply the shampoo onto the palms and emulsify the shampoo in your hands. Apply the shampoo to the scalp using the fingertips and stroke the shampoo down the scalp between the plaits. Avoid vigorous massage techniques as this will matt the hair and the plaiting may become loose. Rinse the hair well to remove all the shampoo. Advise client to return to the salon for the removal service.
Twisting	A light oil may be applied but nothing water-based as this will loosen the twists.	Not to be carried out until the twists have been removed, as they will just loosen.

Keys to good practice

You should advise your clients to cover their hair when they sleep. The plaited and twisted hair should be covered with a scarf or a 'durag'. Don't forget to advise your clients on the products they should be using at home to maintain their plaits or twists in optimum condition, e.g. a moisturising spray for braided hair will add moisture to the hair and scalp, and prevent dehydration.

Removal of plaits and twists

Some clients will remove their plaits and twists at home. However, you should be advising your client to return to the salon for this service, when a deep penetrating conditioning treatment may be carried out. This will help to maintain the hair's condition and prevent future services from becoming limited.

Plaits should be removed carefully by opening up the plait and, taking small sections at a time, undoing the plaited hair with your comb using a picking movement. When all the plaits have been removed, you should then disentangle the hair using a wide-toothed comb. This will also help to remove any braid debris. You must make sure that you support the root area whilst both unpicking and disentangling the hair. The hair can then be gently shampooed and a deep conditioning treatment should be carried out to add moisture to the hair.

Twists should be removed by carefully untwisting the hair, and then disentangling it with a wide-toothed comb. The hair can then be gently shampooed and a deep conditioning treatment should be carried out to add moisture to the hair.

Keys to good practice

If you are cutting off bands used to secure the twists, care must be taken not to cut the hair.

Remember

When removing plaits or twists, hair loss may be apparent. This may not necessarily be due to hair breakage, but the hairs that are normally shed on a daily basis have been contained within the plait or twist and are now free to fall. It is essential that you reassure your client of this.

In the salon

Meleika returned to the salon eight weeks after having cane row braiding in her hair. The braids looked slightly matted and she was complaining of an itchy scalp. Natalie, the stylist, questioned her regarding her home maintenance programme. It became obvious that Meleika had not been carrying out the maintenance programme that she was initially advised to follow. Natalie soon realised that Meleika's itchy scalp was caused by her not using the moisturising spray; therefore her scalp had become dehydrated. The matted hair was caused by her shampooing her hair too vigorously, and not wearing a scarf to bed.

1. As a stylist how can you ensure that the client fully understands the implications of not following your advised maintenance programme?
2. What should Natalie advise Meleika to do next?

Knowledge check

1. State two safety considerations that should be taken into account when plaiting and styling hair.

2. What are the potential consequences of excessive tension on the hair and scalp?

3. Why is it important to condition the hair after any plaiting, twisting or braiding has been removed, and before any other service is undertaken?

4. Why is it important to maintain accurate sectioning when plaiting and twisting?

5. Name 4 different types of added hair that may be used when plaiting and twisting the hair.

6. State the reasons for using added hair when plaiting and twisting.

7. State the potential effects of wearing added hair over a long period of time.

8. What retail products would you advise a client to use at home following a plaiting or twisting service?

Key skills mapping

Key skills have been recognised as those skills that are beneficial not only in a training and work environment, but also for general life. They are skills that will enhance your learning, performance, help you to be flexible, organised and to overcome problems.

There are six separate Key skills specifications:

- communication – speaking; listening; reading and writing
- application of number – using numbers; doing calculations and interpreting results
- information technology – using computers to research, develop and present information with text, images and numbers
- working with others – focuses on how you work with others to achieve shared goals
- improving own learning and performance – focuses on personal, career and learning development
- problem solving – focuses on the skills necessary to recognise and deal with problems.

The last three are generally termed as the 'wider' Key skills. Key skills are set at levels 1–5 for the wider Key skills and communication; and levels 1–4 for information technology and application of number. However as you work towards your hairdressing qualification the highest level of Key skills you will need to achieve is at level 2.

Key skills are useful for everyone, whether you are a school pupil or part of the senior management team in a large company. For anyone to be successful both at work and in everyday life an appropriate level of competence in these Key skills is very useful. As a candidate you can achieve any of the individual Key skills at any level deemed appropriate for you. Unless you already know exactly which level you are at, or your training programme has dictated the level for you, you may be assessed to determine which level for each Key skill is most appropriate for you. For example, everyone working towards the completion of the Advanced Modern Apprenticeship in Hairdressing will have to achieve the application of number and communication Key skills at level 2, whereas I.T. is optional.

Achieving key skills at level 2 is related to achievement of grade A* - C in GCSE's. At the higher Key skills levels candidates will be expected to work with greater autonomy and to decide themselves how and when the skills can be applied in different situations.

To achieve a Key skills accreditation, candidates will be required to produce a portfolio of evidence and to pass externally marked test papers. The portfolio produced must contain evidence of their application of the Key skill within their vocational area. For example, for the communication Key skill, hairdressing candidates can collect evidence of communicating with the use of a visual aid through a consultation using a stylebook or colour chart. This all needs to be annotated on the consultation sheet.

The awarding body will externally moderate the portfolio produced in order to check the quality and to standardise the assessment.

The externally marked tests can be sat at various dates throughout the year and are all multiple-choice papers. If a candidate does not pass the paper initially they can re-sit at a later date.

Relating Key Skills to the NVQ Hairdressing and Barbering level 3 course

While collecting evidence for your NVQ level 3 Hairdressing and Barbering qualification by carrying out services on clients or taking part in any hairdressing related activity, you can simultaneously generate evidence appropriate for a Key skills accreditation.

Although the evidence you produce may not wholly meet the requirements for a Key skills accreditation, you will be able to learn how Key skills are integrated into this vocational area; and how Key skills can enhance your learning and performance.

Communication

C 2.1a Contribute to a discussion about a straightforward subject.

> Units that will help you collect evidence:
> H19, H20, H21, H5 H26, H27, H28, H29, H30, H31, H33 & H35

Evidence of your ability to discuss a straightforward subject can be generated each time you carry out a thorough and effective consultation with a client. Contributing to a discussion is not only about talking, you will also need to show that you are listening to your client and their needs; and helping to move the discussion forward by making suggestions or giving advice.

Remember to inform your assessor that you wish to be assessed and keep your consultation sheets as evidence.

C2.1b Give a short talk about a straightforward subject using an image.

> Units that will help you collect evidence:
> H24, H32 & G11

Whilst completing units H24, H32 & G11, you will be asked to present your evaluation to your colleagues and line manager. Your talk or presentation can be about the show, photoshoot or competition you have just carried out; or the promotional activity that the salon has recently undertaken.

It may be advantageous to practice your talk first to ensure you are fluent on the day and that you speak clearly and to the point. It may also help if you make notes or have prompt cards to help you keep to the point of the talk and to ensure that you keep good time and do not bore your audience!

Remember to include an image in your presentation. For example, you may want to show a collage of the photos taken at the photoshoot, or examples of leaflets used in the salon's promotional activity.

C2.2 Read and summarise information from at least two extended documents about straightforward subjects. One of the documents should include at least one image.

> Units that will help you collect evidence:
> G6, G10 & G11

In order to write the assignments for the following units, you will need to select and read relevant material from various sources. You can collect information from stylebooks, trade magazines, your line manager, other stylists or the Internet. An important part of this unit is to show that you are able to find the relevant information that you need so you will need to read, summarise and structure the information to suit the purpose of the document that you are creating.

Think about the trade magazines you have access to and where you may find other sources of information.

C2.3 Write two different types of documents about straightforward subjects. One piece of writing should be an extended document and include at least one image.

> Units that will help you collect evidence:
> G6, G10 & G11

From the research you have done previously in C2.2, you can now use this information to write your assignments.

As you write up your assignments ensure that you have structured it well, and that the information you are using is relevant and that the way you write is suited to the audience. It is also very important that you check that your spelling, punctuation and grammar are correct and that the message you are trying to send through your document is understandable.

Application of Number

N2.1 Interpret information from two different sources including material containing a graph.

Units that will help you collect evidence:
G6, G10, G11 & H32

Whilst carrying out the following units, you will undertake many different activities, for example:

* checking deliveries of stock
* obtaining information relating to your own retail and technical targets
* obtaining information on the costs of making improvements to the salon.

You will need to show evidence that you have obtained information from two sources, that the information you have obtained is relevant and that you have understood the information presented to you from the graph.

N2.2 Carry out calculation to do with:
   a. Amounts or sizes
   b. Scales or proportions
   c. Handling statistics
   d. Using formulae

Units that will help you collect evidence:
G6, G10, G11 & H32

Using the information you have gained from unit N2.1, you are required to carryout calculations that clearly show your methods and levels of accuracy.

Remember, you must show evidence of comparing data with a minimum of 20 items.

You'd be surprised how many calculations you carry out every day, from the mixing ratios of colour to working out the correct amount of change to give a client!

N2.3 Interpret the results of calculations and present findings. You must use at least one graph, one chart and one diagram.

Units that will help you collect evidence:
G6, G10, G11 & H32

The evidence you have gathered and calculated for N2.1 and N2.2 must now be presented by the use of a graph, a chart and a diagram. This may include, for example, a graph of some type showing your retail and technical targets against the amount of money you have actually taken in both areas. You can use your I.T. skills to produce the graphs, charts and diagrams.

Remember that the above are suggested tasks only, with references to various units to help you identify where you may gather evidence for your Key skills portfolio. Your lecturer may use other tasks and activities; and give you additional guidance through your Key skills accreditation.

Index